Epidemiology for Field Veterinarians

An Introduction

Epidemiology for Field Veterinarians

An Introduction

Dr Evan Sergeant BVSc, PhD, MANZCVS
AusVet Animal Health Services Pty Ltd

Dr Nigel Perkins BVSc, MS, PhD, FANZCVS
AusVet Animal Health Services Pty Ltd

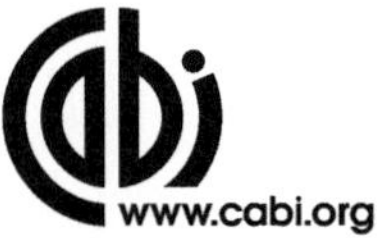

CABI is a trading name of CAB International

CABI
Nosworthy Way
Wallingford
Oxfordshire OX10 8DE
UK

Tel: +44 (0)1491 832111
Fax: +44 (0)1491 833508
E-mail: info@cabi.org
Website: www.cabi.org

CABI
38 Chauncy Street
Suite 1002
Boston, MA 02111
USA

Tel: +1 800 552 3083 (toll free)
E-mail: cabi-nao@cabi.org

A catalogue record for this book is available from the British Library, London, UK.

Library of Congress Cataloging-in-Publication Data

Sergeant, Evan, author.
Epidemiology for field veterinarians : an introduction / Dr Evan Sergeant, Dr Nigel Perkins.
p. ; cm.
Includes bibliographical references and index.
ISBN 978-1-84593-683-9 (hardback : alk. paper) -- ISBN 978-1-84593-691-4 (pbk. : alk. paper) 1. Veterinary epidemiology. I. Perkins, Nigel, author. II. Title.
[DNLM: 1. Epidemiologic Methods--veterinary. SF 780.9]

SF780.9.S47 2015
636.089'44--dc23

2014046558

ISBN-13: 978 1 84593 683 9 (hbk)
ISBN-13: 978 1 84593 691 4 (pbk)

Commissioning editor: Caroline Makepeace
Assistant editor: Alexandra Lainsbury
Production editors: Shankari Wilford and Tracy Head

Typeset by SPi, Pondicherry, India
Printed and bound in the UK by CPI Group (UK) Ltd, Croydon, CR0 4YY

Contents

Contributors

Angus Cameron, BVSc, MVS, PhD, MANZCVS, Senior Consultant, AusVet Animal Health Services Pty Ltd, Lyon, France.
Brendan Cowled, BVSc, PhD, FANZCVS, Senior Consultant, AusVet Animal Health Services Pty Ltd, Milton, New South Wales, Australia.
Jenny Hutchison, BVetBiol, BVSc, MS, PhD, Dip ACVIM, Senior Consultant, AusVet Animal Health Services Pty Ltd, Canberra, Australian Capital Territory, Australia.
Ben Madin, BSc (Vet Biol), BVMS, MVPHMgt, PhD, MANZCVS, Senior Consultant, AusVet Animal Health Services Pty Ltd, Melville, Western Australia, Australia.
Nigel Perkins, BVSc, MS, PhD, FANZCVS, Senior Consultant, AusVet Animal Health Services Pty Ltd, Toowoomba, Queensland, Australia.
Evan Sergeant, BVSc, PhD, MANZCVS, Senior Consultant, AusVet Animal Health Services Pty Ltd, Orange, New South Wales, Australia.

Preface

In a changing world with increasing demand for international trade in animals and animal products, and faced by challenges such as emerging and re-emerging disease threats, climate change, ecosystem health, population growth and ever increasing complexity and capacity for data generation, analytics and real-time information flows, the broad field of epidemiology is becoming both more complex and more relevant for veterinarians.

There are many books devoted to advanced and complex epidemiology applications of interest to the specialized few in areas such as simulation modelling of disease outbreaks, spatial epidemiology, quantitative techniques for analysing large and complex datasets, and risk analysis to name a few. There is little available information providing a grounding in applied epidemiology for veterinarians and animal health professionals working to address animal health problems in the day-to-day field environment.

This book is intended to meet this need. It is written by veterinary epidemiologists with formal training in the discipline and more importantly with extensive experience in applying epidemiologic methods to real-world problems in many different countries and regions around the world.

This book should be of value to private veterinarians and to government animal health staff who have responsibility for investigating, controlling and preventing animal diseases. It also has direct application to those who are tasked with developing policy related to animal health events. We hope this book will be found on the desks and in the hands of busy people working in the field rather than academic libraries.

Acknowledgements

The development of this book and the content has been based on many years of experience across the AusVet team and in particular through preparing and delivering training courses and our involvement in client-funded activities around the world. We acknowledge the input and feedback from many people who have solicited, encouraged, reviewed and participated in these events.

1 What is Epidemiology?

1.1 Introduction

This book provides an introduction to the application of epidemiological methods, including the investigation and resolution of disease problems in animal populations. Different methods are required depending on the problem under investigation and involve the collection, analysis and interpretation of data, as well as the synthesis and interpretation of information arising from data and other sources.

As an epidemiologist, you will often be asked to investigate disease incidents or evaluate and make recommendations on policy or disease management issues. These situations are often complicated by practical, political, economic or management considerations resulting in constraints on the quality of the information and data available for analysis and interpretation, the ability to collect additional data and the time-frame in which a response is required. It is essential that an objective and transparent approach is used in such situations, and that it is flexible enough to make the most of the available data.

This chapter provides an introduction to epidemiology, how it relates to other disciplines, its role in decision making and a brief description of important epidemiological study types. Chapter 2 introduces the concept of an epidemiological approach to thinking and problem solving. Chapter 3 covers the specific application of this approach to the investigation of disease outbreaks and subsequent chapters describe in more detail concepts and methods introduced in earlier chapters.

1.2 Epidemiology and Where it Fits

As animal production systems have intensified, the interaction of disease agents with other factors such as the physical environment, nutrition and genetics has become more complex. This complex interplay among a variety of factors sits in delicate balance while the goal of increasingly efficient production is sought. In such a system, even small changes in some factors can facilitate expression of disease. Resultant morbidity and mortality translate into lost production and reduced profitability.

Increasing urbanization, with consequent encroachment on natural environments, over the last century has contributed to emergence of new diseases, many of which are zoonoses, affecting people as well as animals. Of 335 emerging infectious diseases identified between 1940 and 2004, 60% were zoonoses and more than 71% originated from wildlife populations (Cutler *et al.*, 2010).

The traditional response to emergence of new disease entities is to identify the pathogen and seek interventions that will prevent or cure disease at the individual animal level. This traditional perspective requires developing an understanding of disease processes at the individual animal, organ, tissue, cellular and molecular level. Such an inside-the-animal approach largely ignores the complex interplay between animals, particularly when animals are aggregated in suboptimal environments that favour spread and expression of disease.

Epidemiology provides a complete set of tools for investigating disease occurrence in populations and for developing control and prevention strategies at the population level, often before the biology of the causal organism is clearly understood. A population of animals has attributes beyond the mere summation of its constituent animal units in the same way that the individual animal is more than just the sum of its individual organ systems. In addition, epidemiology looks at higher levels of populations. For example, the aggregation of pens, mobs or ponds on a particular farm may be regarded as a population, as could all the farms in an area such as a province or country. The different perspectives of traditional and population medicine approaches are shown in Fig. 1.1. At the same time, epidemiology often uses information collected as part of more detailed investigations on groups of individuals to make inference about the population from which they arise.

1.3 Diseases in Populations

Epidemiology is the study of patterns and causes of disease in populations. Understanding these issues will in turn contribute to identification of options for control and prevention of diseases. At its simplest, epidemiology is about supporting better decision making to ensure appropriate response or preventative measures for population health.

Suboptimal animal health and production in livestock systems may be approached as a type of disease. It is common to see epidemiologic principles and methods applied to livestock systems to ensure optimal health, welfare and production outcomes.

Most diseases do not occur at random in a population – they follow distinct patterns according to exposure of individuals in the population to various factors associated with the host, agent and environment (see Fig. 1.2). Epidemiologists rely

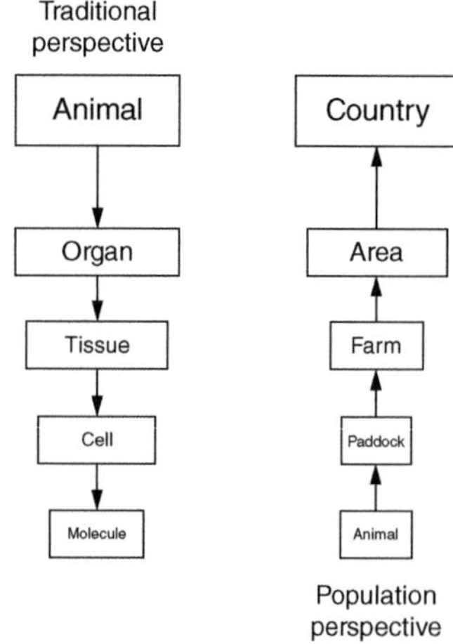

Fig. 1.1. Representation of the relationship between the traditional perspective of investigating disease and a population perspective.

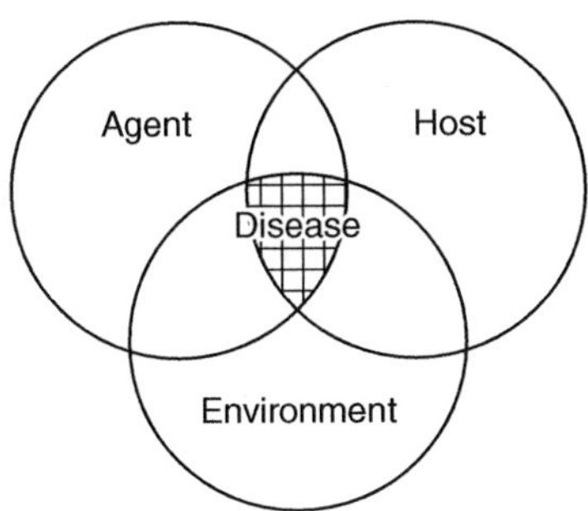

Fig. 1.2. Epidemiology studies the relationships between agent, host and environment resulting in disease occurrence.

on this non-random nature of disease events to generate and test hypotheses about likely causes and risk factors for disease.

Epidemiological studies provide insight not only into those factors operating at the population level but can also raise hypotheses worth exploring further at the individual animal, organ, cellular and genetic level. Thus, the understanding of disease processes operating at the population level requires both a downward (towards the molecular level) and upward (towards the population level) approach to investigation. By using such a bidirectional approach, fresh insights into the mechanisms and control of disease can be obtained.

1.4 Where Does Epidemiology Fit?

Epidemiology is an integrating science with close links to clinical and laboratory medicine as well as biostatistics and health economics. In addition, it is the basic science that underpins state veterinary medicine, biosecurity, preventive veterinary medicine and herd health programmes. Epidemiologists usually use the word disease in its broadest sense to include any health-related condition or event of interest, in addition to clinical illness.

Epidemiology is concerned with (adapted from Thrushfield, 2005, p. 16):

- detecting the existence of a disease or other production problem;
- identifying the causes of disease;
- estimating the risk of becoming diseased;
- obtaining information on the ecology and natural history of the disease;
- defining and quantifying the impact and extent of the problem;
- planning and evaluating possible disease control strategies and biosecurity measures;
- monitoring and surveillance to prevent further disease episodes; and
- assessing the economic impact of disease and control programmes.

1.5 The Role of Epidemiology in Policy Development

Effective animal health policy development requires not only a sound scientific basis, but also a clear understanding of the social and political context in which policy is being made. Successful interventions need to be politically, socially and economically acceptable if they are to be acted upon. Epidemiologists are in an excellent position to take a lead role in providing not only scientific input to policy, but also for integrating the broader 'macro-epidemiological' issues required for successful policy (Hueston, 2003).

Hueston (2003) uses the example of bovine tuberculosis (TB) in white-tailed deer in Michigan, USA. Despite bovine TB being close to eradication in the USA, increased deer populations in areas of north-east Michigan were providing a reservoir of infection that was jeopardizing progress with eradication in the region. The situation was compounded by poor farming conditions and low returns resulting in an increase in feeding of deer for hunting clubs as an alternative source of income. This led to increased deer density and congregations around feeding stations, allowing efficient spread of TB within the deer population.

From a purely disease control perspective this is a relatively simple problem with a simple solution. Stop feeding deer and increase culling to stop transmission. However, this would not solve the underlying social and economic issues that led to the problem in the first place. In fact, resolution of this sort of problem requires consideration and integration of priorities and opinions from a wide variety of groups, including local farmers, public and animal health agencies, wildlife agencies, sporting shooters and hunters, and the public. Failure to consider and integrate the views and needs of all of these groups into any solution is likely to lead to lack of support and eventual failure.

The role of the epidemiologist (and other scientists) in providing technical input is complemented by social and political considerations, so that the decision maker has full information on which to base a decision.

Technical information feeding into policy development should be objective, science-based, and free of biases. In order to achieve this, epidemiologists need to be aware of and apply skills from three broad areas of expertise:

- Cognitive analysis framework. This is a non-statistical approach to assessing available evidence using logical thought processes. This requires a thorough grasp and application of all the basic epidemiological concepts. In many cases, clear logical thought applied to the appropriate observations and information may be all that is required to solve an epidemiological problem.
- Appropriately planned and valid collection of data and information for statistical analysis.
- Statistical data analysis incorporating hypothesis testing where appropriate. A wide range of statistical tools has been developed to help describe patterns in data, and to distinguish random effects from genuine associations. These tools need to be applied within the cognitive analysis framework which provides a more general understanding of the problem. Only in this way will such issues as bias, confounding and lack of biological importance in the face of statistical significance be successfully addressed.
- Communication of the findings of these analyses in an effective manner, appropriate to the needs of the end-user. It is essential to distinguish between that which is known, that which may be inferred or deduced, and that which is not known. The level of confidence associated with the findings needs to be clearly expressed, although it is often difficult for policy makers to grasp these concepts.

1.6 Types of Epidemiological Study

There are many types of quantitative epidemiological study but they can be broadly grouped into observational study, intervention study and theoretical epidemiology as shown in Fig. 1.3. The underlying principles for all types of study are similar. In the process of finding causes of disease, factors which are statistically linked with the disease of interest and suspected to be causal for the disease (known as risk factors) are identified.

The different epidemiological study types rely on different approaches to sampling from the population in order to investigate the relationship between potential risk factors and the outcome of interest. Differences in methodology result in important differences in study characteristics and also in the strength of any inference that can be made from the results. The characteristics of different study types are described briefly below and the advantages and disadvantages of each type are summarized in Table 1.1. For more information on epidemiological study design, readers should consult standard epidemiology texts (Martin *et al.*, 1987; Thrushfield, 2005; Rothman *et al.*, 2008; Dohoo *et al.*, 2010).

1.6.1 Observational studies

In observational studies nature is allowed to take its course, while differences or changes in the characteristics of the population are studied, without intervention from the investigator. There are four common types of observational study: descriptive study, cross-sectional study, case-control study and cohort study.

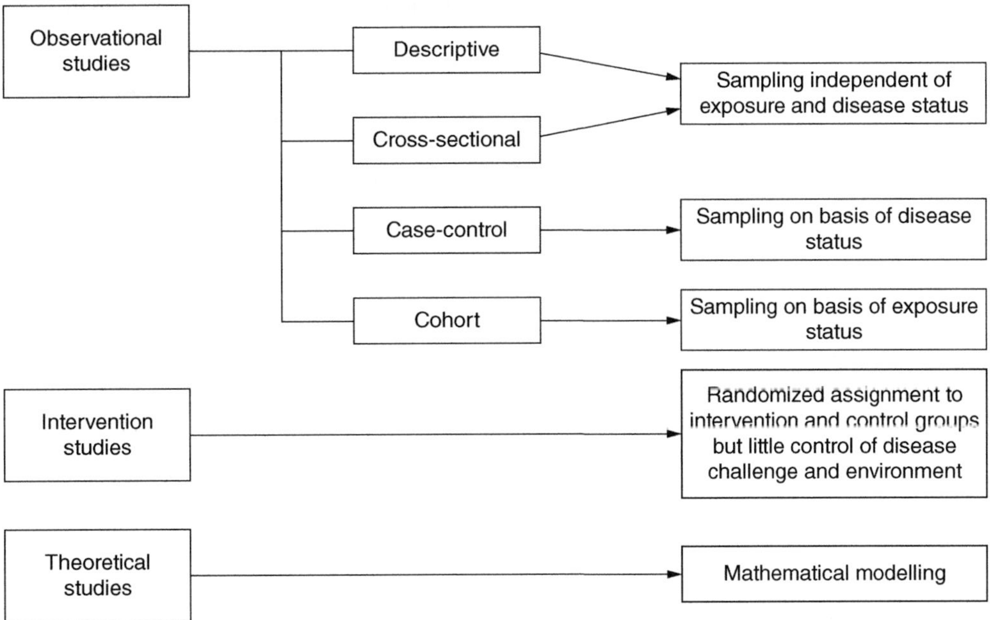

Fig. 1.3. Classification of quantitative epidemiological study types.

Table 1.1. Characteristics, strengths and weaknesses of main study types (adapted from Thrushfield, 2005).

Study type	Characteristics	Advantages	Disadvantages
Descriptive	Observational Describe patterns of disease in the population	Relatively quick and easy Can generate hypotheses on possible risk factors for further investigation Does not require random sampling or high degree of rigour	Does not support hypothesis testing or inference for possible risk factors Is unable to estimate prevalence or incidence or exposure proportions Subject to inherent biases and errors because of the nature of the data
Cross-sectional	Observational Observation at point in time Outcome/exposure not considered in selection	Disease prevalence in exposed and unexposed populations can be estimated Exposure proportions can be estimated Relatively quick and cost-effective Can study multiple factors at once	Unsuited to investigating rare diseases Less useful for acute diseases May be difficult to control potential confounders Incidence cannot be estimated May be difficult to determine causality May be problems with reliability of data/recall for historical data
Case-control	Observational Retrospective longitudinal Selection based on outcome status	Good for rare diseases Relatively rapid and cost-effective Relatively small sample sizes Often use existing data Can study multiple factors at once	May be difficult to establish causality Unable to estimate prevalence or incidence or exposure proportions Rely on access to historical data or recall Difficult to validate data May be affected by variables for which data are not collected Selection of controls often difficult

Continued

Table 1.1. Continued.

Study type	Characteristics	Advantages	Disadvantages
Cohort	Observational Prospective longitudinal Selection based on exposure status	Can calculate incidence in exposed and unexposed individuals Can provide strong evidence for causality	Exposed/unexposed proportions cannot be estimated Large sample sizes, particularly for rare diseases Can only investigate small number of potential risk factors at any one time Long duration of follow-up Relatively expensive and time-consuming Loss of individuals to follow-up
Clinical/field trials	Intervention Longitudinal Randomized selection	Relatively quick Can provide strong evidence for causality Usually strong internal validity Relatively small sample size and usually short duration Unable to estimate incidence/prevalence	May be problems with external validity, particularly to diverse target population Can be expensive depending on the intervention and situation Requires significant cooperation and rigorous management

Descriptive studies

A descriptive study (Fig. 1.4) has the objective of describing the distribution and occurrence of a disease in a population in terms of animal, place and time, without statistical hypothesis testing of possible risk factors. Descriptive studies may generate hypotheses, which can then be further investigated.

Cross-sectional studies

In a cross-sectional study (Fig. 1.5), prevalence of the disease in question is measured and compared among those with and those without the risk factor(s) of interest. A weakness of cross-sectional studies is that evidence for causation is only realistically produced for permanent (sometimes called fixed) factors such as species and sex.

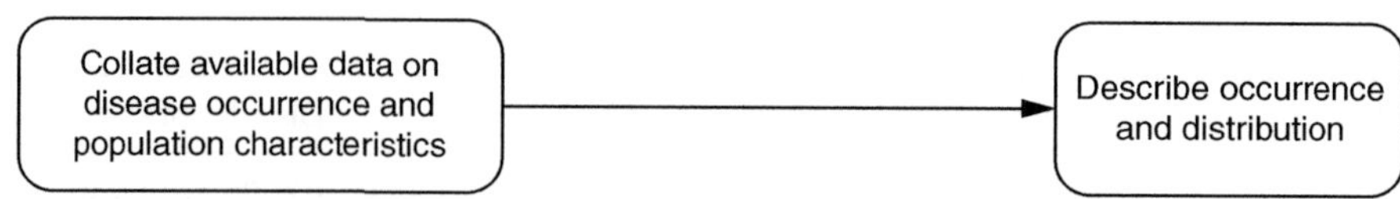

Fig. 1.4. Descriptive studies.

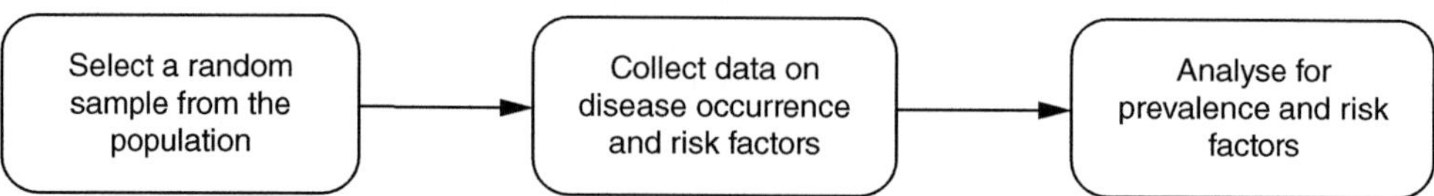

Fig. 1.5. Cross-sectional studies.

For example, you might undertake a randomized cross-sectional study of villages in a country for exposure to foot-and-mouth disease (FMD) virus. This would allow you to estimate the seroprevalence and to identify possible risk factors for exposure to support either follow-up studies and/or planning for future management of FMD.

Case-control studies

In a case-control study (Fig. 1.6), selection is based on whether or not subjects have the outcome (disease) of interest. A case group is selected from animals (or other units) with the disease of interest and a control group is selected from units without the disease. The frequencies of suspected risk factors are then measured for the two groups and compared. Case-control studies are well suited to rare diseases and many suspected risk factors can be compared at the same time. They are relatively quick and inexpensive to perform but are susceptible to many biases and do not yield estimates of the frequencies of disease in the exposed and unexposed populations.

For example, you might undertake a case-control study for FMD occurrence in village livestock. Case villages would be selected from known affected villages while controls would be selected from unaffected villages in the same region. This would allow you to identify village-level risk factors for infection, to support planning for prevention and management of future outbreaks.

Cohort studies

In a cohort study (Fig. 1.7), exposed and unexposed animals without the disease of interest are selected based on exposure to a hypothesized risk factor. The investigator does not assign or impose the factor of interest, but merely observes the course of natural events. After a suitable period of observation, the frequency of the disease of interest is compared between the two groups. Cohort studies can provide a complete description of the development of disease and true incidence rates in exposed and unexposed groups. They are particularly suited to evaluating the importance of specific risk factors identified by earlier, less-informative studies.

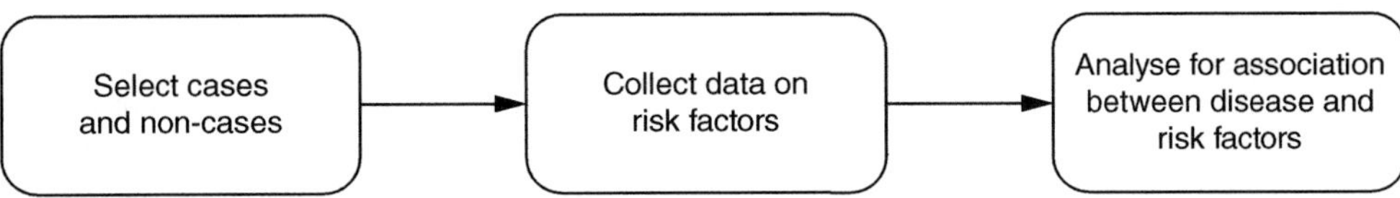

Fig. 1.6. Case-control studies.

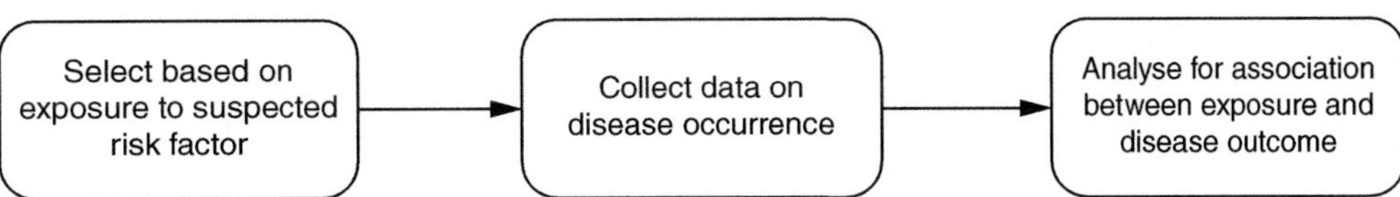

Fig. 1.7. Cohort studies.

The best known examples of cohort studies are numerous studies investigating health outcomes associated with cigarette smoking. Comparison of health outcomes between smokers and non-smokers has allowed researchers to quantify the increase in risk of lung cancer, cardiovascular disease and other health problems associated with increased levels of smoking.

1.6.2 Intervention studies

An intervention study (Fig. 1.8) is in reality an epidemiological experiment imposed at the population level. These are sometimes also called clinical or field trials. This is in contrast to laboratory or pen experiments, which are conducted under much more rigorously controlled conditions. The purpose of an intervention study is to evaluate the effects of some preventive or treatment (intervention) strategy. We commonly think of such studies as pertaining only to testing vaccines or drugs. However, the same methodology is applicable to other interventions such as changes in management or nutrition. Eligible experimental units are allocated randomly to two or more groups, the treatments applied and the outcomes measured and analysed for associations.

For example, mineral deficiencies can often result in poor growth and even death of young sheep or cattle. Often you may suspect that a particular mineral is deficient but be unable to demonstrate this conclusively. One way of achieving this is to run a field trial, comparing growth rates in treated and untreated groups that are similar in all other ways.

1.6.3 Theoretical studies

Theoretical epidemiology studies (Fig. 1.9) are based on mathematical modelling using a computer and are designed to answer what-if type questions in an attempt to extend the limits of existing knowledge. There are a wide variety of modelling methods used, but the primary aim is to reproduce a realistic simulation of disease behaviour

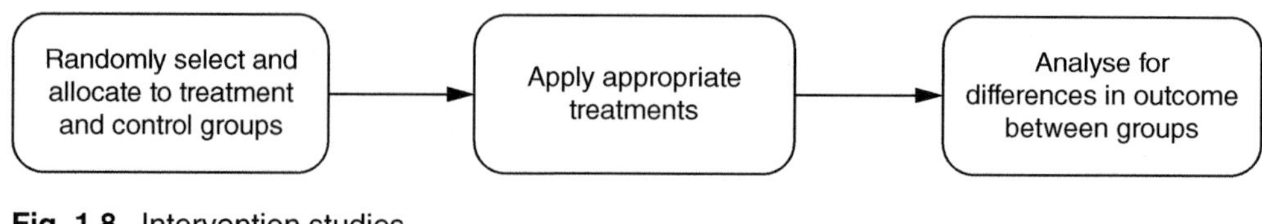

Fig. 1.8. Intervention studies.

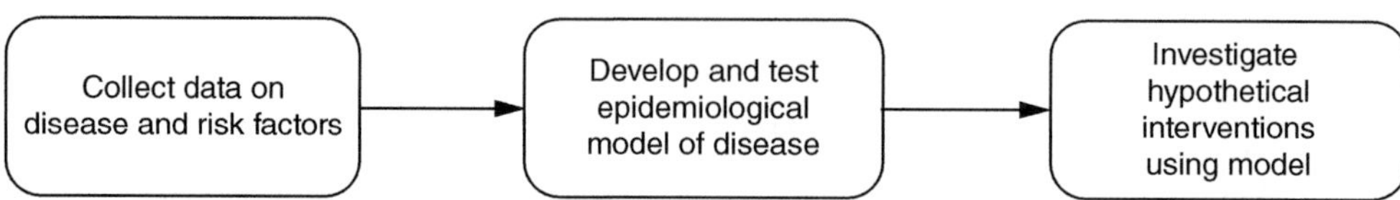

Fig. 1.9. Theoretical studies.

in a population (or whatever other characteristic is being modelled). The major benefits of models are that:

- The process of developing and interpreting the model often leads to valuable insights into disease epidemiology and behaviour that might not otherwise be apparent.
- Models provide a structured and controlled environment in which hypothesized interventions can be tested and evaluated at significantly lower cost than undertaking field experiments or observations to achieve the same result (or for interventions that may not be practical to implement experimentally).

Models are particularly useful in examining the behaviour and impact of infectious diseases as well as the possible effects of a range of interventions. The results from such studies need to be confirmed with follow-up observational or intervention studies wherever possible.

For example, simulation models of the spread of FMD have been used to help understand the behaviour of the 2001 outbreak in the UK and to predict the potential impact of alternative control strategies (Morris *et al.*, 2001).

References

Cutler, S.J., Fooks, A.R. and Van Der Poel, W.H.M. (2010) Public health threat of new, reemerging, and neglected zoonoses in the industrialised world. *Emerging Infectious Diseases* 16, 1–7.

Dohoo, I., Martin, W. and Stryhn, H. (2010) *Veterinary Epidemiologic Research*, VER Inc., Charlottetown, Prince Edward Island, Canada.

Hueston, W.D. (2003) Science, politics and animal health policy: epidemiology in action. *Preventive Veterinary Medicine* 60, 3–13.

Martin, S.W., Meek, A.H. and Willeberg, P. (1987) *Veterinary Epidemiology*. Iowa State University Press, Ames, Iowa.

Morris, R.S., Wilesmith, J.W., Stern, M.W., Sanson, R.L. and Stevenson, M.A. (2001) Predictive spatial modelling of alternative control strategies for the foot-and-mouth disease epidemic in Great Britain. *Veterinary Record* 149, 137–144.

Rothman, K.J., Greenland, S. and Lash, T. (2008) *Modern Epidemiology*. Lippincott, Williams & Wilkins, Philadelphia, Pennsylvania.

Thrushfield, M. (2005) *Veterinary Epidemiology*, 3rd edn. Blackwell Science, Oxford, UK.

2 The Epidemiological Approach

2.1 Introduction

In this chapter we introduce the concept of an epidemiological approach to disease investigation. The epidemiological approach is really about applying a logical, structured and transparent approach to any epidemiological investigation or project. It applies equally well to all types of epidemiological studies but is particularly important when investigating outbreaks of disease where the cause is unknown.

The epidemiological approach may be distinguished from a clinical approach to animal disease that is reliant on clinical examination of sick animals in conjunction with a range of ancillary procedures and information (history, signalment, laboratory testing, and examination of the immediate environment). The clinical approach is reliant on developing a list of candidate or differential diagnoses and narrowing that down to a most likely diagnosis. Control and prevention is then based on existing knowledge about the most likely diagnosis. In situations where there is a lack of available information, where the actual disease is novel or not included in the differential list then the clinical approach may not produce effective response measures.

In many cases, policy makers require rapid decision making, often in the absence of detailed and reliable information. The advantage of an epidemiological approach is that you can often draw some conclusions about the likely cause or risk factors for a disease, even in the absence of detailed data for statistical analysis or identification of the agent involved. In this situation, conclusions may be limited in scope and qualified by the quantity and quality of available data. Often, the main outcome will be interim recommendations for possible control and additional recommendations for further investigation to collect additional data and fill knowledge gaps. We will see an example of this later in this chapter and in Chapter 3, where we discuss applying the epidemiological approach to disease outbreak investigations.

2.2 A Structured Approach

The key to any successful epidemiological investigation is to use a structured approach, being as systematic as possible and always ensuring that the current working hypothesis is that which is most consistent with available data and information. Use of a clear, objective and well-structured approach will ensure that your conclusions and recommendations are easily understood, and that the process of arriving at these conclusions is transparent. This is essential so that you are in a position to defend your conclusions if they are challenged, and so that the basis and limitations of the conclusions are understood by those responsible for implementing any response to your recommendations.

Lack of clarity and structure is more likely to lead to conclusions that are poorly understood or that cannot be readily defended against opposition from detractors. In this situation, confusion and disagreement is likely, and the recommendations may never be acted upon, regardless of their validity.

2.3 Identify the Scope and Responsibilities for the Investigation

The first step in any epidemiological analysis is to define clearly the problem and the scope, context and expected outcomes of the investigation.

This might include determining if there is a disease problem and, if there is, to:

- determine the extent and impact of the problem;
- identify possible and probable cause(s) and source(s) of the problem;
- identify likely risk factors for the disease; and
- make recommendations for control and/or treatment and for future prevention.

Where the analysis is undertaken at the request of a third party (e.g. government policy makers), it is important that any request is clearly documented and that the terms of reference are clear and unambiguous. It is also essential that these terms of reference are used to guide your analysis and conclusions, to ensure that you meet the expectations of your client. Unclear or non-existent terms of reference are likely to result in poor analyses and risk failing to meet the expectations of the client or result in a dispute with the client over whether the analysis has been completed satisfactorily.

2.4 SMART Objectives

Clearly defined objectives and outcomes provide a road-map for your investigation – they tell you where you want to get to, and provide guidance on the steps needed to get there.

For example, if the objective of an investigation is to estimate the prevalence of white spot disease virus in shrimp breeding stock, the study design should be directed at this objective, not at identifying risk factors or looking for other viruses.

SMART objectives are:

- **S**pecific;
- **M**easurable;
- **A**chievable;
- **R**elevant; and
- **T**ime-limited.

Specific objectives are clear and well-defined. There should be no ambiguity or scope for misinterpretation. On completion of the investigation, it should be a straightforward process to determine whether or not the objectives have been achieved.

Measurable objectives allow you to monitor and quantify progress toward achieving them and completing the investigation. Measurable objectives also allow you to know when they have been achieved.

Objectives must be achievable, either with currently available resources and skills or with the required additional skills and resources identified and available externally.

Objectives must also be relevant to the overall project and achieving the required outcomes. Objectives that are not relevant risk wasting effort on producing a result that is subsequently ignored.

Any investigation should include a timeline and milestones to be achieved within the time frame. Failure to specify a time frame risks a project being continually delayed while projects that are perceived to be more urgent (those with specific deadlines) are progressed.

2.5 Operational Issues

During planning, it is also important to address operational issues. Failure to have clearly defined responsibilities and milestones can cause major difficulties at a later date, particularly if there is a dispute over whether the job has been completed, and who is responsible for any aspects that have not been satisfactorily completed.

Important issues to consider include:

- Make sure that the terms of reference are clear and specific and understood.
- Are the project milestones and deadlines clearly defined and reasonable?
- If there are multiple people or organizations involved ensure that it is clear who is responsible for what, and particularly what your responsibilities are. For example, if you are expecting your client to provide data or assistance in some form be sure that this is clearly stated in your agreement with them, otherwise they might regard it as your responsibility to obtain the data.
- If there are costs associated with obtaining data, are these included in the budget?
- What resources will be available and who will provide them?
- Who will direct the project – who is in charge and what is the chain of command?
- How will data be shared and who will do the analysis?
- Who is responsible for project management (physical and financial), communication, collaboration, etc.?
- Who is responsible for collection, filing and collating of material?
- Who is responsible for writing the final report and in what format is it required?
- What other project outputs are required?
- Are the budget and payment schedule clear and appropriate?

2.6 Gathering Existing Data and Information

Once it is clear what is required, the next step is to start collecting information and data for analysis. In this context, the term data is used in its broadest sense, and includes numeric data (able to be subjected to mathematical operations) and non-numeric data (facts) derived from related documents or other observations and that are not suited to quantitative analysis.

Information refers to interpreted outputs from prior analyses or conclusions from prior observations. Raw data can be turned into information through analysis and interpretation of findings.

For example, information gathered in looking at salmonellosis in sheep feedlots may come from a literature search, from which it is concluded that *Salmonella* is orally acquired and exposure dose is important – this may lead to identification of simple measures such as feeding in raised troughs that prevent faecal contamination of feed and ensuring good drainage to prevent slurry build-up. Alternatively, data might be available from feedlot and veterinary records, providing facts about cases (and non-cases) of salmonellosis that have occurred. These data would then need to be collated, summarized and interpreted to generate information from which to draw conclusions.

Relevant data and information might come from a variety of sources, including:

- the client;
- previous studies undertaken;
- scientific literature;
- other researchers;
- expert opinion; and
- other sources, such as farmers, veterinarians, pet owners, industry support workers (e.g. stock agents, feed merchants, etc.) and others.

Depending on the nature of the study, there may be comprehensive data already available and provided by the client for analysis, or it may be up to you to go out and collect any required data from these sources. It is important to document the source and nature of any data you use, and to identify any potential concerns about data quality, completeness and potential biases.

For an outbreak investigation, relevant data could include quantitative data on individual cases of disease, case histories on individual animals (both cases and non-cases), veterinarians' (or others') observations and impressions on cases, laboratory reports on testing undertaken on affected and unaffected animals, as well as potential sources of disease (such as samples of feed, water, soil and environment).

In other cases, the available data could comprise a series of paper files describing the issue of concern and providing relevant historical data. These files need to be read, collated and summarized to put the data into a form that can be easily understood and interpreted.

In many cases, the data will be fragmented or incomplete, and it is important to identify the deficiencies and gaps, and to ensure that any potential biases are addressed in your analysis. Fortunately, it is often still possible to draw important conclusions from incomplete data.

For example, in 1994, an incident occurred in Queensland, Australia where a previously unidentified virus (since characterized as Hendra virus) was responsible for the death of 14 horses and one human (with a second affected human subsequently recovering), associated with a single racehorse stable (Baldock *et al.*, 1996). During the investigation it became apparent that this was a previously unidentified disease and that the aetiology was unknown. However, even before the causal virus was identified, it was possible to determine that it: was probably infectious in nature; was most likely to be directly transmitted; was not highly contagious (either among horses or humans); and that it probably originated from an, as then, unidentified wildlife reservoir (Baldock *et al.*, 1995). Just on 1 year after the Hendra outbreak, flying foxes (fruit bats) were identified as the presumptive natural host of the virus, with about 14% of flying foxes sampled being seropositive (Baldock *et al.*, 1996). The virus was subsequently isolated from uterine fluids of a flying fox (Halpin *et al.*, 1996). Flying foxes were known to feed in trees in a spelling paddock associated with the index case. The specific mechanism of transmission among bats and from bats to horses is still not known.

In fact, perfect data/information to support your analysis is the exception rather than the rule, and in many cases you will be expected to draw conclusions and make recommendations based on less than perfect data/information. When this happens it is essential not only to recognize the limitations of the available data and information, but also to continue with those analyses that the data will support and draw what conclusions you can. In many cases, your recommendations are likely to include collection of additional data to provide further support (or otherwise) for your preliminary conclusions.

2.7 Searching the Literature and Other Sources

For many investigations and analyses it is essential to undertake a literature search, either to support a formal review of the relevant literature as part of the investigation, or to gather additional information to assist in completing the task. A literature search might be useful to:

- identify previous studies that are relevant to the current task;
- gather additional data that might be of use in supplementing existing data for the study;
- develop a differential diagnosis list in a disease outbreak of unknown cause;
- see how others have approached similar tasks; and
- gather additional information to support your conclusions.

With widespread access to the Internet and library services, searching for information is now relatively easy. Most of the relevant veterinary, medical and epidemiological literature is now indexed and readily available through a number of Internet-based search engines.

Some of the commonly used, web-based, scientific databases include:

- Medline/PubMed indexes all major medical, veterinary, epidemiological and associated journals, and is freely available for all users through PubMed (http://www.ncbi.nlm.nih.gov/entrez/query.fcgi).
- Medline is also available through Current Contents and other service providers through institutional library subscriptions.
- ScienceDirect (http://www.sciencedirect.com) provides indexing and search facilities for a wide variety of scientific journals in the physical, life, health and social sciences.
- Biosis previews/Web of knowledge (http://thomsonreuters.com/products_services/science/science_products/a-z/biosis) indexes a wide variety of journals, conference proceedings, books, review articles, etc., in the broad life sciences area. Available through institutional subscription.
- Sciverse Scopus (http://www.scopus.com/home.url) claims to be the world's largest abstract and citation database of peer-reviewed literature and quality web sources, covering a multitude of topics. It is available through institutional subscription and some publishers provide temporary access to reviewers of journal papers.
- Agricola (http://agricola.nal.usda.gov) is the catalogue of the National Agricultural Library of the USA and provides citations and abstracts for an extensive collection of agricultural literature.

- CAB Abstracts (CAB Abstracts) includes over 6.3 million records from 1973 onwards, with over 300,000 abstracts added each year, covering agriculture, environment, veterinary sciences, applied economics, food science and nutrition. Access is via institutional subscription or by time-based payment.
- JSTOR (http://www.jstor.org) indexes more than 1000 refereed journals from a wide variety of disciplines, including aquatic, biological and health sciences and statistics. Available through institutional or individual subscription.
- SIGLE (http://www.opengrey.eu), or System for Information on Grey Literature in Europe, indexes more than 700,000 bibliographical references from the grey literature (research reports, doctoral dissertations, conference papers, official publications and other types of non-refereed publications) produced in Europe. Open access to all users.

More general search engines include:

- Scirus (http://www.scirus.com/srsapp) is a broader search engine covering a wide range of scientific information across disciplines and publication types. Scirus covers not only scientific journals, but also web publications and a range of other non-refereed sources.
- Google Scholar (http://scholar.google.com.au/schhp?hl=en) also supports broad searches of the academic and scientific literature. It allows for searching across many disciplines and sources and ranks documents according to relevance and quality or frequency of citation.
- Google (http://www.google.com) and other Internet search engines can be used, but the content returned is not limited in any way other than by your search. These engines will return news items, personal web pages and any Internet content that is relevant to the search criteria (and some that is not!).

Most search engines search on a series of keywords. These keywords are words that appear in the title or abstract of a paper, or can be specified by the author as being relevant descriptors of the contents of the papers. Searches can also be made on author and publication names. The search engine will return a list of all papers (or other sources) that are indexed under the keyword or name you have entered. For example, entering the search term 'epidemiology' will return all resources indexed under the keyword epidemiology (>1,000,000 on PubMed).

Searches can be refined by adding more terms and constructing logical search statements. Different search engines handle multiple terms differently, often using an advanced search page to set search parameters. In PubMed and Medline, terms can be combined in a search statement using AND and OR logical operators. For example: dogs and hepatitis; Johne's disease or paratuberculosis. If AND and OR operators are combined in one statement, the AND part will be processed first, then the OR, unless the OR is contained in parentheses.

For example: cattle and Johne's disease or paratuberculosis is different to cattle and (Johne's disease or paratuberculosis). The first statement will retrieve all resources for Johne's disease in cattle or paratuberculosis in any species, while the second returns only resources relating to Johne's disease in cattle or paratuberculosis in cattle.

In the information technology age it is almost too easy to search for information on the Internet, and care must be taken to avoid information overload. It is important to compose and refine searches carefully, to make them highly specific for the desired topic. If this is not done, a large number of non-relevant articles are likely to be listed, making it very difficult to identify the important ones for closer scrutiny.

For example, a search on PubMed for Johne's disease returns more than 800 matches. By refining the search to find references about vaccines in cattle (Johne's disease and cattle and vaccine), this list can be reduced to less than 50. Additional terms can be added to further refine the search as necessary.

At the same time it is important not to get too specific, in case important papers have not been indexed on all the terms you have used. For more information about searching PubMed see Mayer (2004), pp. 30–51.

Once a list of potential sources has been identified, selected items can usually be saved to a text file, or often to a reference manager. Abstracts of papers listed on PubMed and Medline are often available online free of charge, but copies of the full papers will usually need to be either purchased online or obtained as downloads or photocopies through a library service (usually government agencies or universities).

A useful feature of Medline through Current Contents (for those with access to this service) is that it is possible to save regularly used searches for re-use or to be run on a weekly basis by the system, with new results each week forwarded as a text file to your email address. This feature is particularly useful if there are subject areas where you wish to stay abreast of the latest developments on an ongoing basis.

2.8 Organize, Analyse, Synthesize and Evaluate the Information and Data

Once the relevant data have been obtained and collated, the next step is to summarize and evaluate the data.

2.8.1 Quantitative data

For quantitative data, the first step is to explore and validate the data (see Chapter 10 on Exploratory Data Analysis for more details).

Important elements of an exploratory analysis are:

- Confirm the validity of the data – was it collected correctly and according to the protocol, were measurements accurate? Can it be validly extrapolated to your study population?
- Verify the data against original records if appropriate.
- Check for missing values and outliers.
- Undertake simple uni- and bi-variate analyses and graphing.
- Identify potential confounders and sources of bias in the data.
- Identify any problems in the data for rectification.

Once the data have been checked and problem records identified or removed, epidemiological analyses can be undertaken.

The specific analyses undertaken will depend on the nature and quality of the data available, but are likely to include some or all of the following:

- descriptive analysis of key variables;
- calculation of proportions of individuals (or groups) with specific characteristics of interest (test results, disease, risk factors, etc.) and associated confidence intervals;

- calculation of odds ratios and relative and attributable risks for disease associated with potential risk factors;
- calculation of mean value and confidence intervals for continuous variables such as weight, milk yield, etc.;
- calculation of median and inter-quartile range for skewed data such as ELISA ratios, metabolite concentrations, etc.; and
- statistical testing and multi-variable analysis for significance of associations identified, where appropriate.

From an epidemiological perspective, estimates and confidence intervals are often more useful for interpreting the results than statistical significance tests. It is important to critically review the results of analysis to ensure that important potential relationships are not overlooked. For example, factors that are biologically important might not be statistically significant if they are either masked by confounding or if the sample size is inadequate. Conversely, a potential risk factor may have a statistically significant association, but be biologically of only minor biological importance because of other factors that are more important (and that may or may not have been identified).

Statistical tests and inference must be appropriate to the nature of the data being analysed; for example, the choice of statistical test for comparison of two groups for a continuous variable, such as body weight, will depend on whether or not the data meet the assumptions of normality and equal variances and whether the groups are paired or independent. In some instances it may be appropriate to transform the data to meet these assumptions or to use alternative non-parametric tests.

It is also important to consider study design and sampling methods during analysis: analytical methods for a cluster-sampling or stratified study design are different from methods used for a simple random sampling design. Similarly, analytical methods for repeated measures on the same individuals or groups are different from methods used for analysis of independent measures. Seek advice for more complex or unusual analyses.

2.8.2 Qualitative data

In many cases, you could be asked to synthesize available information and make conclusions and recommendations with very little (or without any) quantitative data to analyse. In such situations the data are likely to consist of paper files, case reports, subjective observations or other soft data.

Qualitative data are not amenable to the numerical methods used to summarize and make inference from quantitative data. Instead, a qualitative analysis is required, following a series of systematic steps, such as:

- thorough review and summarization of the available material;
- identification of consistent patterns or anomalies in the data;
- identification of strengths and limitations in the data; and
- identification of likely and logical explanations for the observed patterns.

Because the data are qualitative and often of limited scope it is usually not possible to make definitive statements about cause-and-effect or other specific relationships.

However, it is often possible to arrive at a conclusion as to the most likely explanation(s) for the observed patterns.

For example, in the Hendra virus outbreak, there were virtually no quantitative data available for analysis from the initial disease outbreak, and yet a remarkably accurate picture of what happened and the cause and source of the outbreak were generated by critical review and interpretation of the findings of medical and veterinary investigations of affected animals and humans.

2.8.3 Formulate and evaluate hypotheses

Once the data and information have been analysed and reviewed it should be possible to formulate working hypotheses about the likely cause or source of disease outbreaks or about suitable strategies to achieve the objectives of the client. At this stage a working hypothesis is usually a broad statement of likely relationships, rather than the formal null and alternative hypotheses required for statistical significance testing.

Examples of hypotheses could include:

- the nature of the causal agent (e.g. toxin, infectious, viral, bacterial, etc.);
- the source of the agent (e.g. environmental, species jump, introduced animals, endemic infection, etc.);
- the method(s) of transmission (e.g. direct contact, food-borne, vector-borne, etc.);
- why the incident has occurred (e.g. change in herd immunity levels, introduction of new disease, change in management practices, etc.); and
- risk factors for disease (e.g. exposure to specific feed components, or potential sources of infection).

For example, in the Hendra virus outbreak, early hypotheses included the nature of the causal agent (viral), the method(s) of transmission among horses and from horses to humans (direct contact) and the source of infection (wildlife).

Once hypotheses have been formulated, it is important to review and evaluate them. In particular:

- Do they explain the observations?
- Are they reasonable?
- Are there any facts that contradict the hypothesis and how can these be explained?
- Are there any unexplained aspects of the situation requiring further investigation and evaluation?
- What additional data do we need to test the hypotheses, or are there sufficient data already available?

For tasks other than disease investigations, hypotheses will relate to the outcomes required by the client.

For example, you might be asked to evaluate a new diagnostic test and make recommendations on how it could best be used in the management of a particular disease. This task would involve evaluation and analysis of data on test performance and hypotheses would relate to the likely sensitivity, specificity, repeatability and reproducibility of the test.

2.8.4 Draw conclusions

Either from the hypotheses that have been developed or directly from evaluation of the available data and information it should be possible to draw conclusions. These conclusions must be based on a systematic assessment of the findings from the analysis, and should support the development of appropriate recommendations to meet the client's needs.

Any conclusions that are made must:

- be clear and concise;
- be supported by evidence from the data and information reviewed;
- meet the terms of reference or objectives specified by the client; and
- acknowledge any limitations resulting from the nature of the available data or the approach used.

Continuing the previous example of evaluating a new test, it should be possible to draw conclusions about whether the test is more or less useful than existing tests, how it can best be used to achieve the objectives of the programme and any additional work required to improve confidence in the test (e.g. improved estimates of sensitivity under different conditions, test reproducibility in other labs, etc.).

2.8.5 Make recommendations

The final step is to make recommendations on issues identified by the client in the terms of reference or in your objectives. Recommendations might relate to actions to be taken, response measures for the treatment, control and prevention of disease or development of policy. Again, recommendations must be clear and concise and directed at meeting the client's needs. They should also be directed at achieving outcomes for the client and should include recommendations for additional data collection and investigations, if required, to provide greater credence to the conclusions.

In most cases, recommendations will relate directly to the conclusions and will be directed at implementing changes to address specific issues identified in the conclusions.

2.9 An Example: John Snow's Cholera Investigations

In September 1854, Dr John Snow undertook one of the first and best known epidemiological investigations (Snow, 1855; Frerichs, 2001; Frerichs, undated b). At this time, London was in the grip of a major outbreak of cholera, the cause of which was still unknown. Snow hypothesized that the true cause of cholera was drinking of sewerage-contaminated water, rather than being spread by miasma or vapours as was believed by most people at the time. He undertook several investigations in cholera-affected London to support his case.

2.9.1 The Broad Street pump investigation

In his most famous investigation, Snow investigated cases in the Soho district of London, based on collation of cholera fatalities from official death registries. He observed that almost all cases occurred in close proximity to the water pump in Broad Street and that many fewer deaths occurred in households closer to other pumps. He also noted that a number of outlying deaths in surrounding districts could be explained by the fact that the people affected had drunk water from the Broad Street pump shortly before the onset of illness (in one case the woman affected reportedly preferred the taste of the water from Broad Street and sent out for a large bottle of it every day).

Snow also reported that all but five of the 535 residents of the local workhouse remained healthy despite being surrounded by affected households and hypothesized that this was because they had their own pump on the premises and did not drink water from Broad Street. Similarly, workers at a local brewery remained unaffected except for two mild cases. In this case, the workers were allowed to drink the product of the brewery and therefore rarely drank any water, certainly not from Broad Street. In contrast, 18 of about 200 workers in a factory on Broad Street subsequently died of cholera, after drinking from pump water freely supplied in the factory.

Based on his early investigations, Snow convinced the Parish authorities to remove the handle from the pump, and the number of new cases decreased almost immediately, although they were already showing a substantial decline from their peak (see Fig. 2.1). Subsequently, Snow produced a detailed map of the area, based on his investigations, showing the place of residence for all cases where he was able to determine their address, clearly showing the clustering of cases in the vicinity of the Broad Street pump (Fig. 2.2).

Why did this cluster of cases occur? Although Snow was clearly able to demonstrate the association of cholera cases with the Broad Street pump, the source of infection is less clear. However, he did note that the sewer passed within a few yards of the well, at a depth of 22 feet, compared to the well's depth of 28 to 30 feet, through gravel. There were also numerous cesspools associated with houses in Broad Street, also offering potential sources of contamination. In fact, Snow concludes 'Whether the impurities of the water were derived from the sewers, the drains, or the cesspools, of which latter there are a number in the neighbourhood, I cannot tell' (Snow, 1855).

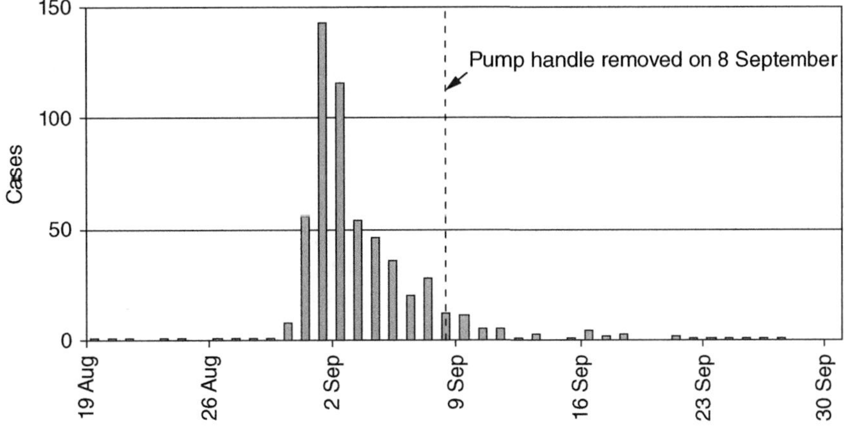

Fig. 2.1. Epidemic curve for John Snow's cholera investigation in Soho in August–September 1854. The handle on the Broad Street pump was removed on 8 September.

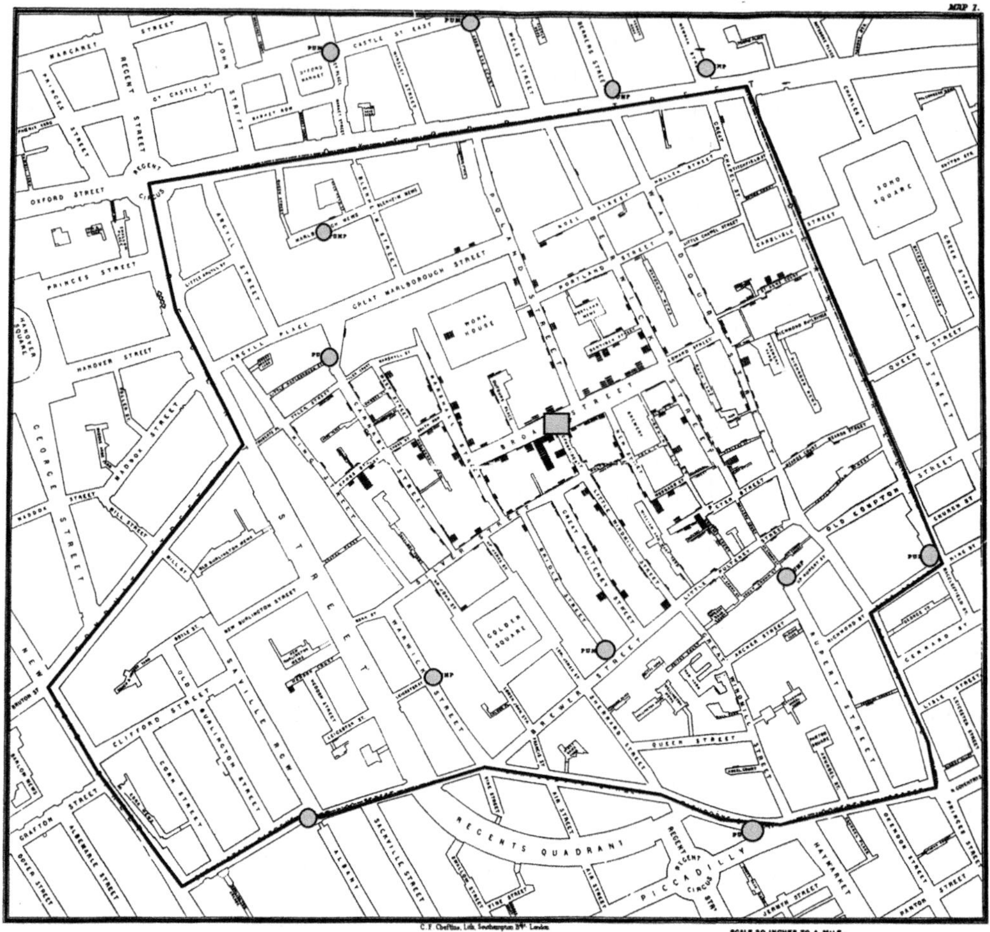

Fig. 2.2. John Snow's map of the 1854 cholera outbreak in London. The Broad Street pump is shown by a central shaded rectangle, other pumps by shaded circles scattered across the map. Cholera cases are shown by black bars at the location where they lived (adapted from Frerichs, undated b; copy of original map published by C.F. Cheffins, Lith, Southhampton Buildings, London, England, 1854 in Snow, John, *On the Mode of Communication of Cholera*, 2nd edn, John Churchill, New Burlington Street, London, England, 1855).

One hypothesis as to the source of the outbreak, put forward by the Reverend Henry Whitehead who also investigated the outbreak, was that the contamination of the well arose from waste water in a cesspool at 40 Broad Street, adjacent to the well (Frerichs, undated a). Whitehead established that an infant at 40 Broad Street became sick on about 28 August and subsequently died from cholera on 2 September. The baby's mother had washed out soiled nappies in a bucket and emptied the water into the cesspool, which was subsequently found to have decayed brickwork, so that contaminated water could seep into the well. He further expressed the opinion that the removal of the handle was critical to preventing a resurgence in cases as the father of the infant also contracted cholera on 8 September (the day the pump handle was removed) and subsequently died. Without the removal of the pump handle the contamination of the well would have increased again and the outbreak renewed (Frerichs, undated d).

2.9.2 The 'Grand Experiment'

At the same time as Snow was investigating the Broad Street cholera outbreak, he also undertook a separate investigation of the association between water source and cholera cases, described as his grand experiment. In 1852, the Lambeth Company, which supplied water to parts of London, moved its water source from downstream of London's sewerage outlet to a cleaner upstream source. Meanwhile, another main water supplier (the Southwark and Vauxhall Company) continued to draw water from downstream.

Taking advantage of this difference, Snow collated cholera death statistics for London during the 1853 outbreak, by sub-district, according to the source of their water. This analysis showed that sub-districts supplied by Southwark and Vauxhall had the highest rate of cholera deaths (114 per 100,000 population), while those supplied by both companies had a lower rate (60 per 100,000) and sub-districts supplied only by Lambeth Company had no deaths recorded. This appears to be the first documented epidemiological cohort study, although the terminology would still not be defined for many decades.

While this provided convincing evidence in support of his hypothesis, Snow was still not satisfied, so during the 1854 outbreak he collected information on the actual supplier for each household where cholera cases were reported, and correlated this with the reported numbers of houses supplied by each company. His analysis showed that in the first 7 weeks of the outbreak, more than 80% (1263/1514) of cholera cases were from households supplied by Southwark and Vauxhall. Additionally, the rate of cases per 10,000 households for households supplied by Southwark and Vauxhall was 8.5 times that for Lambeth households and more than 5 times that for the rest of London (see Table 2.1).

2.9.3 Why are John Snow's investigations significant?

At the time of John Snow's investigation the discipline of epidemiology was in its infancy, although the London Epidemiological Society, of which Snow was a founding member, was formed at about this time (Frerichs, undated c). Similarly, virtually nothing

Table 2.1. Deaths per 10,000 households in the 1854 cholera outbreak in London, by water source.

Water source	Number of houses	Cholera deaths	Deaths per 10,000 households
Southwark and Vauxhall Company	40,046	1,263	315
Lambeth Company	26,107	98	37
Rest of London	256,423	1,422	59

was known about infectious diseases, with the dominant theory of the day being spread of disease through vapours or miasma. Although the causative organism of cholera was first identified by an Italian scientist (Filippo Pacini) in 1854, his findings were largely unnoticed. It was not until 1883, when Robert Koch repeated and publicized the discovery, that *Vibrio cholerae* became widely accepted as the cause of cholera.

Against this background, Snow used his observational skills to develop a hypothesis and then test it, to demonstrate a causal link between water contaminated with human sewerage and cholera. He used simple numerical summaries and spatial representations to demonstrate his findings. However, this was all achieved without access to computers, sophisticated statistical or GIS software, or even to simple statistical methods or epidemiological measures such as relative or attributable risk. More than a century before Hill proposed his criteria for causality (Bradford-Hill, 1965), Snow fulfilled many of these criteria in his investigation (Table 2.2).

Table 2.2. Summary of considerations for causation (adapted from Bradford-Hill, 1965) and Snow's evidence to fulfil these criteria.

Criteria for causation	Snow's evidence
Strength of association – proportion affected higher in exposed than unexposed	Higher incidence in Broad Street residents compared to those closer to other pumps Higher incidence in households supplied from Southwark and Vauxhall compared to Lambeth Company
Consistency of the association on replication – multiple independent studies show similar findings	Consistent findings in both Broad Street investigation and the grand experiment
Specificity of the association – does altering only the factor alter only the effect?	Removing the pump handle may have contributed to the prevention of new cases in the Broad Street outbreak, although a substantial decline was already apparent
Temporal relationship – exposure should precede disease	Snow documented several cases where people (who did not regularly drink from the pump) became sick shortly after drinking water from the Broad Street pump
Dose-response – does greater exposure result in more severe disease?	Snow noted the intermediate incidence in parts of London supplied by both Companies, compared to those with contaminated water from Southwark and Vauxhall and clean water from Lambeth. He also reported several cases in the Broad Street outbreak where people who drank the water were fatally affected, while others in the same household who did not drink the water were more mildly affected
Biological plausibility – is the proposed relationship biologically plausible?	Although Snow does not make the point specifically, the idea of a gastrointestinal disease being contracted from drinking water contaminated with human sewerage is quite plausible, particularly if the miasma theory that was then prevalent is discounted

Continued

Table 2.2. Continued.

Criteria for causation	Snow's evidence
Coherence – does the causal relationship conflict with the known natural history of the disease?	Snow's findings were completely at odds with the miasma theory of disease occurrence that was popular at the time. However, at the time of his investigations the field of microbiology was just starting and virtually nothing was known of the true natural history of cholera, so this conflict is not surprising
Experimental evidence – can it be reproduced experimentally?	Snow relied on a natural experiment, using the differences in cholera incidence in households with different water supplies to demonstrate his findings, as a true controlled experiment was not possible
Analogy – is the relationship similar to other known cause–effect relationships?	At the time of Snow's investigation there were no known cause–effect relationships with which he could make an analogy
Intervention – does elimination of the putative causal factor reduce the incidence of disease?	Removing the pump handle reduced the severity of the outbreak and prevented its prolongation. However, more significantly, cholera incidence in parts of London supplied by the Lambeth Company in 1854 had substantially reduced cholera incidence compared to the 1849 outbreak (prior to moving their intake upstream to clean water)

References

Baldock, F.C., Pearse, B.H.G., Roberts, J., Black, P., Pitt, D. and Auer, D. (1995) Acute equine respiratory syndrome (AERS): The role of epidemiologists in the 1994 Brisbane outbreak. In: Morton, J. (ed.) *Proceedings of the Australian Association of Cattle Veterinarians*, Australian Association of Cattle Veterinarians, Brisbane, Australia, pp. 174–177.

Baldock, F.C., Douglas, I.C., Halpin, K., Field, H., Young, P.L. and Black, P.F. (1996) Epidemiological investigations into the 1994 equine morbillivirus outbreaks in Queensland, Australia. *Singapore Veterinary Journal* 29, 57–61.

Bradford-Hill, A. (1965) The environment and disease: association or causation? *Proceedings of the Royal Society of Medicine* 58, 295–300.

Frerichs, R.R. (2001) History, maps and the internet: UCLA's John Snow site. *Society of Cartographers Bulletin* 34, 3–7.

Frerichs, R.R. (undated, a) Index case at 40 Broad Street. Available at: http://www.ph.ucla.edu/epi/snow/indexcase.html (accessed 12 December 2009).

Frerichs, R.R. (undated, b) John Snow. Available at: http://www.ph.ucla.edu/epi/snow.html (accessed 18 December 2009).

Frerichs, R.R. (undated, c) London Epidemiological Society. Available at: http://www.ph.ucla.edu/EPI/snow/LESociety.html (accessed 18 December 2009).

Frerichs, R. R. (undated, d) Removal of the pump handle. Available at: http://www.ph.ucla.edu/epi/snow/removal.html (accessed 18 December 2009).

Halpin, K., Young, P. and Field, H. (1996) Identification of likely natural hosts for equine morbillivirus. *Communicable Diseases Intelligence* 20, 476.

Mayer, D. (ed.) (2004) *Essential Evidence-Based Medicine*. Cambridge University Press, Cambridge, UK.

Snow, J. (ed.) (1855) *On the Mode of Communication of Cholera*. John Churchill, London.

3 Investigating Disease Outbreaks

3.1 Introduction

A disease outbreak is a short-term epidemic or a series of disease events that are clustered in time and space. In many cases, the cause of the outbreak is unknown, at least initially. The disease events are usually new cases of a known disease occurring at a higher frequency than that normally expected, or cases of a previously unrecognized disease.

An outbreak, by its nature, requires a rapid investigation and implementation of control measures, often before a final aetiological diagnosis can be confirmed. An outbreak investigation is therefore a systematic process to identify risk factors for the disease that can be manipulated to prevent the further transmission of the disease-causing agent, control or stop the outbreak, and prevent future outbreaks.

Prompt and effective investigation of outbreaks is also an essential component of disease surveillance, particularly for new and emerging diseases. Active investigation of disease incidents provides ongoing surveillance for the detection and characterization of new and emerging diseases.

The epidemiological approach to outbreak investigations is based on the premise that cases of a disease are not distributed randomly, but occur in patterns within the population at risk. In fact, the occurrence of most diseases depends on a whole range of factors relating to the host (e.g. breed, species, age), the agent (e.g. strain virulence, methods of transmission, etc.) and the environment (e.g. housing, nutrition, management), rather than just on whether or not an individual was exposed to a pathogen. It is the role of the epidemiologist to analyse these patterns, to understand why the outbreak has occurred and to help meet the primary objective of ending the outbreak.

In this chapter we provide a general discussion of the steps required to investigate an outbreak of disease of unknown cause or where other factors have resulted in an increased occurrence of the disease. In subsequent chapters we provide more detailed description and examples of the specific methods discussed here.

3.2 The Basic Steps

An outbreak investigation usually follows a series of basic steps (adapted from Lessard, 1988). Not all steps are necessarily included in every investigation, nor do they always follow the same sequence. In practice, several steps may be undertaken simultaneously.

The basic steps in any disease outbreak investigation are:

1. Establish or confirm a provisional diagnosis.
2. Define a case.
3. Confirm that an outbreak is actually occurring.

4. Collect data on cases and non-cases.
5. Analyse the data:
   i. Exploratory analysis to verify and check the data.
   ii. Identify potential patterns of disease in time, space and by animal characteristics.
   iii. Descriptive and statistical analysis of any potential risk factors.
6. Formulate working hypotheses in an attempt to identify the type of epidemic, the possible source and mode of spread.
7. Implement control and preventive measures.
8. Undertake intensive follow-up investigations to identify high-risk groups and possible further outbreaks.
9. Report the findings of the investigation with recommendations for dealing with future possible outbreaks of the same disease.

Each of these basic steps is further explained in the following sections. Throughout the following discussion, investigation of Menangle virus infection in an Australian piggery is used as an example (Kirkland *et al.*, 2001; Love *et al.*, 2001).

Menangle virus was first identified in 1997, following an investigation of a serious outbreak of mummified and stillborn fetuses in a commercial piggery at Menangle, New South Wales, Australia. A high proportion of litters born to sows that were pregnant at the time of exposure to the virus were affected, although clinical disease was not noticed at the time of infection. After an extensive investigation the infection was traced to a nearby colony of fruit bats (flying foxes), with a high proportion of bats sampled found to be seropositive for Menangle virus antibodies.

3.3 Confirming the Diagnosis

An outbreak investigation is usually likely to occur in either of two situations:

1. Known aetiological diagnosis: in many situations the aetiological agent causing the outbreak will either be known or identified early in the outbreak (e.g. salmonellosis in dairy cows, anthrax in anthrax-endemic areas, foot-and-mouth disease in endemic countries). In this situation the investigation is directed primarily at identifying factors contributing to the occurrence and extent of the outbreak.
2. Outbreaks where the cause is unknown: where the aetiological agent is unknown, the investigation is directed at establishing an aetiological diagnosis, as well as identifying contributing factors that can be manipulated to control the outbreak.

If a definitive diagnosis for the cause of the outbreak is not known, a provisional diagnosis is often made, based on clinical signs, crude epidemiological patterns and pathological findings. Whenever possible, laboratory tests should be undertaken to verify the provisional diagnosis. Since some laboratory procedures may require weeks, the implementation of control measures is often based on the provisional diagnosis and the identification of risk factors during the investigation.

A definitive diagnosis is usually reached through a process of application of various tests and comparing the results from each. This is combined with the investigator's judgement, a thorough knowledge of the literature, past experience and intuition to organize the observations and reach a diagnosis.

Generally, a test procedure is interpreted to mean a test performed on a specimen in a laboratory. However, the same principles also apply to information obtained from the clinical history, physical examination, gross pathology, etc. A test is any procedure used to assist in determining the cause of disease or whether or not an animal is infected or has been exposed to a particular agent. In making a diagnosis, the investigator needs to have confidence in the accuracy of the method(s) used. An accurate test is both precise and valid. In other words the result is repeatable (a measure of precision) and gives a true measure of the value being measured (sensitive and specific – measures of validity). More formally, precision is defined as a lack of random error while validity is a lack of systematic error or bias. Chapter 7, on Diagnosis and Screening, provides more details on the evaluation and application of diagnostic tests.

Box 3.1 lists a number of ways that a disease might be diagnosed. These methods may be used alone or in combination to arrive at a final diagnosis. However, all of these methods are subject to random and systematic error and this must be taken into account when making a diagnosis.

Because any group of animals is likely to contain a range of pathogens, and even where there is a specific primary pathogen there can be secondary infections, it is also vital that a full range of specimens be taken from a number of animals at different stages of disease (including apparently healthy animals) so that comparisons can be made.

When selecting healthy animals for examination, it is important to obtain them from at least two sources including:

1. From a farm that appears to be experiencing the particular problem.
2. From one or more farms in the same area, but which appear to be free from the disease of interest.

Sampling of large numbers of animals may not always be feasible, but should be done whenever possible, particularly in enterprises with large populations, such as poultry

Box 3.1. Some methods used to diagnose disease.

- History
- Behaviour
- Clinical signs
- Physical examination
- Autopsy
- Molecular biology
- Microbiology
- Serology
- Epidemiology
- Response to therapy
- Production
- Economics
- Biochemistry
- Physiology
- Imaging
- Transmission tests

or aquaculture enterprises. At least ten animals at each stage of disease should be examined but, if resources permit, this number should be extended to as high as 30, or more. Statistical methods can then be used to assist in identifying which pathogen is the most likely to be the primary cause of disease. Failure to sample and test apparently healthy animals for comparison risks concluding a potential pathogen identified in affected animals is causal, when in fact it is also present in unaffected animals and may be completely unrelated to the disease outbreak.

Table 3.1 shows the number of animals that need to be examined to provide data for statistical analysis of association between disease and a finding or a possible causal factor (putative factor). Such analysis can assist in identifying which of a range of possible causes is most likely to be the primary cause.

As can be seen from the dark-shaded boxes, examining 25–30 animals per case and control group will provide 80% power across a pretty wide range of scenarios provided there is a reasonable difference between case and non-case groups.

The light-shaded boxes show the differences in prevalence required for a sample size of approximately ten animals per group.

Where the difference between cases and non-cases is large (top left corner), only small numbers of animals are required to provide a high level of confidence that the observed association is not due to chance. In contrast, very large numbers are required if the difference between groups is likely to be small (diagonal from bottom left to top right).

Table 3.2 provides example findings from laboratory testing for three organisms on samples collected from 30 cases of a particular syndrome and 30 non-cases.

From the above results, and with reference to Table 3.1, Organism 2 is the only one that is statistically associated with an animal being a case, despite Organism 3 being isolated more frequently from cases. The reason for this conclusion is that differences in observed proportions between cases and non-cases for Organisms 1 and 3 are smaller than for Organism 2, so that the sample size of 30 is insufficient to detect a statistical difference in isolation rates in these cases, but is sufficient for Organism 2. This does not prove that Organism 2 is the primary pathogen (as it could be an opportunistic, secondary invader), but by examining a reasonable number (in this case, 30) of cases and non-cases we are much better able to understand the relative importance of the three organisms.

Provisional and definitive diagnoses for Menangle virus were based initially on pathological findings, and subsequently on characterization of the causal agent, as follows:

- Provisional diagnosis:
  - mummified fetuses, stillbirths and congenital defects in piglets;
  - suspected due to an unidentified virus (known viruses excluded).
- Definitive diagnosis:
  - Menangle virus infection.

A variety of virological and pathological studies were used to arrive at these diagnoses. In particular, serological testing for Menangle virus on archival samples collected from 54 sows more than 3 months prior to the outbreak was negative for all samples, compared to 58/59 (98%) positive for samples collected immediately before the first affected litters were recorded.

Table 3.1. Number of animals per group to examine to determine if a particular finding is more common in cases than non-cases (95% confidence, 80% power, equal sizes for case and non-case groups and assuming a two-tailed test).

		Percentage of cases with pathogen									
		100	**90**	**80**	**70**	**60**	**50**	**40**	**30**	**20**	**10**
Percentage of non-cases with pathogen	**1**	4	6	7	9	12	15	21	30	50	121
	10	6	8	10	13	17	25	38	72	219	–
	20	7	10	13	19	28	45	91	313	–	–
	30	9	13	19	29	49	103	376	–	–	–
	40	11	17	28	49	107	408	–	–	–	–
	50	15	25	45	103	408	–	–	–	–	–
	60	20	38	91	376	–	–	–	–	–	–
	70	28	72	294	–	–	–	–	–	–	–
	80	44	219	–	–	–	–	–	–	–	–
	90	93	–	–	–	–	–	–	–	–	–
	100	–	–	–	–	–	–	–	–	–	–

Table 3.2. Hypothetical outbreak investigation of cases and non-case data and status with respect to organism 1, 2 and 3.

	Number (%) of positive		Sample size per group required to detect observed difference
	Cases	Non-cases	
Organism 1	14 (47%)	19 (63%)	408
Organism 2	26 (87%)	14 (47%)	25
Organism 3	27 (90%)	25 (83%)	219

3.4 Define a Case

A case definition is a set of standard criteria for deciding whether an individual unit of interest in the study has a particular disease or other outcome of interest.

It is important when investigating disease on a population basis that consistency of diagnosis is maintained within the particular study, regardless of the method(s) of diagnosis used. This involves developing a case definition, which is applied uniformly to all units in the investigation. Failure to do so will lead to bias (non-random error) in the study. Different case definitions may be developed for different units of interest, for example one for affected animals and one for affected farms.

For example, the investigator may be interested in comparing the occurrence of a particular disease in two different countries. Great care would need to be exercised if in one country the disease was diagnosed based on microbiological findings whereas in the other country a pathological or serological basis was used.

Where large numbers of animals are dying rapidly, a case may be defined as a dead animal. The need to distinguish between the small number of deaths due to other causes is trivial in such situations. However, for many outbreaks, specific criteria must be developed to define a case.

An optimal case definition depends on criteria that can be applied to any potential case in the source population. In many instances, it will be difficult to define a set of criteria that will include all true cases of the disease of interest and exclude all similar, but unrelated conditions. Few cases will show the complete range of disease criteria and there will always be some non-cases that have some criteria (e.g. clinical signs) similar to those of the particular disease being investigated.

The choice of a particular case definition will depend on the objectives and methods used in the investigation and may change during the investigation as new information becomes available. Some examples of case definitions that might be used for highly pathogenic avian influenza (HPAI) investigations are given in Table 3.3.

No matter what case definition is used, it will not be perfect. In fact, case definitions are subject to the same types of errors as screening and diagnostic tests in general, i.e. they are subject to random (lack of precision) and non-random (false negative and false positive) errors. For example, we know that HPAI may produce only mild clinical signs in some cases, particularly in vaccinated flocks. Thus, the first case definition will result in some false negative results where the study unit is an individual animal. False positive results could occur with the first two animal-level definitions, because other avian diseases may also produce clinical signs that are similar to HPAI, or birds may be infected with other influenza viruses that could produce positive serological test results. In any test system, there is always a trade-off between sensitivity (minimizing false negatives) and specificity (minimizing false positives) – as we increase one there is a related decrease in the other.

The case definition may also lead to an appropriate name for the syndrome being investigated. Several different case definitions for epizootic ulcerative syndrome (EUS) of fish are given in Table 3.4.

An appropriate name for the disease described in the first three case definitions would simply be *Aphanomycosis* while an appropriate name for the fourth would be red spot. If the consensus among experts is that EUS is a specific condition involving tissue damage due to *Aphanomyces piscicida/invadans* regardless of the predisposing factors, then it could be called *aphanamycosis* as this implies that *Aphanomyces piscicida/invadans* infection is a necessary (although not a sufficient) cause.

All of the case definitions in Tables 3.3 and 3.4 are legitimate. It should also be noted that the animal case definitions in Table 3.4 range from being very specific (but less sensitive) for the first through to very sensitive (but less specific) for the fourth.

How then should these case definitions be used? It is often useful to have definitions for a suspect case based on field observations (history, clinical signs, gross pathology, etc.) and a confirmed case based on laboratory findings especially where it may take some

Table 3.3. Examples of case definitions for highly pathogenic avian influenza (HPAI) in poultry.

Study unit	Case definition
Animal	An individual bird exhibiting specified clinical signs consistent with HPAI
	A bird with a positive result in a serological test for influenza A virus
	A bird with a positive result for H5N1 virus in a PCR or virus isolation test
Flock	A flock in which greater than a specified percentage of birds have clinical signs consistent with HPAI
	A flock in which greater than a specified percentage of birds are seropositive for influenza A virus
	A flock in which one or more birds have had a positive result for H5N1 virus in a PCR or virus isolation test

Table 3.4. Examples of case definitions for epizootic ulcerative syndrome (EUS) in fish.

Study unit	Case definition
Animal	A fish with necrotizing, granulomatous dermatitis and/or myositis and/or granulomas in internal organs with *Aphanomyces piscicida/invadans* found within the lesion
	A fish with one or more granulomas with *Aphanomyces piscicida/invadans* found within the lesion
	A fish with lesions in which *Aphanomyces piscicida/invadans* can be found
	A fish with one or more surface lesions, each of which could be described as a red spot
Pond	A pond with one or more fish meeting the selected case definition for an individual animal
River	A river with one or more fish meeting the selected case definition for an individual animal

time to confirm cases. Where a previously unrecognized and potentially serious syndrome is being investigated, it is advisable initially to use a very broad case definition (high sensitivity but lower specificity) to minimize the risk of missing any cases. In this instance, a revised definition that is more specific can be applied later when time permits.

Different case definitions may be more appropriate depending on the objective of the application. For example, say we are interested in the early detection of aphanomycosis in an area because the disease has never been reported and we think it is exotic. In this situation, we are interested in early detection and would want to know about any fish that could possibly be a case (i.e. we want a very sensitive case definition). We would probably choose the 'red spot' definition to identify suspect cases and then subject these to laboratory examinations aimed at detecting *Aphanomyces piscicida/invadans*. If we found evidence of the fungus, we would then have a confirmed case.

Further discussion of the approach to development of a case definition is given by Stephen and Ribble (1996), using marine anaemia in farmed Chinook salmon as an example.

Case definitions used in the Menangle virus investigation were:

- for fetuses, piglets that were mummified or stillborn with deformities; and
- for litters, any litter with six or fewer pigs born alive (some litters were born with up to six live piglets and up to six mummified fetuses).

3.5 Confirm the Outbreak

Confirming that an outbreak exists may seem superfluous, but in many instances it is required, particularly where the disease is already endemic. The challenge here is determining what is normal and when the level of disease is higher than normal. By definition, an outbreak or epidemic exists when the current incidence is in excess of the usual incidence of cases in the population determined to be at risk. The term excess is obviously imprecise. This is usually not an issue for large, rapidly spreading epidemics but can pose a problem for slower-developing epidemics, vector-borne diseases that can occur over a wide geographic area or diseases that are endemic in the population.

For example, on many dairy farms, a certain level of mastitis is expected, but an unexpected increase in the number of cases will lead to severe production losses and treatment costs if not recognized early. Similarly, a poultry farm may regularly monitor the number of deaths that occur, but would not consider an outbreak to have occurred until there was a rise in the number of deaths above normal levels.

For diseases that are not normally known to occur in a particular population, a single case could be regarded as an outbreak. For example, Nipah virus is endemic in fruit bats in much of Asia and causes sporadic disease in the human population in Bangladesh each year. However, in other countries cases in animals and humans are not normally known to occur and any cases would be regarded as constituting an outbreak, as occurred in pigs and humans in Malaysia in 1998. Similarly, small numbers of cases of bovine spongiform encephalopathy (BSE) that have occurred in countries such as Denmark, Canada and the USA were considered as outbreaks and treated as such.

For diseases that already occur in the population, or which have a similar presentation to diseases that already occur, it is more difficult to determine whether an outbreak is occurring. In this case, it is important to compare the current incidence or prevalence with long-term trends, or to use production indices as an indicator of disease-related changes in production over time. It is also important to confirm whether an apparent increase in endemic disease occurrence is due to known causes or is there a new disease occurring that is confusing the situation? Methods for investigating long-term trends in disease occurrence are discussed further in Chapter 5, Patterns of Disease in populations.

For the Menangle piggery, an outbreak was confirmed to be occurring, as measured by several indices:

- The percentage of case litters jumped from <10% prior to the onset of the outbreak to >30% in the first full week of the outbreak.
- The percentage of case litters peaked at 65% during the outbreak, well above the normal level of <10%.
- Case litters continued to occur at a greater than normal rate for 15 weeks.

3.6 Data Collection

Data collection and recording is a critical step in any disease outbreak investigation. Relevant data can come from a number of possible sources, including from the farmer's records, from direct observation and measurement of animals and from the results of laboratory investigation.

Electronic capture of the data is important to facilitate subsequent collation and analysis. Ideally, this should be in a purpose-built database, but in many cases time and resource will not support development of a database, so spreadsheets will often be the method of choice. Other forms of data recording (e.g. word-processing documents or text files) are unsatisfactory because the resulting data are not amenable to analysis without being further transcribed into a suitable format, providing additional work and the opportunity for errors to occur.

During data collection, it is important to ensure that data are collected on both cases and non-cases (e.g. on animal characteristics or laboratory testing). It is also important to collect detailed descriptive data on the population(s) at risk, to provide denominators for calculation of attack rates and other descriptive measures. When collecting and recording data, it is also important to use consistent coding (e.g. of animal characteristics) to facilitate analysis. Individual animals should be clearly and consistently identified to allow correlation of data or results from different sources. Ideally, data should be either collected electronically (e.g. from farm or laboratory systems) or entered directly into whatever data management system is used by the person collecting the data, to minimize data entry and transcription errors. With the availability of personal digital devices and laptop computers, remote collection and entry of data at the site of the outbreak is now a very real possibility.

3.7 Data Analysis

3.7.1 Exploratory data analysis

The first step in any data analysis is to explore, verify and clean the data. This step is described in detail in Chapter 10, Exploratory Data Analysis, and summarized briefly here.

The main aims of exploratory data analysis (EDA) are to familiarize yourself with the data, to identify and correct any errors or missing values and to help identify a strategy for more elaborate analyses. Essentially, EDA is an iterative process that includes manipulating the data into a format that is suitable for further analysis, checking data quality, summarizing the data into graphs and tables and where necessary correcting errors, ensuring consistent coding and terminology and aggregating data or transforming it to facilitate subsequent analyses.

At the end of the exploratory analysis you should have a dataset that is ready for further analyses.

Epidemiologists study patterns of disease occurrence in populations, so it is important to characterize the outbreak in terms of time, place and animal characteristics, particularly for diseases where the cause is obscure. In some instances, the unit of study may not be an animal. Rather it may be some aggregation of animals such as a pen, mob or whole farm even. The characterization must be done in such a manner that analyses can inform answers to the following kinds of questions:

1. What is the exact time period of the outbreak?
2. Given the diagnosis, what is the probable period of exposure?
3. Is the outbreak most likely from a common source, propagated or both?
4. Is the outbreak still spreading or has it peaked and started to decline?
5. What are the significant features of the geographical distribution of cases?
6. Are there any particular groups of animals that appear to be at greater risk than others?
7. Which animals have the highest and which have the lowest risk of disease?
8. What are the relevant attack rates in different groups of animals?
9. Are there clusters of disease in time and/or space that might help explain why the disease has occurred?

Temporal, spatial and animal patterns of disease are discussed briefly below and in more detail in Chapter 5 on Patterns of Disease.

3.7.2 Temporal patterns

Variation in the frequency of occurrence of cases of a disease over time is called its temporal pattern.

There are three basic time spans used to describe temporal patterns:

- an epidemic period, which is of variable length depending on the duration of the particular epidemic;
- a 12-month period to describe seasonal patterns; and
- an indefinitely long period of years to identify long-term trends.

Knowledge of seasonal patterns and long-term trends is important when deciding whether or not an epidemic exists in the present period and in predicting future epidemics.

The temporal pattern of an outbreak is described in terms of its epidemic curve (see Fig. 3.1). The epidemic curve is a graph plotting the number of cases of the disease in question against the time of onset of each case, either as a bar graph or frequency polygon. The first case identified for a particular outbreak is referred to as the index case. For infectious diseases, identifying the index case is important as information

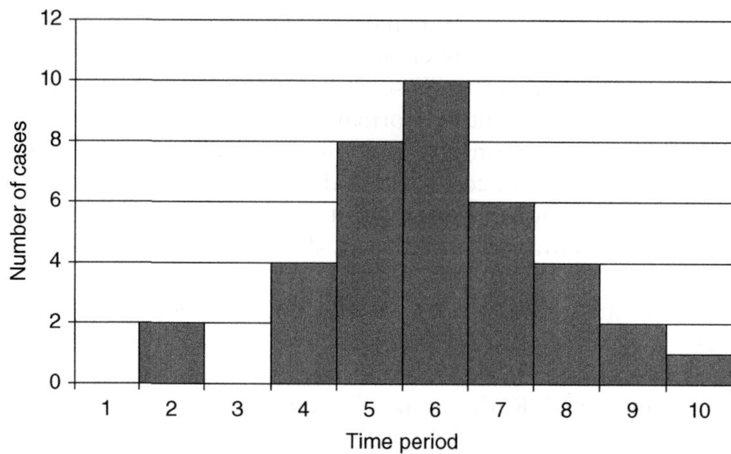

Fig. 3.1. Example epidemic curve.

about the index case can be valuable in ascertaining the source of the outbreak and the incubation period.

For Menangle virus, temporal patterns were analysed on a weekly basis, because many piggery records are maintained as weekly averages and the epidemic extended over a >20-week period. In addition to the percentage of affected litters per week, average litter sizes and numbers of piglets that were live, mummified or stillborn were plotted, providing a comprehensive picture of the temporal pattern. All indices showed a very rapid rise from week 15 (of the calendar year), when the outbreak started, to week 21, when case numbers peaked. This pattern is strongly suggestive of a propagating epidemic with a rapidly spreading agent and relatively short incubation period (see Fig. 2 from Love *et al.*, 2001 for a graphical representation of these patterns).

3.7.3 Spatial patterns

Describing the outbreak in terms of place may assist with finding the source of the outbreak. It is often useful to consider place and time together. This can be done by drawing a plan of the spatial layout of the farm (or population), recording the location and dates when cases occurred. Such a diagram may also give a lead to whether the outbreak is a common source or propagating.

For example, Fig. 3.2 shows the layout of households in a Thai village, overlaid with the occurrence of cases of foot-and-mouth disease. From this map, it is apparent that this is a propagating epidemic, with the index case identified by a circle, a small number of secondary cases identified in week 2 and additional cases in week 3. It also appears that infection has spread locally from the index case to a number of nearby households, as well as to some more remote households, where there has also been local spread. The initial spread was perhaps through utilization of common grazing, allowing close contact between early cases and susceptible animals from elsewhere in the village. This was probably followed by local spread among clusters of households and perhaps from infected animals moving on laneways through the village.

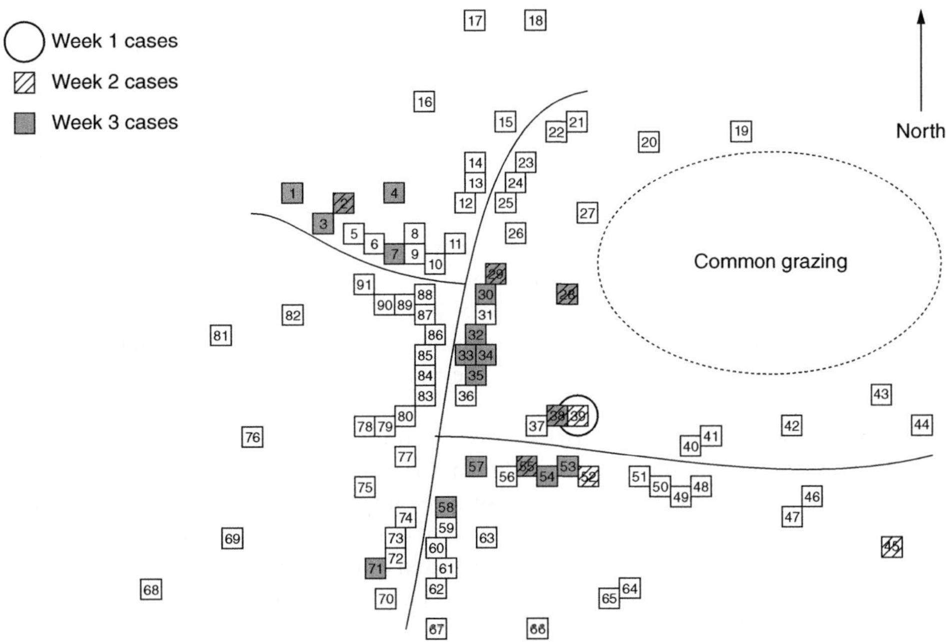

Fig. 3.2. Spatial representation of the spread of foot-and-mouth disease over a 3-week period in a Thai village (adapted from Cleland *et al.*, 1991).

For larger scale epidemics, spot maps are useful and GIS systems may be required to track large-scale epidemics. Where epidemics last for an extended period it is often useful to produce maps at daily, weekly or monthly intervals to monitor progress of the epidemic and identify patterns of spread.

For the Menangle virus outbreak, the piggery comprised four separate management 'Units'. Unit 1 was about 200 m from Unit 2, while Units 2 and 3 and 3 and 4 were each separated by about 50 m (see Fig. 1 in Kirkland *et al.*, 2001). Although all units were affected, 44% of litters were affected in Unit 2, compared to 28%, 26% and 37% for Units 1, 3 and 4, respectively. Analysis also showed that Unit 3 was affected first, in week 15. Other units were subsequently affected in weeks 23 (Unit 2), 24 (Unit 4) and 27 (Unit 1). It was also observed that a fruit bat colony (the hypothesized source of infection) was in close proximity to Units 3 and 4. Unit 1 was furthest from the hypothesized source and was the last unit to be affected, while Units 3 and 4 were closest to the hypothesized source.

3.7.4 Animal patterns

Although the word animal is used here, we should really refer to cases and non-cases and their characteristics to embrace the wider definitions where cases might be pens, cages, ponds, mobs, whole farms, villages or even some higher level of aggregation. For simplicity, this discussion is restricted to animals only.

Age, sex, geographical origin and genotype are frequently associated with varying risk of disease. However, it should be kept in mind that animal patterns can be closely linked to temporal and spatial patterns of disease. For aggregations of animals such as mobs, cages and farms, the total number of animals in the aggregation and the stocking density are commonly associated with varying risk of disease. Animal (or unit) characteristics are not limited to fixed characteristics such as species, breed, age or sex. Any exposure to potential risk factors for disease should also be considered under animal characteristics. For example, important risk factors could include nutritional or management differences.

To describe patterns of disease by animal types, it is first necessary to outline what measures of disease frequency are used in outbreak investigations. The basic measure of disease frequency in outbreaks is the attack rate (AR), which is a special form of incidence rate where the period of observation is relatively short. An attack rate is the number of cases of the disease divided by the number of animals at risk at the beginning of the outbreak.

Where different risk factors for the disease under investigation are to be evaluated, attack rates specific for the particular factor are calculated and compared.

For example, in the foot-and-mouth disease example shown in Fig. 3.2, 8 of 21 buffalo <1 year old were affected for an attack rate of 0.38 or 38% (Cleland *et al.*, 1991). In contrast, 34 of 158 buffalo >1 year old were affected (attack rate = 0.215 or 21.5%). This suggests that young animals were almost twice as likely to be affected as older animals.

For the Menangle virus example:

- The percentage of affected litters in Unit 3 (the first affected unit) increased from an average of 6.6% prior to the outbreak to 64% at the peak and an average of 28% during the outbreak.
- Percentages of affected litters varied among units from 26% in Unit 4 to 44% in Unit 2.
- Farrowing rates were reduced more in older sows (Units 3 and 4).
- The percentage of case litters was higher in younger sows (Units 1 and 2).
- However, age of sows was also confounded by spatial distribution in the piggery.

3.7.5 Analysing potential risk factors

Once the data for temporal, spatial and animal-level factors has been collated, it should be analysed to understand patterns and identify potential risk factors. The most commonly used measures for comparing disease risk among groups are relative risk (or risk ratio) and attributable risk. Relative risk (also called risk ratio) is the ratio of the risk of disease or death among the exposed group compared to the unexposed. Attributable risk is the difference in risk that is explained by the characteristic or risk factor under study. These are discussed in greater detail in Chapter 6 on Measuring Disease Frequency.

Relative and attributable risks provide measures of the biological importance of the risk factor, whereas statistical significance testing or confidence intervals tell you whether the observed result is likely to have occurred due to chance or not. Risk factors can be statistically significant but have little biological impact if the relative risk is low.

A relative risk greater than 1 (or positive attributable risk) indicates an increased risk compared to the reference group, while a relative risk less than 1 (or negative attributable risk) indicates a reduced risk (i.e. the factor is protective). Relative risk cannot be negative, but can range from 0 to positive infinity. It is common practice (but not essential) to use the group with the lowest attack rate as the reference group for calculating and attributable relative risk, so that relative risk is >1 and attributable risk is positive. The higher the attack rate difference and the further the relative risk from 1, the more impact the specific factor has on the risk of disease. Methods are also available for calculating confidence limits and for statistical significance testing for relative and attributable risks. The analysis becomes more complicated if there is evidence of interactions and confounding among factors. Stratified and multi-variable analyses can be used to investigate these phenomena.

Factor-specific attack rates and corresponding relative and attributable risks for such factors as species, age, sex, feed, mob, management system, etc. can be computed and arranged in an attack rate table as shown in Table 3.5. An attack rate table is simply a tabular presentation of attack rates for different risk groups, accompanied by relative and attributable risk values for comparison between groups. Table 3.5 shows an attack rate table for an investigation of stillbirths in a group of young cattle, with the attack rates expressed as percentages. The second last column is the relative risk or risk ratio (RR), which is the ratio of the attack rates, and the last column is the difference in attack rates (the attributable risk).

In the example in Table 3.5 the highest relative risk is 2.3, indicating that younger heifers (14 months) were at 2.3 times the risk of having a stillborn calf compared to older (17 months) heifers. However, this has to be interpreted with caution, as the attack rate for older heifers was 15.5%, suggesting that other factors may also have been involved in causing this problem. Examination of the other relative risks list shows them all to be less than 2, suggesting that these factors are not very important. Therefore, from the data provided we can determine that younger heifers are at increased risk of stillbirth, but that there are probably additional factor(s), for which we do not have data, that are contributing to this problem.

For the Menangle virus outbreak, attack rates varied between units, but all units were affected to some degree. As a result, relative risks ranged from 1.0 (Unit 4 = reference group) to 1.7 (Unit 2) and did not contribute greatly to further understanding of the outbreak.

3.7.6 Statistical analysis

Once potential risk factors have been identified and their importance assessed in attack rate tables it may be useful to undertake further statistical analyses. Before

Table 3.5. Attack rate table for risk factors for stillbirths in a group of Hereford heifers.

Factor	Levels	Stillborn	Live	Total	Attack rate	Relative risk	Attributable risk
Age	14 months at joining	14	25	39	35.9%	2.3	20.4%
	17 months at joining	16	87	103	15.5%		
Sire breed	Hereford	22	78	100	22.0%	1.0	0.8%
	Angus	7	26	33	21.2%		
Sex of calf	Female	18	48	66	27.3%	1.7	10.9%
	Male	11	56	67	16.4%		
Type of birth	Assisted	16	41	57	28.1%	1.7	11.6%
	Normal	14	71	85	16.5%		

discussing statistical analysis further, it is important to differentiate the roles of statistical analysis and descriptive measures of disease such as attack rates and relative or attributable risks.

Attack rates and relative risks describe the biological importance of a risk factor such as how much disease is occurring, how much of it is due to exposure to the particular risk factor and what impact would eliminating the risk factor have on the amount of disease?

Statistical testing on the other hand tells you if the observed relationship is likely to be due to chance or not – is the apparent relationship real or not?

This distinction is important to understand, because potential risk factors can have a high relative risk but be statistically not significant or vice versa, depending largely on sample size. Therefore, it is important to always consider high relative risk values (say >3) as being worth further investigation, even if they are not statistically significant.

Detailed descriptions of statistical methods are beyond the scope of this book. However, simple methods such as the Chi-square test are available to test for significance of relative and attributable risks and stratified analysis (Mantel-Haenszel) or multiple logistic regression analysis are available for where confounding might be occurring. Confounding occurs when an apparent relationship between the factor of interest and the outcome is due to a second factor that is related to both the first factor and the outcome. An introduction to statistical principles and basic statistical methods is provided in later chapters.

3.8 Establish a Working Hypothesis

Based on the analysis of time, place and animal data, working hypotheses are developed for further investigation and to plan an initial response to control the outbreak. These may concern one or more of the following:

- whether the outbreak is common source or propagating;
- if a common source, whether it is a point or multiple exposure;
- the mode of transmission – contact, vehicle or vector; and
- possible risk factors for exposure/infection.

Any hypothesis should be compatible with all the facts.

Corrective action can be taken based on the more realistic hypotheses. For example, epidemiological analysis of outbreaks of white spot disease in pond-reared shrimp in Asia led to a hypothesis that sustained high levels of salinity could trigger an outbreak. Based on this hypothesis, careful monitoring of salinity levels and the ability to exchange water when required are management options to help prevent further outbreaks triggered in this way.

Whenever possible, hypotheses that are generated during the investigation should then be formally tested to confirm (or deny) their validity. This may be by:

- formal statistical testing of the available data;
- controlled treatment trials to test hypothesized treatments; or
- collection and analysis of additional data to enable formal testing of the hypothesis.

Based on these hypotheses it may also be possible to draw up a hypothesized path model or causal web for the outbreak, showing how the various factors interact to cause the disease. This process helps to understand the disease process and can often lead to an improved understanding of the relationships between hypothesized risk factors. Consideration of these relationships will often help identify points where intervention can be made to control and/or prevent the disease occurring.

For Menangle virus, based on the observations during the outbreak, it was hypothesized that:

- The outbreak was a propagating epidemic of a previously unidentified virus causing infertility, stillbirths, mummified fetuses and congenital deformities.
- The probable source of infection was from a fruit bat colony, either on fly-past or entry to sheds or laneways.
- Spread within the piggery occurred via close contact and fomites during acute infection and at farrowing.

An obvious conclusion from this was that the easiest way to prevent future outbreaks was to prevent any contact between pigs and fruit bats by enclosing and screening all sheds and laneways.

Sera and faeces were collected from fruit bats from the nearby colony, to test the hypothesis that the bats were the source of this virus. Positive serum samples were obtained 40 of 80 (50%) bats, but virus was unable to be isolated from faeces from 55 bats.

3.9 Implement Control and Preventive Measures

Hopefully, the investigation should lead to the identification of causal factors involved in the outbreak and their relationships, so that control measures can be implemented and the outbreak terminated. The information gained will also ensure that the risk of similar occurrences in the future is reduced. Strategies to stop the epidemic must be put in place as soon as possible and will often be undertaken in the absence of conclusive findings.

In some cases, it will not be possible to stop an outbreak once it starts, but the detailed investigation of one or more outbreaks should provide valuable insight into possibly important component causes and support the development of strategies to prevent future outbreaks.

Actual measures implemented will depend on the individual circumstances, but could include one or more of the following:

- specific treatments;
- vaccination;
- changes in nutrition, feed ingredients and/or management factors;
- isolation or quarantine;
- surveillance of the affected population and other at-risk populations for evidence of further spread and new cases;
- changes in environment and/or housing;
- safe destruction and disposal of contaminated waste or other infectious materials;
- disinfection and decontamination; and
- salvage sale or slaughter of animals.

Based on the findings from the various investigations it was not deemed possible to prevent continuing spread of the virus at the time of the outbreak. Instead, it was decided to undertake a staged eradication programme once the main epidemic had burned out, including:

- progressive eradication from the four production units;
- segregation, depopulation and staged repopulation of units;
- sheds and walkways flying-fox-proofed to prevent re-introduction; and
- serological testing to monitor progress.

Successful eradication was achieved and subsequently demonstrated by ongoing monitoring of the population.

3.10 Further Investigations and Follow-up

Additional investigations can include clinical, pathological, microbiological and toxicological examinations as well as additional epidemiological studies. Epidemiological follow-up includes detailed analysis of existing data, identification of additional cases on existing or other premises and undertaking of additional specific studies to formally test some of the hypotheses that have been generated, as discussed above. Flow charts of management and movement of animals and feedstuffs may be required as part of this process.

Feeding trials may be required where toxins are suspected as well as transmission experiments and treatment or vaccination trials for possible infectious agents.

Follow-up should also include ongoing monitoring of the outbreak and the effect of recommendations. Analysis and review of outbreak data should be a continuing process and review and modification of recommendations may be required as new findings emerge.

During the Menangle virus investigations, a wide range of additional investigations were undertaken, including:

- detailed pathological, serological, microbiological and virological examination of affected and unaffected pigs to determine the likely cause and to rule out known infections and other diseases;
- cross-sectional serological survey of all units/sheds to determine the extent and progress of infection;
- surveys of pigs and piggeries in contact to determine whether infection had spread beyond the Menangle piggery;
- testing of archived sera (from this and other piggeries nationwide) to demonstrate that it was a new infection not previously present in the Australian pig population;
- interview and testing of piggery workers and others potentially exposed in order to evaluate public health risks;
- serology on other species as potential sources; and
- serology and virus isolation on fruit bats to support the hypothesis that they were the likely source.

3.11 Reporting

A final report should document the findings of the investigation. For small outbreaks, this may take the form of a brief discussion with the farm manager outlining the important features and actions required to prevent future occurrences. Important results or recommendations requiring urgent action may also be delivered verbally to minimize delays. However, it is wise to always produce some form of written report so that a permanent record of events exists for future use. For new or unusual conditions, findings should be published in the scientific literature.

The primary aim of the report is to document the findings and recommendations arising from the investigation for the client and for future reference. The report should also address the original objectives of the investigation (see Chapter 2). The report should be clear, concise and readable, using simple language and examples and avoiding jargon and technical terminology wherever possible. Key elements of the report include the following.

3.11.1 Summary

For lengthy reports a brief summary at the start, providing the key findings and recommendations, may be appropriate.

3.11.2 Background/Introduction

This should provide a brief discussion of the background to the investigation, including a summary of the history and clinical signs and background information provided by the client.

3.11.3 Objectives

It is important to clearly document the objectives of the investigation, as originally agreed with the client. This provides a reference point for evaluation of the results and recommendations to ensure that the investigation has achieved the desired outcome and met the expectations of the client.

3.11.4 Methods

A description of the approach taken to the investigation is valuable both for future reference and also so that the client can understand what was done during the investigation.

3.11.5 Results

Include a summary of the results, including epidemic curves, output of spatial and temporal analyses, relevant attack rate tables and laboratory results and summaries of data analysed and statistical tests. Avoid including excessive irrelevant data, such as lengthy details of all the tests that were done and their results unless they are relevant to the outcome. Also include case definitions and the definition of the population at risk.

A discussion of the financial impact can also be included, if appropriate. More detailed data or results may be included as appendices.

Usually it is helpful to include a brief discussion and interpretation of results, unless their interpretation is self-evident.

3.11.6 Conclusions

This section should include an overall interpretation and synthesis of the results, leading to the development of hypotheses as to the likely cause, potential risk factors and possible control and preventive measures.

3.11.7 Recommendations

Provide a clear and simple series of recommendations for the client to implement. Where possible, identify those recommendations that will have the greatest potential impact and return on investment, to assist the client in deciding which recommendations to implement in situations where it might not be financially or practically feasible to implement all recommendations. A financial analysis of the cost and potential benefits of specific recommendations may be appropriate, particularly where significant expenditure is required to implement the recommendations.

Recommendations may include direct actions to control the current outbreak or prevent future recurrences, as well as recommendations for further investigations required to clarify or confirm interim findings. Recommendations may also be for interim actions based on preliminary findings, with further actions to depend on the outcome of additional investigations.

3.11.8 Appendices

Appendices should include copies of laboratory and other external reports, details of more complex analyses where these might be required, large tables of detailed information that are not required in the body of the report and any other material that may be relevant but is either too detailed or takes up excessive space for inclusion in the main report.

For Menangle virus, the findings from the investigation were eventually published in the *Australian Veterinary Journal*, providing a permanent record of the investigation.

References

Cleland, P.C., Chamnanpood, P. and Baldock, F.C. (1991) Investigating the epidemiology of foot and mouth disease in northern Thailand. In: Kennedy, D.J. (ed.) *Epidemiology Workshop: Supplement to Epidemiology at work. Proceedings 176*, The University of Sydney Postgraduate Committee in Veterinary Science, Sydney, Australia, pp. 17–32.

Kirkland, P.D., Love, R.J., Philbey, A.W., Ross, A.D., Davis, R.J. and Hart, K.G. (2001) Epidemiology and control of Manangle virus in pigs. *Australian Veterinary Journal* 79, 199–206.

Lessard, P. (1988) The characterization of disease outbreaks. *The Veterinary Clinics of North America: Food Animal Practice* 4, 17–32.
Love, R.J., Philbey, A.W., Kirkland, P.D., Davis, R.J., Morrissey, C. and Daniels, P.W. (2001) Reproductive disease and congenital malformations caused by Menangle virus in pigs. *Australian Veterinary Journal* 79, 192–198.
Stephen, C. and Ribble, C.S. (1996) Marine anemia in farmed chinook salmon (*Onchorhynchis tshawytshca*): development of a working case definition. *Preventive Veterinary Medicine* 25, 259–269.

4 Causality

4.1 Introduction

There is a great deal of information in the scientific literature related to causality or causation. Discussion of causality often requires care and attention to precise meanings or definitions of particular words and occasional philosophic interludes into related topic areas. This section attempts to provide a relatively simple and practical summary of causality in the context of veterinary epidemiology.

A cause can be described as something that has the capacity to influence or make a change in an outcome of interest such as disease state in animals. Causal factors are generally expected to be associated with occurrence of change in the outcome of interest in some measurable way, to precede the change in time, and to be responsible for or contribute to the change in the outcome (Susser, 1991). In this section we shall use the occurrence of disease as the major change or outcome of interest.

4.2 Sufficient, Necessary and Component Causes

A cause is an event, condition or characteristic that plays an essential role in producing an occurrence of the disease in question.

A cause (or combination of component causes) may be considered sufficient if the presence of the cause inevitably produces disease (Rothman and Greenland, 2005).

It is widely recognized that change in disease state or in health or production outcomes in animal populations are almost always the result of multiple causal factors operating together to produce a sufficient cause. The individual causes may be called component causes. A necessary cause is defined as a component cause that must be present in any group of causes that comprise a sufficient cause (Rothman, 1976). The counterfactual interpretation of this means that regardless of what other causes are operating, if a necessary cause is not present, the disease will not occur.

It is rare for a single cause to be both necessary and sufficient. Thrushfield (2005) provides the example of exposure to high levels of gamma radiation, which in turn will lead to radiation-related disease.

A common example of a necessary cause is the presence of a specific microorganism in cases of infectious diseases, such as foot-and-mouth disease, avian influenza or rabies.

Figure 4.1 shows three sufficient causal mechanisms, each in turn comprised of component causes. The relative importance of component causes in contributing to the disease outcome may be represented by the proportion of the pie allocated to any one cause. This reinforces the notion that some component causes may play a more important role than others in contributing to the occurrence of disease. Causes that are relatively more important may be expected to be contributing to occurrence of more disease cases than less important causal factors.

Many diseases are considered to have complex causal webs or multifactorial aetiology that may or may not have necessary component causes. An example is bovine respiratory disease (BRD), where numerous infectious and non-infectious component causes may be present in any particular individual. Another example is salmonellosis in sheep (see Fig. 4.2), where a number of factors related to the agent, host and environment interact to result in development of disease.

Component causes in a causal web may interact in a variety of sometimes complex ways with some causes acting to modify the effect of other component causes.

An important finding in complex causal associations is that interfering with the effect of one or few key component causes may have a substantial protective impact on disease frequency. In such cases it is not necessarily critical to identify or describe the complete causal web to be able to implement effective preventive measures.

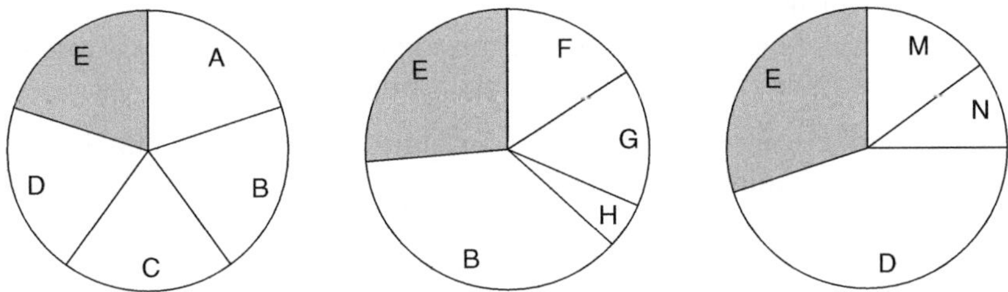

Fig. 4.1. Use of pie charts to demonstrate three separate sufficient causal mechanisms, each made up of multiple component causes identified by letters. There is one candidate necessary cause (E) that is the only component cause found in every sufficient causal mechanism (adapted from Rothman and Greenland, 2005).

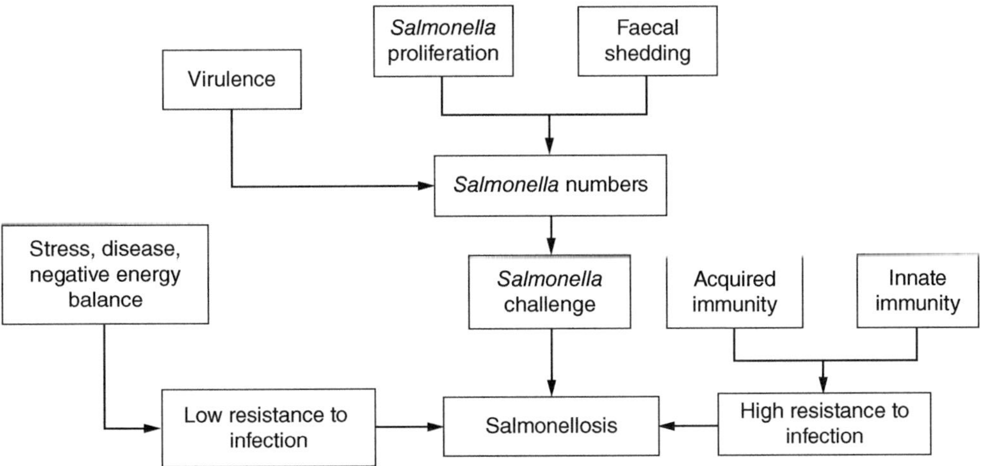

Fig. 4.2. Causal web of factors contributing to occurrence of salmonellosis in sheep (Makin *et al*., 2009).

4.3 Causal Criteria

For many years, the traditional view of causality was deterministic (i.e. agent X produced effect Y). Specificity of both cause and effect was implied. The development of the Henle-Koch postulates (Koch, 1892) reinforced this view and was helpful in formulating the link between microorganisms and disease.

1. The organism must be present in every case of disease.
2. The organism must not be present in other diseases.
3. The organism must be isolated from tissues in pure culture.
4. The organism must be capable of inducing disease in experiments.

However, in light of development of disease epidemiology and natural history, Koch's postulates were considered too restrictive in thinking about causality. For example, Koch's postulates do not adequately allow for situations such as:

- involvement of multiple aetiologic factors;
- multiple effects of single causes;
- occurrence of a carrier state;
- quantitative causal factors (amount of exposure rather than presence/absence); and
- non-agent factors (e.g. age, sex, breed, environment).

The epidemiologist interprets causality in quite a wide sense. This is somewhat different to the more traditional Henle-Koch view of the role of cause being restricted to aetiological agents with all other contributions being designated as contributing or predisposing factors. An epidemiological definition of a cause of a disease is an event, condition or characteristic that plays an essential role in producing an occurrence of the disease.

This broader perspective of causality led to the development of causal criteria or considerations, as proposed by Evans (1976) and Bradford-Hill (1965) and summarized in Table 4.1. Causal criteria provide lists of characteristics that can be used to judge whether a particular factor might be causal or non-causal, recognizing that such lists may provide food for thought but may not necessarily allow classification of putative causes in every case. Thrushfield (2005) considers Evans' criteria as being consistent with modern concepts of epidemiology.

4.4 Diagrams of Causation

Causal diagrams involve drawing plausible pathways to show potential causal factors and how they interact with each other, to influence the outcome of interest. Causal diagrams provide a stimulus for critical thinking about underlying biological relationships, clarify assumptions, provide a visual medium for communicating and discussing causality, identify gaps in understanding and inform subsequent statistical analyses.

It is important to note that causal diagrams are based on underlying mathematical and graphical theory with quite specific terminology and formal methods for development and interpretation (Greenland and Pearl, 2011). However, informal diagrams may be easily constructed based on limited understanding of the formal rules and still provide useful input into understanding relationships amongst putative causal factors

Table 4.1. Causal criteria from Evans (1976) and Bradford-Hill (1965).

Evans' criteria for causation	Bradford-Hill criteria and brief explanation	
Prevalence of the disease should be higher in those exposed to the putative causal factor than in non-exposed	Strength of association	Strong associations with higher risk ratios are more likely to be causal than a weak association
Exposure to the causal factor should be more common in those with disease than those without disease, when other factors are held constant	Consistency	Consistently finding an association between a putative cause and a disease outcome in multiple studies by different investigators
Number of incident cases of disease higher in animals exposed to the cause than in animals not exposed, as shown in prospective studies	Specificity	If a factor is only associated with a specific disease it was said to be specific and considered more likely to be causal
Temporal patterns of disease should follow exposure to the cause with a distribution of incubation periods on a bell-shaped curve	Temporality	The causal factor should precede the outcome it is proposed to be causing
A spectrum of host responses should follow exposure to the cause along a logical biological gradient from mild to severe	Biological gradient	A dose-response association is supportive of a causal relationship
A measurable host response to the cause should regularly appear after exposure, and be absent before exposure, or should increase in magnitude if present before exposure. This pattern should not occur in animals not exposed	Plausibility	Is the association biologically plausible?
Experimental reproduction of the disease should occur with higher incidence in animals exposed to the cause than in those not exposed, under experimental or natural conditions	Coherence	The proposed causal association should not contradict current scientific knowledge
Elimination or modification of the putative cause or of the vector carrying it should decrease the incidence of the disease	Experiment	A causal association is more likely if it is supported by results from controlled, randomized trials
Prevention or modification of the host's response on exposure to the putative cause should decrease or eliminate the disease	Analogy	A causal association may be more likely if there are other examples of causal associations for analogous exposures and outcomes
The whole thing should make biologic and epidemiologic sense		

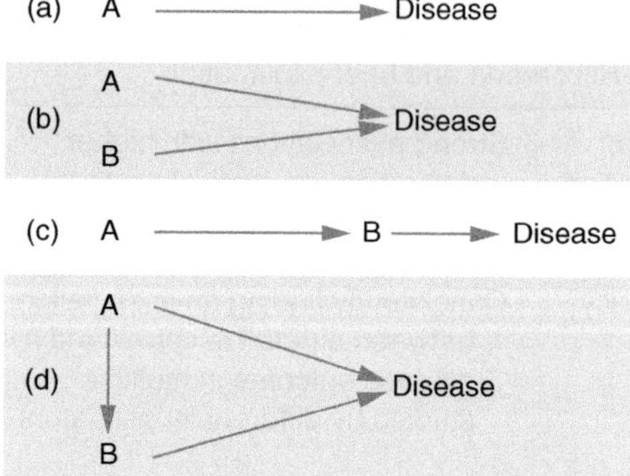

Fig. 4.3. Path diagrams illustrating direct and indirect causality: (a) direct causality between A and disease; (b) direct causality between A and B and disease; (c) A is an indirect cause of disease and B is a direct cause; B is also called an intervening cause; (d) A has both a direct and indirect causal association with disease (adapted from Thrushfield, 2005).

and other factors that may be non-causal or confounding. Diagrams are usually based on simple principles. They generally start at one side (the left in conventional Western writing styles) and move to the right in causal order. Lines are used to link one factor to something else that it causes or modifies, with arrows to indicate the direction of causality.

Causes can also be classified as direct or indirect, as shown in Fig. 4.3.

A direct causal factor has no other factor intervening between it and the outcome of interest.

In addition, if considering causality at an individual animal level, direct causes must be measured at the individual animal level (Martin *et al*., 1987).

An indirect cause has an intervening direct cause acting between it and the outcome of interest.

As an example of this, poor ventilation in a live export ship may be associated with increased risk of respiratory disease in livestock but this would be considered an indirect cause of disease in individual animals because it is measured at a different level.

4.5 Association or Causation

An association is a relationship, a linkage in occurrence, or a dependency between two variables. An association without additional information does not imply that the factor is causal, just that there is a relationship between the factor and disease occurrence.

To evaluate an association that we suspect might be a causal association, we look at several pieces of information:

1. The chance that the observed association occurred just because of random variation (the p-value).
2. The possibility that the so-called cause and effect are related intrinsically in some non-causal fashion (night and day go together).
3. The chance that there was bias (systematic or non-random error) in the study.
4. The causal criteria described above.

These four considerations are described in detail below.

4.5.1 Random variation

Random variation results from within- and among-animal variation and measurement errors that occur due to imprecision (lack of perfect repeatability) in the measuring equipment or people using the equipment.

Because there are many usual sources of ordinary, anticipated random variation, we do not expect that all samples from the same population will have exactly the same mean or that factors will have the same frequency of occurrence. Rather, we anticipate and accept that there will be some variation due to random error.

Statistical hypothesis testing is used to determine whether an observed difference between groups may be due to random variation or whether it may be attributed to some other non-random effects.

4.5.2 Intrinsic non-causal relationships

Not all associations are causal even if they are statistically significant.

Some non-causal associations are described as intrinsic. Night and day are associated in a regular repeating pattern that has no random variation. Most people who have a left hand also have a right hand. There is no causal relationship between the two hands – the association is simply intrinsic. Another example of a non-causal association is the use of suntan lotion and drowning.

4.5.3 Bias

The concept of bias is introduced briefly here. Bias is a systematic (non-random) error in the data resulting from inadequacy in the study design or measuring instruments and procedures. It is not a matter of random variation or imprecision. The term validity refers to a lack of bias.

While you can work hard to protect against bias, you can never rule bias out completely as an explanation for an association. However, if you are satisfied that bias seems reasonably unlikely, you can go on to consider the information provided by the causal criteria. Actually, the criteria incorporate judgements about bias, so in fact many of these pieces of information are considered simultaneously.

4.5.4 Causal criteria

After ruling out chance, intrinsic relationships and bias as a possible explanation of an association, it is usual to consider the possible causal factors as risk factors for disease.

Risk factors are those characteristics of some individual study units, which, on the basis of epidemiological evidence, are associated with increased risk of disease. Risk factors may be either causal or non-causal, depending on the outcome when the causal criteria are applied. Non-causal risk factors are sometimes called risk markers. For example, being nearer the ocean may be a risk factor for shrimp farms experiencing a

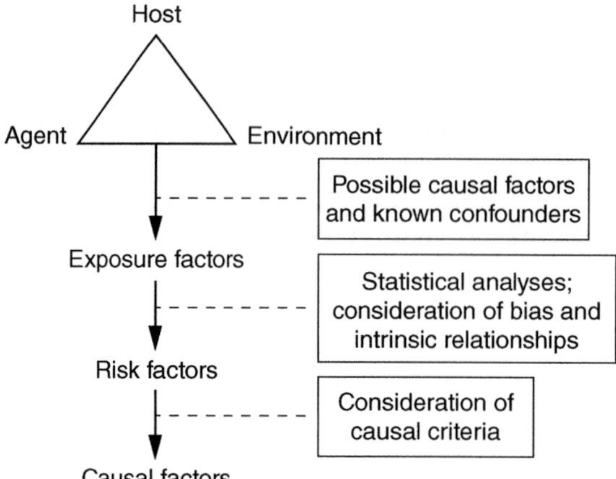

Fig. 4.4. Evaluating associations to identify causal factors.

white spot disease outbreak, but it may or may not be a cause. The process of considering the causal criteria and deciding if a risk factor is causal or not is subjective and requires impartial judgement on behalf of the investigator.

This whole process of evaluating associations to identify causes is summarized in Fig. 4.4.

4.6 Confounding

Confounding is an important issue in epidemiology and refers to the situation where there is mixing of associations between factors. Assume we have a risk factor (F), which has a causal association with the disease of interest (D). Then we have a third factor (C), which is a confounder.

In order for C to act as a confounder for the relationship between F and D, a number of criteria must be in place, as summarized below and graphically in Fig. 4.5:

- There must be an association between C and D:
  - C may be a cause of D;
  - C may have a non-causal association with D;
  - C must not be caused by D, meaning that C must not be a consequence of disease.
- C must have an association with F:
  - C may be a cause of F;
  - C may have a non-causal association with F;
  - C must not be caused by F.
- C must not be an intervening factor along the causal pathway from F to D.

Figure 4.6 provides an example of confounding from a study by Willeberg (1979). In this study there was found to be an apparent association between presence of fan ventilation and respiratory disease in housed pigs. However, further analysis demonstrated that there was a genuine association between herd size and occurrence of respiratory disease (larger herds were more likely to have respiratory disease) and also that larger herds were also more likely to have fan ventilation. Once this was accounted

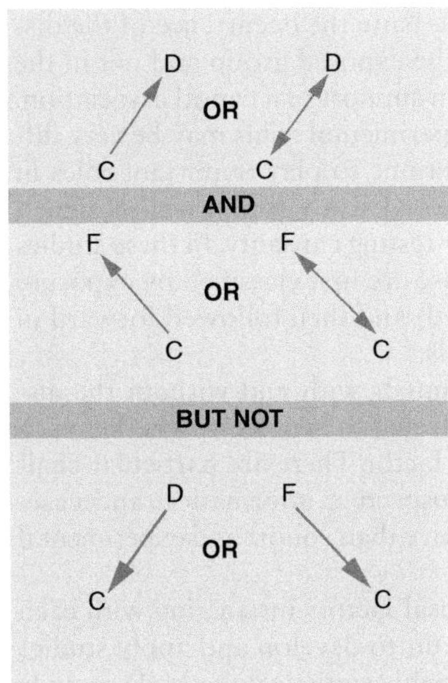

Fig. 4.5. Conditions for C to be a confounder for the F–D relationship (adapted from Woodward, 1999).

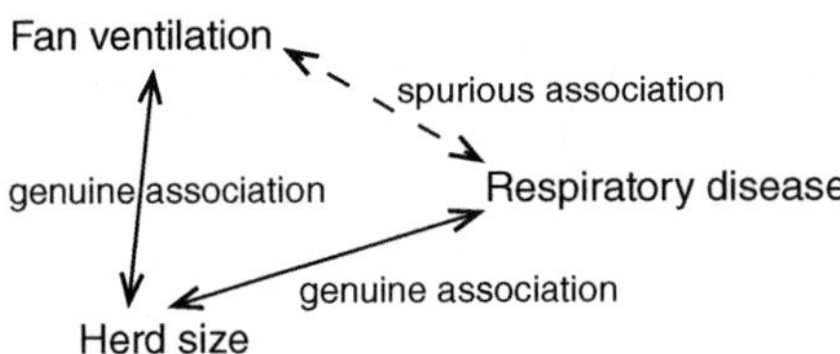

Fig. 4.6. Example of confounding, where the apparent relationship between fan ventilation and respiratory disease in pigs is confounded by herd size (Willeberg, 1979, adapted from Thrushfield, 2005).

for in the analysis the apparent relationship between fan ventilation and respiratory disease disappeared. In this example, herd size is the *confounder*, while the relationship between fan ventilation and respiratory disease is *confounded*.

4.7 Statistics and Causality

Statistical association is a measure of whether an association (between cause and effect) is stronger than one might expect due to chance alone.

Demonstration of a statistically significant association between cause and disease provides a useful approach to assessment of strength of association but does not provide proof of causation. Statistical associations may occur without any causal link or they may reflect bias in subject selection or measurement, or confounding between a non-causal factor (A) and some other factor (B) may result in factor (A) being erroneously misclassified as causal.

A randomized clinical trial offers the most direct way to test causality by assigning disease-free individuals into two groups, with one group to be exposed to the putative causal factor(s) while the other group remains as a comparative unexposed or control group. The groups are then followed to measure the occurrence of the disease or outcome of interest. If the disease occurs in the exposed group and not in the unexposed group then this provides strong evidence in support of a causal association.

There are many situations where randomized experimental trials may be very difficult to perform and observational studies must continue to play important roles in understanding and assessing causality. In observational study types, well-designed cohort studies provide the most effective potential for testing causality. In these studies individuals that are free of the defined outcome/disease are first classified by exposure to the putative causal factor (exposed or non-exposed) and then followed forward in time to record occurrence of disease in the individuals.

Case-control studies involve identification of animals with and without the disease of interest and then historical information is collected to determine whether each individual was exposed or not to the putative causal factor. There are particular challenges and opportunities for bias in collecting retrospective information and case-control studies are generally considered to be less effective than cohort and experimental studies at assessing causal associations.

In situations with large numbers of potential causal factors interacting with each other across large scales in time and space, it is difficult to develop and apply studies to assess causation (Plowright *et al.*, 2008). Multivariable statistical methods provide the ability to assess relative importance of numerous putative risk factors including assessment of interactions between factors. Plowright *et al.* (2008) describe the use of a combination of plausible hypothesis generation through approaches such as causal diagrams, and inferential statistical analyses to test specific associations that may be raised as hypothetical links in initial causal diagrams. Causal diagrams are identified as a visual approach that can facilitate communication and exploration of various possible relationships. The authors also describe the use of multiple separate analytical approaches in an attempt to triangulate conclusions about causality by looking for consistent findings from separate datasets or different methodological approaches. Examples of this sort of approach are commonly seen in outbreak investigations where field observational studies are combined with focused experimental trials that may test quite specific hypotheses, all informing a general understanding of causality.

References

Bradford-Hill, A. (1965) The environment and disease: association or causation? *Proceedings of the Royal Society of Medicine* 58, 295–300.

Evans, A.S. (1976) Causation and disease: the Henle-Koch postulates revisited. *Yale Journal of Biology and Medicine* 49, 175–195.

Greenland, S. and Pearl, J. (2011) Adjustments and their Consequences – Collapsibility Analysis using Graphical Models. *International Statistical Review* 79, 401–426.

Koch, R. (1892) Ueber bakteriologische Forschung. *Verhandlungen des X. Internationalen medizinische kongresses*. Translation: Rivers, T.M. (1937) Viruses and Koch's postulates. *Journal of Bacteriology* 33, 1–12.

Makin, K., House, J., Perkins, N. and Curran, G.I. (2009) *Project LIVE.123: Investigating mortality in sheep and lambs exported through Adelaide and Portland*. Meat and Livestock Australia, Sydney, Australia.

Martin, S.W., Meek, A.H. and Willeberg, P. (1987) *Veterinary Epidemiology*. Iowa State University Press, Ames, Iowa.

Plowright, R.K., Sokolow, S.H., Gorman, M.E., Daszak, P. and Foley, J.E. (2008) Causal inference in disease ecology: investigating ecological drivers of disease emergence. *Frontiers in Ecology and the Environment* 6, 420–429.

Rothman, K.J. (1976) Causes. *American Journal of Epidemiology* 141, 90–95; discussion 89.

Rothman, K.J. and Greenland, S. (2005) Causation and causal inference in epidemiology. *American Journal of Public Health* 95(S1), S144–150.

Susser, M. (1991) Philosophy in epidemiology. *Theoretical Medicine* 12, 271–273.

Thrushfield, M. (2005) *Veterinary Epidemiology*. Blackwell Science, Oxford.

Willeberg, P. (1979) The analysis and interpretation of epidemiological data. *Proceedings of the 2nd International Symposium on Veterinary Epidemiology and Economics*, Canberra, pp. 185–198.

Woodward, M. (1999) Chapter 4: Confounding and interaction. In: *Epidemiology Study Design and Data Analysis*. Chapman and Hall/CRC, Boca Raton, Florida.

5 Patterns of Disease

5.1 Introduction

A basic premise of epidemiology is that, in a population of animals, or groups of animals (herds, ponds or farms), disease does not occur randomly in animal groups, over time or in space. Although the transmission of disease among individuals involves chance events, the resultant effect at a population level is to produce distinct patterns which can be described and analysed by the epidemiologist to gain insight into the cause and behaviour of disease with a view to prevention or control.

To begin to understand why we see patterns at the population level, we need to understand the behaviour of disease in the individual animal and how disease agents move from animal to animal and farm to farm. In later chapters we will learn how to more formally analyse disease patterns.

In this chapter we explore some basic disease principles that result in the patterns that are seen in populations.

5.2 Unit of Study

We can examine patterns of disease by looking at individual animals or some other unit of study that is an aggregation of animals (an animal group), sometimes assumed to be randomly mixing for the purposes of disease transmission. Examples are farm, herd, flock, shed, tank, cage, pond, village, district, province, state, etc.

Before talking about patterns of disease, it is therefore important to understand the concept of unit of study. In medical epidemiology and with many livestock and aquatic animal diseases, the unit of study may be the individual person or animal. Thus, a medical epidemiologist may be interested in identifying factors that make some people more susceptible to influenza than others. However, in many cases, the unit of study can be aggregations of individuals, so that an epidemiologist might be interested in risk factors for the occurrence of foot-and-mouth disease at the farm or village level, rather than in individual animals. The unit of study is the biological unit of primary concern in an epidemiological investigation and may be individual animals or aggregations of animals at various levels.

For example, it may be observed that in a particular village outbreak of foot-and-mouth disease, disease appears to be more common in young cattle than in older cattle. Here the unit of study is the individual animal and the characteristic that seems to be associated with disease is the age of the animal.

However, the unit of study can also be an aggregation of individuals such as a farm or village. Extending the foot-and-mouth disease example, it may be observed that some villages experience a greater number of cases than others. An epidemiologist is interested in identifying factors associated with a higher prevalence of disease. These factors can then be manipulated to help control the disease in future outbreaks.

5.2.1 Characteristics of the unit of study

When describing patterns of disease and relating those patterns to characteristics (or factors) of the unit of study, it is important that the chosen characteristics are relevant to the chosen unit of study. For example, the characteristics of species, sex and age are relevant where the unit of study is the individual animal but are not relevant where the unit of study is the farm or pond. Examples of different units of study and characteristics appropriate to each are shown in Table 5.1, in hierarchical order. By this we mean that a number of animals are contained in a management unit such as a pen, mob, pond or cage and then a number of management units make up a farm, a number of farms make up a village or locality and so on.

A characteristic that is relevant to a certain level in the hierarchical order is assumed to apply equally to all units lower in the hierarchical level. For example, if the unit of study is the pond and if we wish to know if the size of the pond affects disease occurrence, then it is assumed that the size of a particular pond affects all fish equally in that pond.

5.3 Population Matters

Epidemiologists are primarily concerned about the patterns of disease in populations. Therefore, it is important to understand and differentiate the populations that can be involved in any epidemiological investigation. The population at risk is the population of individuals susceptible to a particular disease and who have some likelihood of exposure.

When considering the natural history of a disease, or describing the occurrence of a disease in a population, the population of concern is the *population at risk*. This refers to the population of individuals susceptible to a particular disease and who have some likelihood of exposure. The population at risk includes non-diseased individuals as well as diseased, and provides the denominator for prevalence and incidence calculations. The population at risk does not include individuals that are not at risk of the disease, because of either innate or acquired immunity.

Table 5.1. Some possible units of study in hierarchical order with examples of relevant characteristics applying to the particular unit of study.

Unit of study	Examples of relevant characteristics (livestock)
Animal	Species, sex, age, breed, weight
Management unit: pen, pond, cage, mob, paddock	Size, soil type, stocking density, stage of production, pasture type
Farm	Location, size, source of stock, production method, other enterprises
Village/locality	Location, number of farms, geographic and climatic factors, farming practices
District/region	Location, state, size, government services, geographic and climatic factors

For example, in an outbreak of pregnancy toxaemia in sheep, the population at risk is all pregnant female sheep on the farm. Male sheep, desexed males and non-pregnant females are not part of the population at risk.

If the unit of study is defined as a pen or farm of animals, then the population at risk is the population of farms (or management units) that are susceptible to the disease, not the individual animals.

For example, when investigating a particular disease within a single farm, the at-risk population may be all the animals on that particular farm or it may be limited to a particular subset of animals on the farm such as animals of a particular age or management group. On the other hand, if an outbreak of classical swine fever were to occur in Australia, the at-risk population would be regarded as the entire pig population in Australia (including feral pigs).

5.4 Natural History of Disease in Individuals and Populations

The progress of disease in an individual animal over time (without intervention) as it occurs in the natural situation (rather than a controlled situation such as in a laboratory or tank experiment) is known as the natural history of disease. The natural history begins with exposure of the host to the disease agent and progresses through to either recovery or death. The epidemiologist is interested in using population-based methods to identify the important factors affecting this natural history, with the intention of identifying possible methods of prevention and control.

Using infectious diseases as an example, the simplest starting point is a host animal that is capable of being infected and that is currently susceptible to infection with the infectious agent.

Exposure refers to interaction or contact between the infectious agent and the host. Not every animal that is exposed will get infected. Infection typically means that the infectious agent is present on or within the host animal and is capable of surviving and replicating.

Once an animal is infected there is usually a period of time before the animal develops any clinical signs of disease. This is called the incubation period.

Animals that develop signs of disease may recover, become a carrier, or die depending on the disease.

In some diseases, infected animals may never develop clinical signs of disease while in other diseases almost all infected animals may develop signs of disease.

Some diseases are capable of producing persistent infection or carrier states in infected animals. Animals may show little or no signs of infection but may be capable of shedding the infectious agent. These carrier animals pose a risk to susceptible animals.

Recovered animals may develop immunity to the infectious agent so that if exposed again they do not become infected. Immunity may last a lifetime for some diseases while for other diseases it may be shorter and as immunity wanes, animals may become susceptible to infection again.

These different stages of disease are collectively referred to as the spectrum of disease and are illustrated in Fig. 5.1.

5.4.1 Incubation period

With infectious diseases, we refer to the incubation period, which is the time period from exposure to infection through to when clinical signs are first manifested.

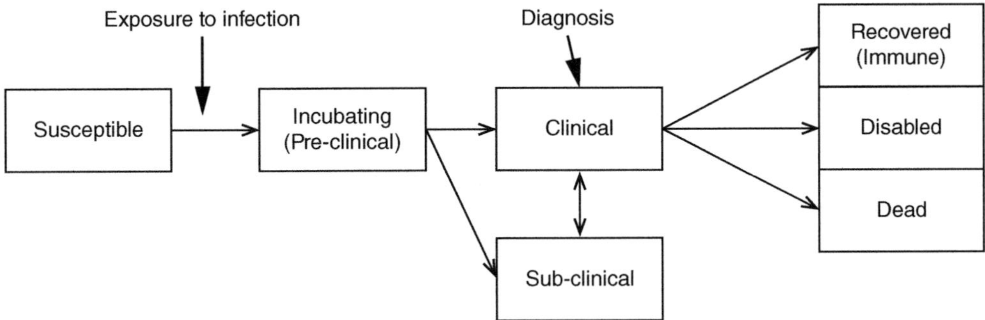

Fig. 5.1. Spectrum of a disease simplified into a number of discrete states or stages through which an individual progresses with time.

For physical agents such as toxins we usually refer to the induction period or latent period to mean a similar thing. For gastrointestinal parasitic diseases, the term prepatent period is used to mean the time from initial infection to when parasite eggs are passed in the host's faeces.

When an infectious disease agent is first introduced into a susceptible population, there will be very few animals in the clinical and subsequent states. As the epidemic progresses, the number of animals with clinical disease will increase and then slowly decrease while the number of susceptible animals will decrease and the number of recovered animals will increase (assuming no mortality). This phenomenon is shown in Fig. 5.2.

It is very important to remember these basic concepts when using diagnostic tests and estimating their usefulness in populations. Often a particular test is useful to detect an infected animal at one stage of disease but not another. Its overall usefulness on a population basis will therefore depend on the proportion of individuals in the population of interest in the various stages of disease at the time that samples were taken. For example, from Fig. 5.2, we can see that if we were to use a test that detected recovered animals (e.g. an antibody detection test) at Day 4 of the epidemic, we would find that only 5% of the animals had recovered. However, by Day 12 almost 90% of the animals have recovered.

5.4.2 Infectivity, pathogenicity and virulence

The terms infectivity, pathogenicity and virulence all relate to the severity of a disease in a population, but each operates at a different point in the natural history of the disease. These terms also need to be understood when considering the progress of an infectious disease in a population. The definitions for each of these terms as they are used in epidemiology are shown below:

- Infectivity refers to the percentage (or proportion) of susceptible individuals exposed to a particular agent who become infected.
- Pathogenicity refers to the percentage of infected individuals who develop clinical disease due to the particular agent.
- Virulence refers to the percentage of individuals with clinical disease who become seriously ill or die.

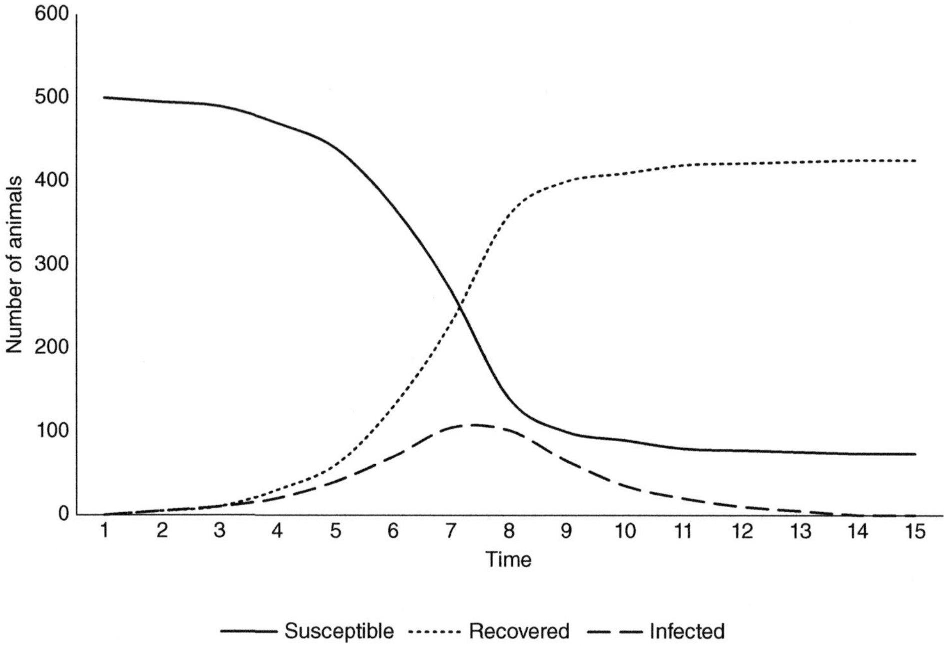

Fig. 5.2. Epidemic pattern in a population of susceptible individuals following the introduction of a directly transmitted infectious agent that begins by affecting a single animal (Reed-Frost model).

For example, Q fever (due to *Coxiella burnetti* infection) is highly infectious but has a generally low pathogenicity in animals (does not cause much disease). On the other hand, foot-and-mouth disease is highly infectious in cattle and also highly pathogenic (most exposed animals develop clinical disease) but with low virulence (few cases die), whereas rabies is both highly pathogenic (most infected individuals get sick) and highly virulent (most subsequently die).

5.4.3 Herd immunity

Progress of a disease in a population is also affected by herd-immunity effects. From a population perspective, herd immunity is the immunologically derived resistance of a group of individuals to attack by disease based on the resistance of a large proportion, but not all, of the group. Herd immunity may arise from innate immunity (although this may not always have an immunological basis), natural infection or vaccination.

Herd immunity will slow the rate of transmission of a disease within a population, with the magnitude of the effect depending on the level of herd immunity. If herd immunity is high, infection may fail to establish or can be eliminated from the population. It is not necessary for all individuals in a group to be immune to eliminate infection. The level of herd immunity (proportion of immune animals in the population) must simply be sustained at a level that exceeds a critical threshold value. This results in the concept that if a minimum critical proportion of animals can be kept immune to infection, a disease can be eliminated from the population.

5.5 Transmission, Spread and Maintenance of Infection

To understand how disease patterns are created, we must understand how disease agents (organisms) move around in the population – from animal to animal, farm to farm, etc. We also need to know how agents can persist in a population and not be easily detected.

5.5.1 Transmission and spread

The chain of infection is the series of mechanisms by which an infectious agent passes from an infected to a susceptible host. To move around in a population, a disease agent must escape from infected hosts and find new susceptible hosts. This is summarized in Fig. 5.3.

The terms transmission of disease and spread of disease have related meanings but are used for different purposes in this text although these terms are often used synonymously.

Transmission refers to the movement of infection from an infected animal to a susceptible animal within an infected population.

Spread refers to the movement of infection from an infected population or subpopulation to a susceptible population or subpopulation.

5.5.2 Methods of transmission and spread

Interest in how a particular disease agent moves around will focus on different mechanisms depending on the unit of interest of the epidemiological investigation. For example, the most fundamental level of interest is transmission from animal to animal. However, within a particular farm there may be interest in methods of spread from one management group to another. At a higher level again, the interest will be in methods of spread from farm to farm. Finally, quarantine authorities are interested in mechanisms of spread from country to country.

Methods of transmission can be broadly classified as direct transmission or indirect transmission, and these can be further categorized as summarized in Table 5.2.

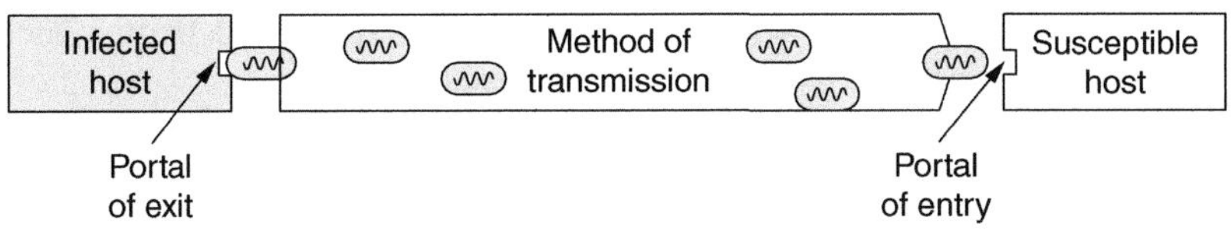

Fig. 5.3. Chain of infection for infectious disease agents.

Table 5.2. Methods of transmission for infectious diseases.

Direct transmission or spread		
Horizontal transmission	Direct contact	
	Contact with discharges (vomitus, faeces, etc.)	
	Cannibalism	
Vertical transmission	Transmission through egg or sperm	
Indirect transmission or spread		
Airborne transmission	Droplet nuclei (~<5 µm)	
	Dust (~>5 µm)	
Vector	Mechanical vector	Arthropods, birds, or other animal or aquatic species
	Biological vector	
Vehicle transmission	Fomites	Vehicles, personnel, equipment
	Animal products	

A vector is an insect or other living organism that transports infectious material from an infected animal or its wastes to a susceptible animal or its immediate surroundings.

A fomite is an inanimate object that is capable of transmitting infection to a susceptible animal.

5.5.3 Maintenance of infection

When active in a population, an infectious agent must be able to survive in host animals and the external environment or vectors and reservoirs. In most instances, within the host animal, defence mechanisms will either eventually terminate the infection or the host will die. However, in some cases, infection will persist and the host will appear relatively normal. Such animals are said to be *carriers*.

A carrier is an animal that is capable of transmitting infection but shows no clinical signs.

A carrier can be incubatory, convalescent or chronic. Carriers are very important in the maintenance of infectious diseases in populations.

5.5.4 Disease reservoirs

Some infectious agents such as foot-and-mouth disease virus can infect more than one host species. In such instances, persistence of infection in a particular area is facilitated by the presence of a range of host species of varying susceptibility to disease. A particular host species is said to be a reservoir host when it is the host species in which the disease agent normally lives and persists in a population and from which it can spill over to other species of hosts and cause disease.

For example, Hendra and Nipah viruses are both viruses that occur commonly in fruit bats with little if any disease in bats but may cause severe disease when they infect other species such as humans (Hendra and Nipah), horses (Hendra) and pigs (Nipah). Fruit bats are therefore a reservoir host for these viruses for other species.

More generally, a disease reservoir is any animal, plant or environment or combination of these in which an infectious agent normally lives and multiplies and upon which it depends as a species for survival in nature. A disease reservoir can be a source of infection for susceptible hosts of different species. An outbreak of disease in a susceptible population may occur when circumstances permit effective contact to be made with the reservoir of infection. Some infectious agents can also persist in a population by surviving for long periods of time within vector species.

In the external environment, infectious agents are exposed to variations in temperature, humidity, concentrations of various chemicals (e.g. oxygen, salinity) and sunlight. The period of survival of an agent in the environment will depend on the particular set of conditions existing at the time. Some agents have the capability to produce resistant forms in response to harsh environments and thus persist for longer periods of time. For example, anthrax forms highly resistant spores, which can persist in the environment for many decades, and some helminths and protozoa form protective cysts and can survive for long periods of time within the host.

5.6 Ecology of Disease

To investigate disease in natural populations, we need to understand the relationships among the hosts, agents and natural environments. These relationships determine the eventual observed pattern of disease both in time and space. For example, climate has a large impact on the geographical distribution of animal species, disease agents and potential disease vectors. The study of the relationship among animals, plants and their environment in nature is known as ecology. Ecology of disease extends this basic concept to include pathogens (agents of disease).

Ecology of disease is the relationship among animals, pathogens and their environment in a natural situation without intervention.

When humans intervene in natural ecological relationships such as by intensively farming livestock or encroaching on natural wildlife habitat, organisms that may have been present but not previously caused significant disease may become more apparent in the population.

This relationship is often termed the epidemiological triad and can be expressed as a Venn diagram as shown previously in Fig. 1.2. What this diagram shows is that it is not until a particular set of conditions relating to the agent, host and environment come together that disease will occur.

5.6.1 Agent, host and environment factors

Some of the components or factors belonging to each of these are shown in Table 5.3.

5.7 Patterns of Disease by Animal or Other Unit of Study

The epidemiologist uses methods that document the patterns of disease in populations and by analysing these patterns, a better understanding of the cause of disease can be obtained. Although disease patterns are traditionally thought of as occurring in time

Table 5.3. List of factors related to agent, host and environment.

Agent	Host	Environment
Infectivity	Species	Climate/weather
Pathogenicity	Genotype	Water system
Virulence	Phenotype	Water quality
Immunogenicity	Age	Food
Antigenic variation	Sex	Geology
Survival	Nutritional status	
	Physiological status	
	Pathological status	

(temporal patterns) and place (spatial patterns), we can also extend this concept to include the identification and analysis of patterns as they occur according to the characteristics of the unit of study (animals, herds, farms, etc.).

Some species, sex or age-class of animal can be more affected by disease than others even though they share a similar environment.

For example, foot-and-mouth disease may be more common in younger animals than older animals and in cattle rather than sheep and goats. Footrot in sheep is more common (and more severe) in some breeds of sheep than others. Johne's disease in cattle is more common in dairy farms than in beef farms in Australia and many other countries.

Many disease agents cause more severe disease in immature animals than adults, though this is not always the case. If the reasons for these differences can be understood, then it may be possible to design prevention and control strategies.

For example, extensively reared (free-range) poultry are generally considered to be at greater risk of contracting avian influenza through contact with wild birds or contaminated water or environment. Increasing biosecurity on free-range flocks (to reduce likelihood and degree of contact) may be one way of reducing the number of outbreaks of avian influenza.

In another example, the unit of study was the individual animal (a cow) and a herd of calving cattle included a mixture of two age groups, one joined at 14 months of age and the other joined at 17 months of age. During calving there was an unusually high number of calves born dead, and further investigation found that cows joined at 14 months were about twice as likely to have a dead calf as those joined at 17 months. Increasing the age at joining is one measure that could be used to help improve calf survival.

5.8 Patterns of Disease by Time

Analysis of the pattern of disease occurrence over time can often provide useful hints as to likely cause and possible control measures. The timing of onset of cases of disease in a population tends to follow one of four patterns.

1. Cases may occur in a sporadic fashion; that is they do not seem to be associated with any other identifiable factor, nor with each other (e.g. non-specific abortion in cattle).

2. Cases may occur regularly at a fairly constant level. The disease is often referred to as being endemic. It virtually always occurs, often at low levels (e.g. mastitis in dairy cows, internal parasites in sheep).
3. Cases may occur in time clusters, a pattern typical of outbreaks or epidemics (e.g. foot-and-mouth disease in cattle or pigs, white spot syndrome in prawns).
4. If an epidemic takes international proportions and affects a large proportion of the population, it is termed a pandemic. Typical pandemics include influenza in humans, parvovirus in dogs and rinderpest in cattle prior to recent eradication. White spot syndrome in prawns could possibly be described as pandemic in parts of Asia.

5.8.1 Epidemic curves

The epidemic curve is a useful summary of the temporal pattern of disease events that also provides a visual display of the scale or magnitude of the event and the rate at which new cases are occurring.

The epidemic curve represents in a graphic form the onset of cases of the disease, either as a histogram, a bar graph or a frequency polygon. The frequency of new cases (or outbreaks) is plotted on the y-axis over a time scale on the x-axis. A typical epidemic curve may be conceived of as having four and occasionally five segments as displayed in Fig. 5.4.

5.8.2 Different types of epidemic curve

Epidemic curves for sporadic, endemic and epidemic diseases are shown in Fig. 5.5. For sporadic disease, most time periods have no cases, with occasional periods experiencing small numbers of cases. For the endemic disease, the number of cases fluctuates between time periods but remains at a fairly stable level, while for the epidemic disease, the number of cases increases sharply from its initial endemic level and then declines slowly back to that level.

5.8.3 The shape of the curve

An epidemic is said to occur when the frequency of cases (or outbreaks) in a population clearly exceeds the normally expected level for a given area and season. The slope

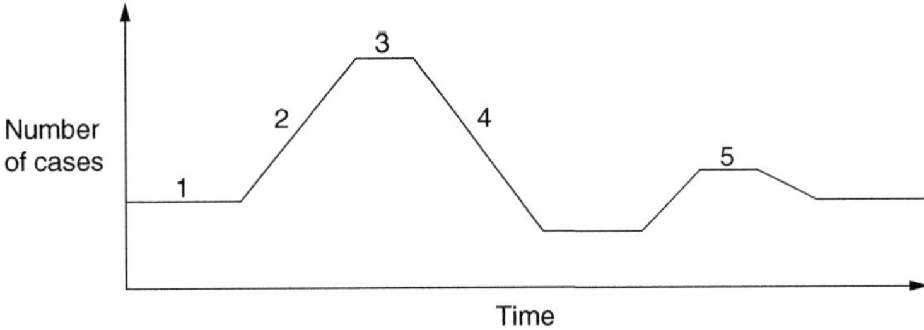

Fig. 5.4. Five stages of an epidemic curve.

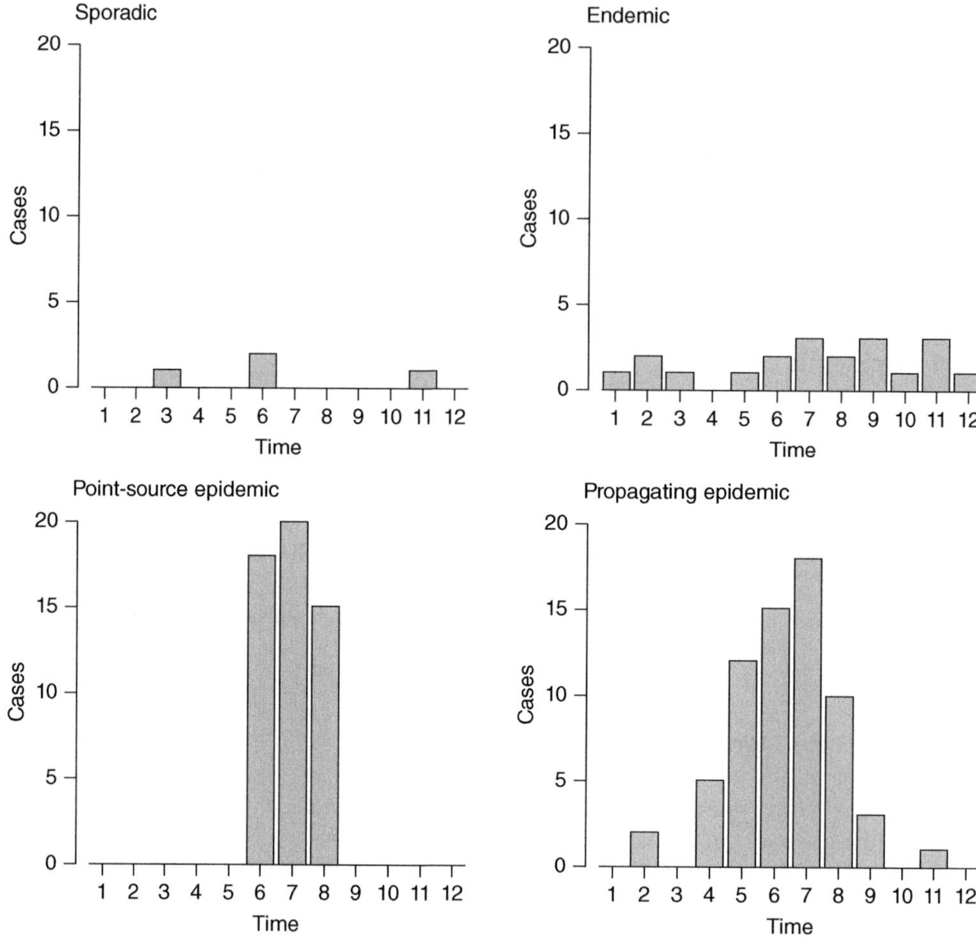

Fig. 5.5. Comparison of epidemic curves for sporadic, endemic, point-source and propagating epidemic diseases.

of the ascending branch of the epidemic curve can reveal something about the type of exposure or about the mode of transmission of the disease agent. If transmission is fast and effective the slope of the ascending branch is likely to be steeper than if transmission is slow or if the incubation period is long.

The length of the plateau and slope of the descending branch are related to the availability of susceptible animals, which in turn depends on many factors such as stocking densities, introductions into the population, the changing importance of different mechanisms of transmission and the proportion of immunes in the population at risk.

Exposure of a large number of animals to an agent at once or within a short period of time (e.g. through exposure to a common source) results in a point-source epidemic, typically a feed- or waterborne disease. Most often toxins are associated with this type of outbreak but it is also possible for food or water spread of infectious agents to produce a point-source epidemic if a large proportion of the population is exposed at once. The ascending branch of the corresponding curve would be almost vertical before reaching its peak. When the disease agent is transmitted via contact or vectors the ascending branch is more gradual and the resulting curve is typical of a propagating epidemic. The slope of the curve also depends on some agent characteristics such as its ability to survive outside the host; on some host factors such as contact rates, population density, etc.

A point-source epidemic is one where many animals (units) are exposed to the source of disease (agent or toxin) over a very short period of time, resulting in a very steep ascending branch of the epidemic curve.

A propagating epidemic is one where transmission occurs among individuals in the population, so that the ascending branch ascends more gradually.

The interval of time chosen for graphing the cases is important to the subsequent interpretation of the epidemic curve. The time interval should be selected on the basis of the incubation or latency period of the disease and the period over which the cases are distributed. The appropriate time interval may vary from several hours (e.g. some acute intoxications) to a month or more (e.g. infectious agents with a long incubation period). A common error in this regard is the selection of a time interval that is too long. Overly long intervals obscure subtle differences in temporal patterns, including secondary peaks resulting from animal-to-animal transmission. A rule of thumb is to make the interval between one-eighth and one-quarter as long as the estimated incubation period.

It may be wise to make several epidemic curves based on different graphing intervals and then select the one that best portrays the data. However, it should be remembered that in many disease outbreaks in animals, the time of onset of illness is often obscure and compromises must be made when making epidemic curves.

The duration of an epidemic is influenced by:

- the number of susceptible animals exposed to a source of infection that become infected;
- the period of time over which susceptible animals are exposed to the source;
- the minimum and maximum incubation periods of the disease; and
- the level of contact between infected and susceptible animals.

Outbreaks involving a large number of cases, with opportunity for exposure limited to a day or less, of a disease having a maximum incubation period of a few days or less, usually have an epidemic curve which approximates a 'normal' distribution. Such epidemic curves usually indicate a common source origin with exposure over a short period relative to the maximum incubation period of the disease.

5.8.4 Population dynamics

The extent of the plateau and the slope of the descending branch in an epidemic curve is mainly a function of the availability of susceptible animals in the population. This in turn may be a function of such things as herd immunity, or some intervention such as vaccination or treatment. In addition, the contact rate among animals will also exert a major impact on the rate of spread. In a population experiencing an outbreak of an infectious disease, individuals may be classed as:

- susceptible;
- resistant;
- immune;

- incubating ± infective;
- diseased ± infective;
- dead;
- convalescent ± infective ± immune; or
- recovered ± immune.

During the course of an epidemic, individuals may move through a number of these states. Consequently, the numbers of individuals in any one category will not remain constant.

5.8.5 Main and secondary peaks and index case

A secondary peak in an epidemic curve is usually due to introduction of susceptible animals into the previously epidemic area, or movement of infected animals from the epidemic area and contact with susceptible animals.

The main peak of the curve is at times preceded by a smaller peak, which could represent the index case(s) (the first case to occur in the epidemic). The interval between this first peak and the beginning of the next or main peak could indicate the incubation period. For example, in Fig. 5.5d, the incubation period is likely to be about two time periods. Identifying the index case can also be important in identifying the source of an outbreak.

In a closed population the pattern of disease may be easily appreciated, but when the population structure changes the pattern often becomes far more complex. For example, in most livestock populations there are births and introductions that often increase the number of susceptible animals; and deaths, culls and harvesting that decrease the number of immune animals. Furthermore, intervention by methods such as quarantine, treatment, vaccination or removal of a toxic source will potentially change the shape of the epidemic curve.

5.8.6 Why do epidemics occur?

Some of the reasons for the occurrence of outbreaks or epidemics due to infectious disease agents are listed below. There are probably many others:

- Recent introduction of the agent into a susceptible population. For example, measles outbreaks occur periodically when the virus is re-introduced into a susceptible population.
- Recent introduction of a susceptible group of animals into an infected area. For example, introduction of unexposed heifers into a herd containing a bovine pestivirus carrier animal.
- Recent increase in virulence or amount of the agent. For example, mutation of avian influenza viruses into highly pathogenic strains and into strains capable of infecting humans.
- Change in the mode of transmission of the agent. For example, bovine tuberculosis has persisted and caused new foci of infection in New Zealand and the UK following wildlife species (possum and badgers) emerging as new reservoirs of infection.
- Change in host susceptibility or response to the agent. For example, early in the AIDS epidemic, many people died as a result of aberrant infections as a result of

the failure of the immune system to control infections adequately that would normally (in the absence of the AIDS virus) be readily controlled and eliminated.

- Factors causing increased host exposure or involving new portals of entry. For example, Hendra and Nipah virus infections have emerged in recent decades in humans, horses and pigs following encroachment of agriculture on bat habitats.

5.8.7 Longer term patterns in the temporal distribution of disease

If data on disease occurrence are collected over longer periods of time it may be possible to look for patterns or trends over varying time periods, such as cyclic fluctuations, seasonal variations or long-term (secular) trends as opposed to erratic or random fluctuations that have no recognizable pattern. Examples of these trends are shown in Fig. 5.6.

Cyclical trends are recurrent patterns (increases or epidemics and decreases in incidence) that may occur over months or years due to underlying changes in the epidemiologic triad that have an influence on disease risk and expression. Examples might include cyclic variations in population immunity that may lead to epidemics of

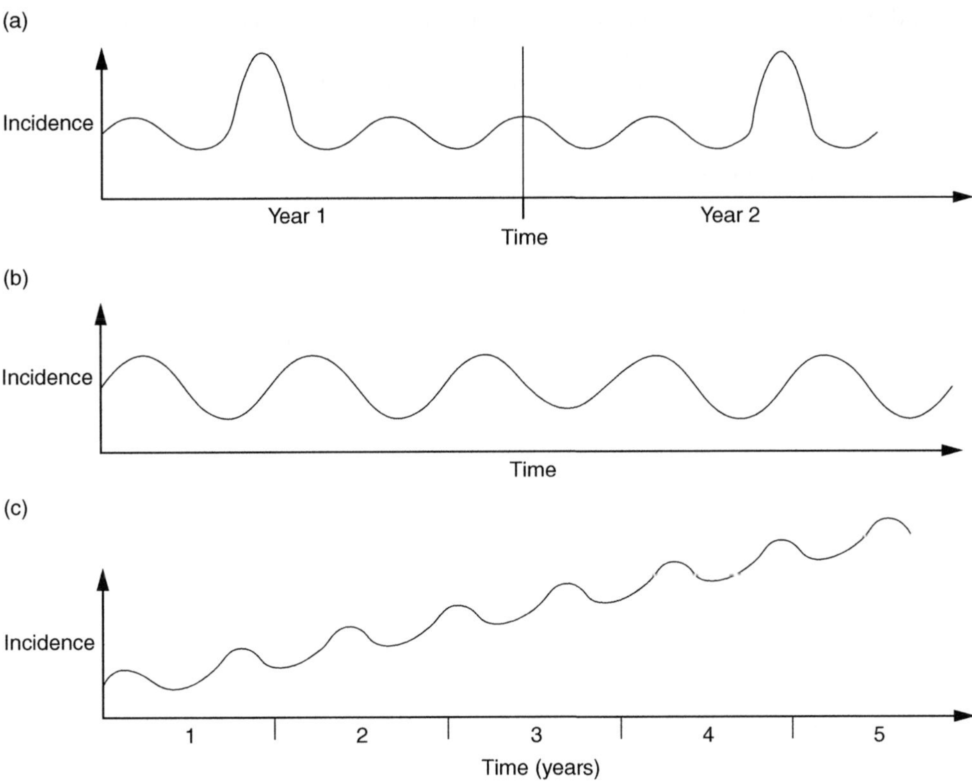

Fig. 5.6. Temporal patterns in the distribution of disease: (a) cyclical fluctuation; (b) seasonal variation; and (c) long-term (secular) trend.

disease followed by a period of very little disease until population immunity wanes and animals are then susceptible to another epidemic. Seasonal patterns of disease are a special case of cyclical variation where disease occurrence may be associated with seasons of the year.

There may also be trends in disease occurrence that only become apparent when many years or decades of data are viewed. These are referred to as long-term or secular trends and may reflect long-term changes in factors contributing to disease risk, or impacts of disease control mechanisms. Caution is urged in interpreting disease data collected over longer periods of time since there may be many reasons for an apparent change in disease frequency including changes in infectivity or pathogenicity of the infectious agent, changes in host susceptibility or population size, changes in the case definition or application of a different diagnostic test. In some situations an apparent change in disease frequency over time may actually be due to changes in detection or reporting and may not reflect any real change in the underlying incidence of disease in a standardized population.

Cyclical fluctuation exists when the variations occur at rather regular intervals; these intervals are usually longer than seasons.

Seasonal variation exists when the ups and downs occur at periodic intervals, coinciding with seasons (where seasons are as short as a week or as long as a year, depending on what biological phenomenon one is measuring).

Long-term (secular) trends are long-term changes where, in addition to short-term ups and downs, the curve either climbs or declines more or less steadily over an extended period of time, usually years.

Erratic variations occur in a totally unpredictable fashion.

5.8.8 Identifying temporal patterns

The types of time variations shown in Fig. 5.6 may not always be obvious from the curve in its raw form. Cyclical and seasonal fluctuations can sometimes be identified by plotting moving averages of the raw data. The long-term (secular) trend can be represented by a straight line, which can be obtained using least squares regression. Rolling averages can be used to smooth out random variation and help identify seasonal or cyclical patterns. Time series analysis is a set of statistical methods used to detect formally whether any of these types of variations exist and to determine the effect of each.

5.8.9 Other representations of temporal patterns

Estimated dissemination ratio

The estimated dissemination ratio (EDR) is a simple and easily calculated measure that provides useful information on the rate of spread in an outbreak and that is calculated in turn only from case frequency data (number of new cases).

EDR is calculated by the number of new cases in a defined window of time (7-day period) divided by the number of new cases in the previous window.

Where the EDR is greater than 1 the epidemic is continuing to expand and where the EDR is less than 1 the epidemic is declining.

EDR is very useful in outbreak situations where data may be limited. Caution is required in interpreting EDR when there are few cases occurring since a very small change in the number of cases in a window may result in a large apparent change in the EDR and the EDR plot can become erratic and difficult to interpret. Figures 5.7 and 5.8 show the epidemic curve and corresponding EDR curve for the 2007 equine influenza outbreak in Queensland, Australia (Kung *et al.*, 2011).

5.8.10 Mathematical models

A variety of mathematical models can also be applied to disease data to describe disease occurrence and understand risk factors and the impact of various control measures.

The simplest modelling approach is the SIR (susceptible-infected-recovered) model and various extensions including the addition of an exposed category in an SEIR (susceptible-exposed-infected-recovered) model or an approach assuming that infected animals that recover are immediately susceptible again (SIS; susceptible-infected-susceptible model). See Fig. 5.2 for an example of a simple SIR model of a disease epidemic in a susceptible population. These models rely on assumptions about the

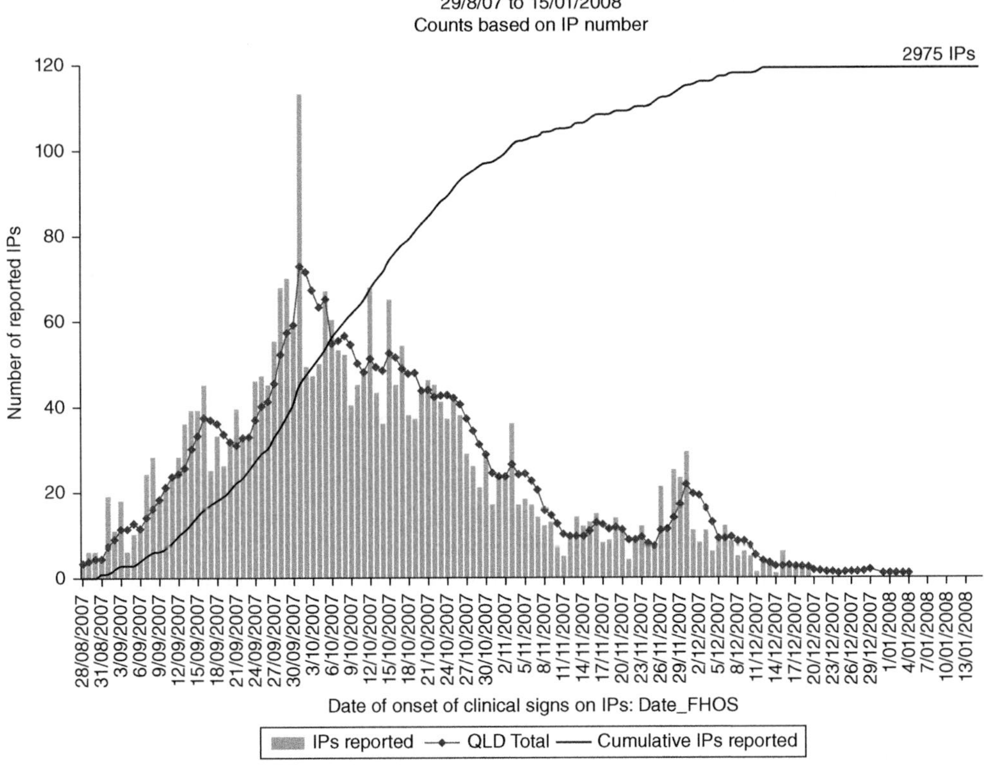

Fig. 5.7. Epidemic curve for 2007 equine influenza outbreak in Queensland, Australia (Kung *et al.*, 2011).

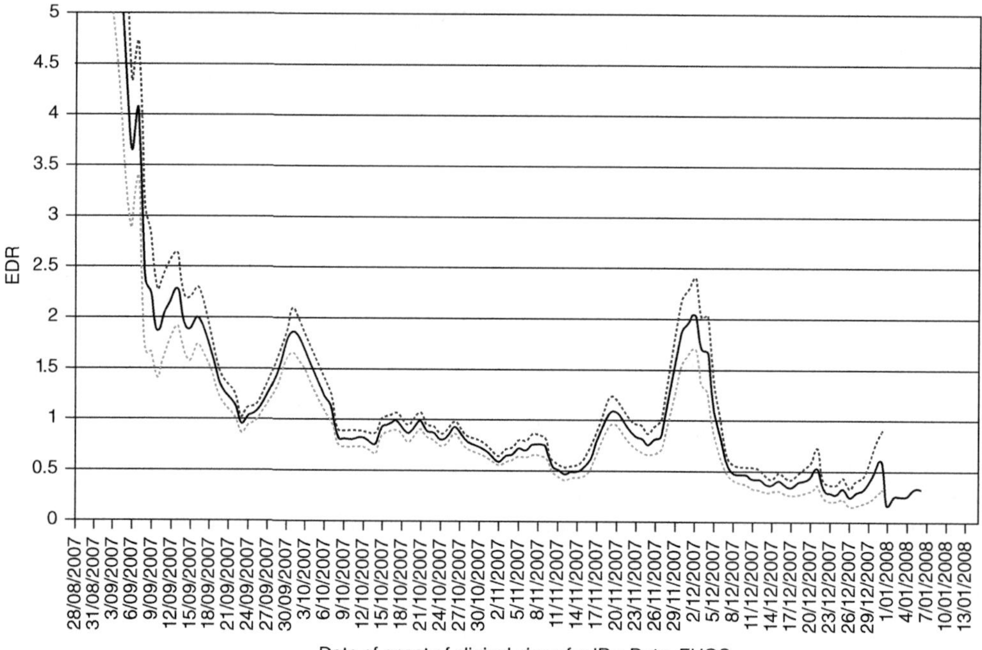

Fig. 5.8. EDR curve for the 2007 equine influenza outbreak in Queensland, Australia (Kung *et al.*, 2011).

proportion of a population in each of the relevant classes and estimations of the rates of transition between the classes.

SIR model outputs provide useful contributions at the population level about our understanding of patterns of disease, including in particular (Keeling and Danon, 2009):

- The importance of the basic reproductive ratio (R_0) as a fundamental parameter driving the pattern of an epidemic.
- Most epidemics end with a proportion of the population not having been infected and therefore remaining susceptible.
- Effective vaccination of susceptible individuals induces immunity and reduces the pool of susceptible individuals, and as the level of vaccinates rises a threshold is reached when further spread is prevented and the epidemic is controlled. It is not necessary to vaccinate every individual to prevent an epidemic and this has supported the concept of herd immunity. In a modelling situation, the proportion of the population that must be vaccinated to control an epidemic is dependent on R_0 and can be calculated as $1-1/R_0$.

R_0 is defined in the context of infectious disease epidemiology as the expected number of secondary individuals infected by a single infected individual during the entire infectious period for that individual, in a population that is entirely susceptible (Heffernan *et al.*, 2005). The effective reproductive ratio (R) is defined as the number of secondary cases infected by a single infected individual in a population that is not entirely susceptible (i.e. that is composed of a mixture of susceptible and non-susceptible hosts).

If R is greater than 1, the disease is continuing to spread in the population. If R falls below 1, each infected individual is infecting on average less than one other individual and this is consistent with a disease that is being cleared from the population. Measuring R therefore provides useful information in assessing the risk of spread in a disease outbreak and also assessing the impact of control measures.

There may also be erratic or random variation in the epidemic curve – unpredictable change. Plotting smoothed averages is one way of looking for patterns over time.

Over time infectious disease models have become increasingly complex, providing increased realism and predictive capacity, generally at a cost of requiring increasing effort to parameterize model inputs and difficulties in validating models. Stochastic, individual-based models have the capacity to model individual subject behaviour and interaction for every subject in a defined population and may provide detailed spatio-temporal outputs describing patterns of disease under various assumptions, including methods of control or prevention.

Infectious disease models have two distinct roles, prediction and understanding. Predictive models are attempting to predict future disease behaviour in specific situations and may serve to inform development of policies or response strategies. It is important that predictive models be as accurate as possible and therefore they are often complex because of the requirement to incorporate more parameters and assumptions to model complex relationships between various input parameters. Models may also be designed to increase understanding of the impact of various parameters on disease behaviour in an idealized and defined world that may have less direct resemblance to real-world situations than in predictive models (Keeling and Rohani, 2007).

5.9 Patterns of Disease by Place

Just as an epidemic curve provides a visual display of clustering of disease cases in time, representing cases as points on a map can provide a visual display of clustering in space. Spatial clustering of disease cases can provide insights into possible exposure and transmission mechanisms for a disease outbreak. Cases may be clustered at a single point or distributed in a spatial pattern that provides clues to exposure (along a road, valley or adjacent to a flowing stream or water source). For example, point exposure to soil deficiencies of toxins may be spatially limited to one paddock or pen. Spatial patterns may also be associated with movement of animals (sale-yards), distribution of vector (arboviruses) and farm management practices (one farm affected).

Spatial variation or patterns can be evaluated at varying scales: local (paddock, pond or farm), district, state, national or regional levels. Simple maps may be hand-drawn crude representations or involve manual placement of dots on an existing map. Developments in digital mapping software, GPS devices and availability of digitized map files provide powerful tools for spatial depiction and analysis of disease occurrence and risk factors.

Computerized mapping and statistical methods for spatial analysis permit formal analysis of spatial patterns where large amounts of data are involved. Examples of the real-world application of spatial epidemiology in disease outbreak response activities are provided in a special issue of the *Australian Veterinary Journal* devoted to the

2007 equine influenza virus outbreak in Australia (Garner *et al.*, 2011; Kung *et al.*, 2011; Moloney, 2011; Moloney *et al.*, 2011).

Chapter 15, Spatial Epidemiology, on Geographic Information Systems and disease mapping provides more detail on spatial presentation and analysis of animal health data.

5.9.1 Plot both cases and non-cases

When plotting or mapping diseases it is important to also plot non-cases, so that the whole population at risk can be visualized. Plotting of only cases can lead to incorrect interpretation of possible reasons for the apparent disease distribution. This is because occurrence of cases may be more frequent in some areas simply because there are more animals or farms at risk in those areas and not because there is any change in causal factors for the disease. Unless you know the overall distribution of farms, you do not know whether this pattern has occurred because of some particular risk factor in that area, or because that area happens to be where all the farms are located.

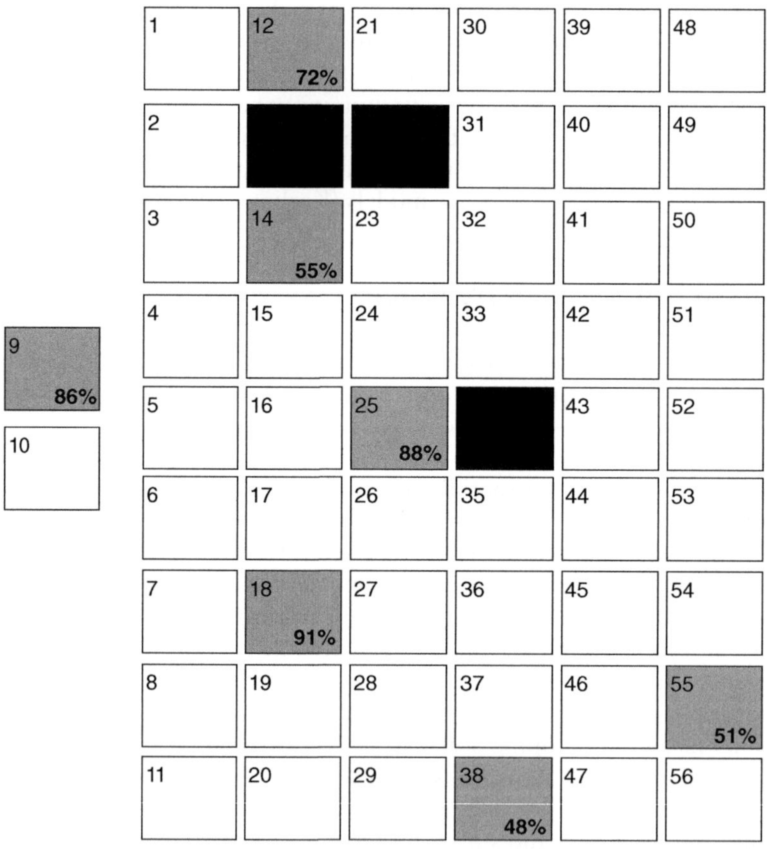

Fig. 5.9. Feedlot layout showing shaded pens with excessive mortality, blacked out pens that are empty and unshaded pens with normal mortality (adapted from Schwabe *et al.*, 1977, p. 39).

If information can be obtained on both cases and non-cases then mapping prevalence or incidence is much more informative than mapping just cases of disease.

As another example, Fig. 5.9 shows the layout of a feedlot experiencing sudden excessive mortalities in some pens (from Schwabe *et al.*, 1977). The diagram shows affected pens (light shading), pens with no cattle (blacked out) and pens with nil or low mortality (unshaded). All pens (other than those with no cattle) were stocked with between 400 and 800 animals and affected pens are shown with the cumulative percentage mortality for the 2 days of the outbreak. Looking at this representation, there does not appear to be any clear spatial pattern in this outbreak.

References

Garner, M.G., Scanlan, W.A., Cowled, B.D. and Carroll, A. (2011) Regaining Australia's equine influenza-free status: a national perspective. *Australian Veterinary Journal* 89(Suppl. 1), 169–173.

Heffernan, J.M., Smith, R.J. and Wahl, L.M. (2005) Perspectives on the basic reproductive ratio. *Journal of the Royal Society Interface* 2, 281–293.

Keeling, M.J. and Danon, L. (2009) Mathematical modelling of infectious diseases. *British Medical Bulletin* 92, 33–42.

Keeling, M.J. and Rohani, P. (2007) *Modeling Infectious Diseases in Humans and Animals*. Princeton University Press, Princeton, New Jersey.

Kung, N., Mackenzie, S., Pitt, D., Robinson, B. and Perkins, N.R. (2011) Significant features of the epidemiology of equine influenza in Queensland, Australia, 2007. *Australian Veterinary Journal* 89(Suppl. 1), 78–85.

Moloney, B.J. (2011) Overview of the epidemiology of equine influenza in the Australian outbreak. *Australian Veterinary Journal* 89(Suppl. 1), 50–56.

Moloney, B.J., Sergeant, E.S.G., Taragel, C. and Buckley, P. (2011) Significant features of the epidemiology of equine influenza in New South Wales, Australia, 2007. *Australian Veterinary Journal* 89(Suppl. 1), 56–63.

Schwabe, C.W., Riemann, H.P. and Franti, C.E. (1977) *Epidemiology in Veterinary Practice*. Lea & Febiger, Philadelphia, Pennsylvania.

6 Measuring Disease Frequency

6.1 Introduction

Measuring the amount of disease is important to assist management or understanding of disease. For example, knowing the amount of disease allows one to determine how large a disease problem is, to compare the amount of disease between groups or to monitor the success of a disease control programme.

Measuring disease can be done in many ways. For example, by counting disease events or by calculating the proportion of a population that is affected. It is also possible to compare the amount of disease between groups with ratios, and this can be useful to examine the effect of risk factors.

This chapter focuses on how to measure the frequency of disease and is a fundamentally important part of epidemiology.

6.2 Counting in Epidemiological Studies

Epidemiologists take a counting approach to measuring the different facets of disease. The other important characteristic of epidemiology that must be remembered is that the interest is in the natural populations in which the particular diseases are operating.

Counting is used in epidemiological studies to understand and/or describe the following:

1. The mechanism(s) of spread of the disease and disease distribution or patterns by time, location, feeding habit, use of the animal, etc.
2. The impact of the disease on the study population and the risk of a given animal in the population having the disease or condition.
3. The implementation and effect of a control programme to prevent or eradicate a disease from the population.

Counts of individual events of a certain disease may be used to evaluate the workload, cost, or the magnitude of resources required to provide adequate health care.

Counts of disease cases are often expressed as a fraction of the number of animals susceptible to the disease. The latter group of animals is called the population at risk (PAR).

For example, the PAR for retained placenta in cattle would be all cows and heifers that calve in the herd; for porcine parvovirus, the PAR would be serologically negative gilts and sows. The population at risk for Monodon Baculovirus infection are *Penaeus monodon* species of prawns.

6.2.1 Population at risk

Before we can start counting, we must first define the following.

1. The population at risk (see Chapter 5, Patterns of Disease): the population at risk is defined by where it is (geography), when (time period of interest), what it is like (description of the population by species, breed, age, sex, etc.) and susceptibility to the condition of interest.
2. The unit(s) of study (see Chapter 5, Patterns of Disease): are we observing individual animals, pens of animals, herds, villages, farms, etc.?
3. A case definition (see Chapter 3, Investigating Disease Outbreaks): this is a clearly defined description used to distinguish cases (animals, herds, farms, etc.) from non-cases. In some situations there may be multiple case definitions, depending on circumstances.

6.2.2 What do we count?

Disease or health events can be expressed in many different forms, depending on the case definition used. For example:

- Clinical cases – the number of: cows with clinical signs of Johne's disease;
- Subclinical cases – the number of apparently healthy chickens that are culture-positive for salmonellosis;
- Animals with certain characteristics – the number of cows that conceived on the first breeding or the number of ewes that have two or more lambs; and
- Combinations of the above – the number of cows with clinical signs of Johne's disease and that are seropositive to paratuberculosis.

As outlined above, the criteria for cases may be clinical, biochemical, haematological, serological, etc. Care should be taken to determine which criterion or combination of criteria best describes the disease to be studied or controlled (the case definition).

For example, definitive diagnosis of Johne's disease might require either histopathological confirmation or positive culture of faeces or tissue specimens. A diagnosis based on clinical signs of diarrhoea and wasting would not be sufficiently specific criteria for a definitive diagnosis.

Counting is also often applied at the group level, such as pens, farms, herds, etc. In this case you would have a case definition for a case herd (or pen, etc.), rather than just for an individual.

In addition to counting the disease events or cases, we also count the number of animals (or other units) without the disease in the study population (i.e. non-cases). Non-cases are any units that do not meet the definition for a case.

For the above example, if a case of Johne's disease is defined as an animal that has clinical signs of diarrhoea and wasting AND either has typical histological lesions in gut tissues OR is positive on culture of faeces or tissues then non-cases are any animals that fail to meet this definition. Non-cases either do not show any clinical signs (possibly despite the presence of the organism), or show clinical signs but are negative on both histopathology and culture (or are uncultured).

6.3 Ratios, Proportions and Rates

So far, we have talked about counting of cases and non-cases. Once we have these numbers, we also need to understand how to use them to better understand the disease we are investigating. There are several ways in which we can combine these numbers to allow us to make meaningful judgements about them.

6.3.1 Ratios

A ratio expresses the relationship between two independent numbers. The denominator usually does not include the numerator. Ratios can be expressed as fractions, but are often expressed simply as the ratio of the two numbers, as shown below:

Ratio = a/b or $a{:}b$, where a is not part of b

Examples:

- The ratio of boars to sows in a pig herd is 1:20.
- Feed to weight gain ratio is 2.5:1.

6.3.2 Proportions

A proportion is a fraction in which the numerator (frequency of disease or condition) is included in the denominator (population). This fraction can be multiplied by 100 in order to create percentages.

Proportion = a/b, where a is part of b, or $a/(a+b)$ where a is not part of b

Examples:

- The proportion of pregnancies ending in abortions on a dairy farm is 5/65 or approximately 9%.
- The proportion of grower pigs (in a particular herd) with lameness is 2%.

6.3.3 Rates

A rate expresses the relationship between a population at risk and the event under study *over* a specific time period.

Rate = a/b where a is part of b per unit time = risk rate; or

a is the number of cases and b is animal time at risk = true rate.

Examples:

- The rate of milk fever in a dairy herd was 10/420 calving cows per year.
- The incidence rate for foot abscess in baby pigs was 2.9 cases per 1000 pig days at risk.

6.4 Epidemiological Elements of Rates

Rates have a number of important epidemiological features.

1. The frequency of occurrence of the event. For example, the number of cows infected with mastitis, the number of new cases of foot abscess occurring per week during the observation period.
2. The population at risk or non-cases at risk of having the disease (differentiation between recovered animals and susceptible animals is important for many diseases). For example, the number of lactating cows that do not have mastitis at the start of the observation period.
3. Time period of the event:
   i. The external time component is the whole time period of the study in relation to calendar time. For example, a study of lameness in dairy cows was undertaken during the months of August through November (inclusive).
   ii. The internal time component is the time relative to a specific event. For example, the number of days or weeks post-calving.

6.5 Crude, Specific and Adjusted Rates

Morbidity (illness) and mortality (death) rates may be classified as crude rates or specific rates (host-attribute-specific and/or cause-specific). In this section the term rate is being used as a general descriptive term to cover rates, ratios and proportions, depending on the circumstances.

Disease rates and proportions such as prevalence and incidence can be expressed as crude rates, specific rates or adjusted rates.

6.5.1 Crude rates

A crude rate is a rate expressed for the entire PAR (e.g. crude mortality rate).

The advantage of crude rates is that they are easy to calculate and to explain. They have the disadvantage that they ignore the potential influence of various host and management factors (e.g. 5 dystocias per 134 calvings).

6.5.2 Specific rates

A specific rate is a rate expressed for a specified subpopulation of the PAR, based on one or more characteristics such as age, breed or sex.

For specific rates, both the numerator and denominator must have the specified characteristic (e.g. age-specific mortality rates: cases and non-cases counted separately for each age group, so that mortality rates can also be calculated for each age group).

Specific rates allow comparisons of subpopulations but are more difficult to explain. They also make it harder to compare populations composed of multiple subgroups (like herds and flocks) (e.g. 4 dystocias per 32 heifers calving; 1 dystocia per 102 cows calving).

6.5.3 Adjusted rates

An adjusted rate (or standardized rate) is a rate calculated by adjusting the rate for each population to match a 'standard' population structure for the characteristic of interest.

Adjusted or standardized rates are used to compare disease rates between populations with different age, sex and/or breed structures. To calculate the adjusted or standardized rate for a population, specific rates are calculated for each level of the selected characteristic and then weighted by the proportion of the similar specific groups in the standard population.

The standard population may be whatever structure you choose, but sensibly, should approximate the structure for the overall population (e.g. when comparing rates of different districts within a region the chosen standard population structure should be similar to the regional population structure).

Table 6.1 provides an example of the application of adjusted rates. In this example, the actual data for the two farms show a substantial difference in the overall percentage of cases – 16% for Farm 1 compared to 25% for Farm 2. However, when the data are standardized to a hypothetical 'standard' structure of 25% of animals <2 years, 50% 2–5 years and 25% >5 years, it is apparent that the adjusted (or standardized) rates are exactly the same at 17.5%. In this example the apparent difference in percentages of cases is because of the different age structures between the two farms, not to any inherent difference in risk between the farms. The actual case percentages for each age group are the same.

6.6 Measures of Morbidity (Illness) in a Population

The key measures of the frequency of disease occurrence are prevalence and incidence.

Table 6.1. Example of application of adjusted (or standardized) rates to two farms with apparently differing case percentages due to different underlying age structures.

	Farm 1		Farm 2	
Age (years)	PAR	Cases	PAR	Cases
Actual				
<2	30	3	20	2
2–5	50	5	30	3
>5	20	8	50	20
	100	16	100	25
Case %		16		25
Standardized				
<2	25	2.5	25	2.5
2–5	50	5	50	5
>5	25	10	25	10
	100	17.5	100	17.5
Case %		17.5		17.5

6.6.1 Prevalence

The prevalence of a condition is the proportion of existing cases of disease present in a population at a given point in time.

Prevalence = number of cases/PAR

For example, the prevalence of arthritis in adult pigs equals the number of cases of arthritis in adults divided by the total number of adults in the population. The prevalence of tuberculosis-infected cattle farms equals the number of infected farms divided by the total number of farms (with cattle).

It is important to note that the denominator may include both susceptible and resistant animals and therefore does not always represent the PAR.

Occasionally, prevalence and incidence are combined into a single measure known as period prevalence. This is a measure of the total number of cases at the start of the time period plus new cases that occurred during the time interval of interest. This measure should be avoided in general.

6.6.2 Incidence

The incidence is the number of new cases that arise in a population over a specified period of time.

Incidence = number of new cases in a given time period/total PAR

Unlike prevalence, incidence reflects risk, or the likelihood of an individual animal contracting the disease in a given period of time. Incidence can be calculated as a risk rate (or cumulative incidence) or a true rate (incidence density).

In addition, attack rate is often used instead of incidence rate in outbreak investigations.

6.6.3 Cumulative incidence

The cumulative incidence (CI) is the number of animals that contract the disease in a defined period divided by the number of healthy animals at risk at the beginning of start of the time period.

The length of the period has a large influence on the cumulative incidence: the longer the period, the higher the cumulative incidence. Therefore, it is essential that the relevant time period is quoted as part of the cumulative incidence, for example 1% per month, or 10% per year.

If animals are lost to follow-up (due to mortality or culling), one can use the average number of animals as the denominator by taking the number at the start of the period plus the number at the end divided by two, which is the same as the number at risk minus half the number of withdrawals.

6.6.4 Incidence rate

The incidence rate (IR; also called incidence density) is the number of new cases of disease in a population during a certain period divided by the total number of animal-time-units at risk for all animals in the PAR. The time units may be animal-years, animal-weeks or any other suitable time unit. Only healthy animals contribute to the denominator because only healthy animals are at risk of contracting the disease under observation. However, a case can contribute to animal time at risk up until the point when it becomes a case.

The relation between CI and IR is:

$$CI(t) = 1 - e\ (-IR * t)$$

where e is the base to the natural logarithm (2.71828183) and t is the time unit of concern. When the expected CI is smaller than 0.10 (10%), the formula is approximately equal to:

$$CI(t) = IR * t$$

The relationship between IR and prevalence is:

$$P/(1 - P) = IR * D$$

where P/(1–P) is the ratio of the proportion of diseased to healthy animals and where D is the average duration of disease. When P is small ($\sim< 0.05$ or 5%) the above formula reduces to:

$$P = IR * D$$

6.6.5 Attack rate

Attack rate (or perhaps better called attack risk) is a specific type of incidence rate that applies to outbreaks or situations where the period of observation is relatively short. An attack rate is the number of cases of the disease divided by the number of animals at risk at the beginning of the outbreak (the outbreak covers a defined time interval).

Attack rate = number of animals affected/number of animals exposed

For example, the attack rate can be used to measure mortality due to highly pathogenic avian influenza virus infection in chickens. If, over a 10-day period, 3500 of the 5000 chickens in a flock die, the attack rate is 0.7 or 70%.

Table 6.2 provides a comparison of the key features of incidence rate, cumulative incidence and prevalence.

Some important issues to remember

1. Incidence is a dynamic measure of disease whereas prevalence is only a static measure of disease.
2. Incidence and prevalence are related. The prevalence of disease in a PAR reflects both the incidence of new cases of disease and the duration of disease in individual cases:

Prevalence = incidence × duration under certain conditions.

Table 6.2. Comparison of measures of disease frequency.

	Incidence rate	Cumulative incidence	Prevalence
Numerator	New cases occurring during a period of time among a group initially free of the disease in question	New cases occurring during a period of time among a group initially free of the disease in question	Existing cases at a point in time
Denominator	Sum of time periods during which individuals could have developed disease	All at-risk individuals present at the beginning of the period	All at-risk individuals examined, including cases and non-cases
Time	From beginning of follow-up until disease occurs for each individual	Duration of period of observation	Single point in time
How measured	Prospective cohort study	Prospective cohort study	Cross-sectional study
Interpretation	Rapidity with which new cases develop over a defined time period	Risk of developing disease in defined time period	Risk of having disease at a particular point in time

3. Changes in the incidence or the duration of a disease will change the prevalence. The incidence rate is usually greater than prevalence if the disease is short in duration and/or fatal. Prevalence is usually greater than the incidence if the disease is chronic in nature.

4. True rate describes the average speed at which the event of interest occurs per unit of animal time at risk. It is often called incidence rate. True rate has no meaning on the individual level. However, it can be interpreted on a population basis.

5. Risk rate (cumulative incidence rate) provides a direct estimate of the likelihood of an animal experiencing the event of interest during the internal time period. Risk rate has a meaning on an individual basis as well as on a population basis.

6. Counting the PAR (i.e. the denominator):

i. With prevalence, the total number of animals examined during the time you counted the frequency of disease is the denominator.

ii. With incidence rates, however, we are looking at a population over a period of time; therefore, the number of animals at risk can change. There are a number of ways to deal with this problem, but the two most common are:

- Use an estimate of the population, either by counting the population at a time midway in the time interval, or by taking the average of the population at the beginning and end of the time interval.
- Calculate the population on each day of the time interval and arrive at the number of animal-days-at-risk (incidence density rate).

6.7 Measures of Mortality (Death) in a Population

6.7.1 Measures of mortality in the general (healthy) population

1. Crude death rate:

$$\frac{\text{NUMERATOR}}{\text{DENOMINATOR}} = \frac{\text{deaths in a given time}}{\text{total population at risk}}$$

2. Cause-specific death rate (a measure of the risk of death from a specific cause):

$$\frac{\text{NUMERATOR}}{\text{DENOMINATOR}} = \frac{\text{deaths in a given time due to the disease of interest}}{\text{total PAR}}$$

3. Age/cause-specific death rate (limits numerator and denominator to specific age/ cause of interest):

$$\frac{\text{NUMERATOR}}{\text{DENOMINATOR}} = \frac{\text{deaths in a given time in the group of interest}}{\text{total PAR for the group of interest}}$$

6.7.2 Measures of disease attributes among the ill or dead animals

1. Case recovery rate (actually a proportion rather than a true rate):

$$\frac{\text{NUMERATOR}}{\text{DENOMINATOR}} = \frac{\text{number of cases recovering}}{\text{total cases for which outcome known}}$$

2. Case fatality rate (a proportion rather than a true rate):

$$\frac{\text{NUMERATOR}}{\text{DENOMINATOR}} = \frac{\text{number of cases dying}}{\text{total cases for which outcome is known}}$$

3. Proportional mortality rate: The proportion of total deaths attributable to a specific cause:

$$\frac{\text{NUMERATOR}}{\text{DENOMINATOR}} = \frac{\text{deaths due to specific cause of interest}}{\text{total deaths in population}}$$

6.8 Comparing Disease Frequencies

Since incidence rates reflect risk, then the incidence rates (or attack rates) of two different groups may be compared in a ratio called the risk ratio or relative risk (RR). The RR compares disease among individuals of the one group to another group. Relative risk and a number of other commonly used measures can be used to compare disease frequency between risk groups in the population.

6.8.1 Relative risk

The relative risk (or risk ratio, relative incidence rate ratio, etc.) is the ratio of the incidence rate (IR) in the exposed group to the IR in the unexposed group.

You can use cumulative incidence, incidence density or attack rate for the calculations, as long as you use the same type of measure in both parts of the ratio. Since RR is the ratio of incidences, RR cannot be calculated for case-control studies (because incidence cannot be calculated in case-control studies). Table 6.3 shows the calculations required to calculate relative risk from an attack rate table or 2×2 table.

RR can vary from zero to infinity. RR is an estimate of how much more likely disease is to occur in the exposed group compared to the unexposed group and has a null value (no association or no increase in risk) of 1, which is equivalent to equal incidence rates. If RR is >1 the factor increases the risk of disease. If RR is <1 the factor decreases the risk of disease. However, a confidence interval for the estimate should always be calculated and the value can only be considered to vary significantly from 1 if the confidence interval does not include 1. As a rule of thumb, RR values greater than about 3 (or less than about 0.33) are considered potentially biologically important.

For example, Table 6.4 shows data and RR calculation for one risk factor (ate vanilla ice cream) as part of an outbreak investigation of a food-borne illness (from Oswego – An Outbreak of Gastrointestinal Illness Following a Church Supper: http://www.cdc.gov/eis/casestudies/xoswego.401-303.student.pdf):

Table 6.3. Calculation of relative risk from an attack rate table.

	Diseased	Not diseased	Total
Exposed	*a*	*b*	*a*+*b*
Not exposed	*c*	*d*	*c*+*d*
Total	*a*+*c*	*b*+*d*	*a*+*b*+*c*+*d*

$$\text{Incidence}(\text{exposed}) = \frac{a}{a+c}$$

$$\text{Incidence}(\text{unexposed}) = \frac{c}{c+d}$$

$$\text{Relative risk} = \frac{a/(a+c)}{c/(c+d)}$$

Table 6.4. Example of RR calculation for a food-borne disease outbreak investigation.

Ate ice cream?	Diseased	Not diseased	Total
Yes	43	11	54
No	3	18	21
Total	46	27	75

$$\text{Incidence}(\text{exposed}) = \frac{43}{54}$$

$$\text{Incidence}(\text{unexposed}) = \frac{3}{21}$$

$$\text{Relative risk} = \frac{43/54}{3/21} = 5.6$$

The interpretation of this result is that people who ate vanilla ice cream were almost six times more likely to become sick than were those who did not eat ice cream. In fact, 95% confidence limits for the RR estimate are 1.96 to 16, suggesting that this difference is likely to be statistically significant. We could also use a Chi-square statistical test to see if this relationship is significant.

6.8.2 Odds ratio

The odds ratio (OR) is a measure of the strength of association that is very useful in epidemiological studies of all types (cohort, case-control, cross-sectional). As the name implies, this is a ratio of the odds of exposure:non-exposure in disease-specific groups or the ratio of the odds of disease:no disease in exposure-specific groups.

Using the same notation for the cells of the 2×2 table in Table 6.3, as we used for the relative risk we get:

$$\text{Odds ratio} = \frac{a/b}{c/d} = \frac{ad}{bc} \text{ or } \frac{a/c}{b/d} = \frac{ad}{bc}$$

For the ice cream example in Table 6.4, OR = (43/11) / (3/18) = 23.5.

The OR is interpreted in a similar manner to the relative risk: values >1 indicate increased risk, while values <1 indicate a protective factor. Just like a RR, the null value of the OR is 1, and the OR has no units. The OR's significance can also be tested using a Chi-square statistical test or confidence intervals. In the above example the 95% confidence interval is from 5.8 to 94.

The interpretation is that the odds of developing disease were 23.5 times greater for those that ate vanilla ice cream compared with those that did not eat vanilla ice cream.

Comparing the RR and the OR, if the disease is rare a number of approximations start to hold true:

- a is small compared to b;
- c is small compared to d;
- $(a+b)$ approximates b; and
- $(c+d)$ approximates d.

Therefore, if the disease is rare, the OR approximates the RR. As a general rule of thumb the OR is considered to be a reasonable estimate of the RR as long as the disease is rare (CI <10% but the approximation becomes better as the disease becomes rarer).

In this particular example the odds ratio (23.5) and the relative risk (5.6) are very different because the outcome, food poisoning, was common in this outbreak.

6.8.3 Attributable risk

Attributable risk (AR; also called risk difference) is the absolute difference between the two incidence rates.

$$AR = IR_{exp} - IR_{unexp} = (a/(a+b)) - (c/(c+d))$$

The AR tells us how much of the disease in the exposed group is attributable to being exposed. It implies the rate of disease that could be prevented if the exposure were removed completely from the population. If you get a negative AR, the AR is telling you the rate of disease that was prevented by the exposure. The AR has the same units as the IR and can theoretically vary from –1 to +1; the null value is zero. Remember that the RR has no units and has a null value of 1.0.

For our ice cream example:

$$IR_{exp} = 0.8 \text{ and } IR_{unexp} = 0.14, \text{ so } AR = 0.8 - 0.14 = 0.66$$

Our interpretation is that the amount of food poisoning above the background rate that is associated with exposure to ice cream is 0.66.

On a cautionary note, there are several variations on the AR difference that have different interpretations. A common variation is the attributable fraction (AF) among the exposed, which expresses the AR as a fraction of the IR among the exposed; this measure indicates the proportion of disease in the exposed that could have been prevented had exposure not occurred. For the ice cream example this would be 0.66/0.8 = 0.825 (82.5%). Attributable risk and attributable fraction can also be calculated at the population level, indicating the rate of disease in the PAR that is due to the exposure. Population AR and AF are not discussed further here.

Significance of the AR can be tested in several ways. The simplest is with the Chi-square test that can also be used for the RR and OR. Attributable risk and the various variations on it are more commonly used in human epidemiology and are relatively uncommon in veterinary epidemiology.

6.9 Biological Importance versus Statistical Significance

RR, AR and OR all provide measures of the biological importance of a risk factor. That is, they provide an estimate of how much exposure to the risk factor increases the rate or amount of disease in a population. Thus a RR or OR that is far from 1 indicates a much higher (or lower) risk due to the risk factor than a RR or OR close to 1.

In contrast, statistical significance only tells us the probability that the observed result would have occurred due to chance alone – it tells us nothing about the biological importance of the risk factor. Statistical significance tells us how reliable, rather than how important, a result is.

A risk factor may have a statistically significant effect in a particular study, but not be biologically important, or vice versa. A potentially important relative risk (>3) that is not statistically significant may be a result of a lack of power in the study (sample size that is too small) and indicates that further research should be undertaken to further investigate the risk factor. On the other hand, a risk factor may be statistically significant but of relatively low biological importance if it is only a small contributor to a complex disease, particularly if the sample size in the study was high.

For example, in a hypothetical screening trial for a new cancer treatment, 0/4 mice treated with the new product died, compared to 4/4 mice that were not treated. The result was statistically significant ($p = 0.014$, Fisher's exact test) and may indicate a potentially valuable new drug. However, the result could have been much different! If one treated mouse had died, the p-value becomes non-significant and the drug might

Table 6.5. Hypothetical data for the relationship between sire breed and stillbirths in Hereford and Angus-cross cattle.

Sire breed	Stillborn	Live	Total
Angus	16	34	50
Hereford	25	125	150
Total	40	160	200

$$\text{Incidence}(\text{exposed}) = \frac{16}{50}$$

$$\text{Incidence}(\text{unexposed}) = \frac{25}{150}$$

RR = 1.9

be discarded, even though there is an apparent difference in proportion mortality (4/4 controls died compared to 1/4 treated mice). In this example the small sample size is having an effect on the ability to assess the findings and it reinforces the importance of using adequate sample sizes in experiments.

In a hypothetical example shown in Table 6.5, an investigation of stillbirths in a herd of 200 Hereford heifers, in which about 20% of calves were stillborn, found that Angus-cross calves were about 1.9 times more likely to be stillborn than pure-bred calves (RR = 1.9), and that this increase in risk was statistically significant ($p = 0.03$). How important is sire breed as a risk factor for stillbirth in this study? In fact, only 25% of all calves were Angus-cross, and there were more stillborn pure-bred Hereford calves than Angus-cross, indicating that while sire breed may have contributed to the increased risk for cross-bred calves, some other unidentified factor(s) was of greater importance overall.

7 Diagnosis and Screening

7.1 Introduction

Clinicians and pathologists devote substantial time to arriving at the correct diagnosis when investigating disease. The diagnosis is usually reached through a process of clinical examination and assessment and the application of various diagnostic tests. Competent investigators use good judgement, a thorough knowledge of the literature, past experience, diagnostic tests and intuition to organize their observations and reach a diagnosis.

In this context, a test is usually taken to mean a test performed on a specimen in a laboratory. However, in a broader sense, any procedure used to provide information that assists in arriving at a diagnosis (or decision about the status of an animal or group of animals) can be considered a test. Therefore, although the principles discussed in this chapter relate primarily to laboratory-based tests, they also apply to information obtained from the clinical history, physical examination, gross pathology and any other procedures or examinations used to help arrive at a diagnosis.

Box 3.1 provides a summary of methods that may be used to diagnose disease.

This chapter discusses the important epidemiological characteristics of tests and their practical application and interpretation in epidemiological studies and surveillance activities. The epidemiological evaluation of tests is also briefly discussed.

7.2 Screening versus Diagnosis

A distinction is usually made between the use of tests for screening and diagnosis. Screening begins with apparently healthy individuals whereas diagnostic testing begins with animals showing signs consistent with the disease in question. Screening tests are used for the presumptive identification of unrecognized disease in apparently healthy populations. A screening test should have both high sensitivity and precision, be easy to perform and of low cost if a large number of individuals are to be tested. A screening test is not intended to be diagnostic: individuals who return a positive result in a screening test should be subject to a more thorough investigation to establish a diagnosis.

On the other hand, diagnostic tests are used to confirm a diagnosis in animals presenting with signs of the disease of concern. Diagnostic tests usually require a high specificity to minimize the likelihood of animals being incorrectly diagnosed with disease.

Screening tests are used to screen healthy animals for disease, whereas diagnostic tests are used to confirm a diagnosis in diseased animals.

Key characteristics of tests used for screening and diagnosis are summarized in Table 7.1.

7.3 Accuracy of Test Procedures

The accuracy of a test can be measured in two ways: validity and precision. An accurate test is both precise and valid. In other words the result is repeatable (a measure of precision) and also gives a true measure of the value being measured (sensitive and specific – measures of validity). More formally, precision is defined as a lack of random error (high repeatability) while validity is a lack of systematic error or bias (high sensitivity and specificity). A test can be precise without being valid and vice versa.

The concepts of precision and validity are most easily understood by thinking of shooting at a target as shown in Fig. 7.1.

7.4 Precision

Tests performed on presumably identical material under apparently similar conditions are expected to produce very similar but not identical results. This variation is attributed to unavoidable random error inherent in every test procedure because factors that may influence the result of a test cannot all be completely controlled. When interpreting test results, this variability must be taken into account.

There are many different factors that contribute to the variability of a test procedure, including:

- uniformity of test material;
- transport and storage of test material;
- reagents;
- equipment and its calibration;

Table 7.1. Comparison of characteristics of screening and diagnostic tests.

Screening	Diagnosis
Applied to healthy population	Applied to sick individual
Seeks unrecognized disease	Differentiates among likely diseases
High sensitivity	High specificity
Large numbers tested	Small numbers tested
Low cost important	Cost not so important

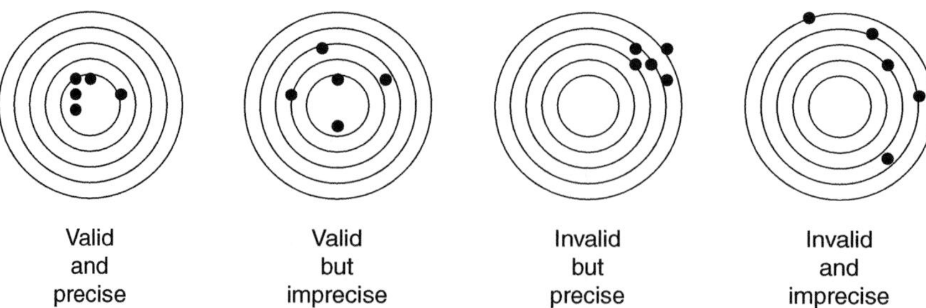

Fig. 7.1. Validity and precision in test procedures.

- operator; and
- environmental conditions such as temperature, humidity, light, air pollution.

Precision is a general term used to describe the variability between repeated tests on apparently identical material. A test with a high level of precision has low variability and vice versa.

7.4.1 Assessing precision

Two complementary measures are used to assess the precision of test methods: repeatability and reproducibility.

Repeatability refers to a test being performed on the same sample(s) under conditions that are as constant as possible in the one laboratory by one operator using the same equipment over a short period of time. An example is replicate wells on the one plate in an ELISA procedure.

Reproducibility is the ability of a test on the same sample(s) to give consistent results in repeated tests under widely varying conditions in different laboratories at different times and by different operators.

Thus, repeatability and reproducibility are two extremes, the first measuring the minimum and the second the maximum variability in results due to random error. Reproducibility provides a measure of the robustness of a test: that is, how well it performs under varying conditions of environment and equipment.

Several measures of precision can be used for measurements made on a continuous scale. These include the error standard deviation, determined from duplicate measurements for each specimen, coefficient of variation (error standard deviation as a percentage of the mean) and the line of identity (where the fitted regression line for the duplicate measurements is compared to the line of identity that has a slope of 1 and passes through the origin). Statistical control charts on positive or negative control samples can also be used to monitor test repeatability over time (see Fig. 7.2). For qualitative measures, the kappa statistic can be used to assess the level of agreement of repeated tests conducted on the same samples.

7.5 Test Validity

The validity of a test procedure is a measurement of the amount of bias in a test result and is quantified by the test's diagnostic sensitivity and diagnostic specificity.

7.5.1 Sensitivity

The diagnostic sensitivity of a test is the proportion of animals with the disease (or infection) of interest that test positive (i.e. proportion of true positives). This contrasts with the laboratory definition of analytical sensitivity, which is the ability of an analytical method to detect very small amounts of the material (such as an antibody or antigen). Sensitivity is also defined as the conditional probability that a test will correctly identify those animals that are infected (Pr T+|D+).

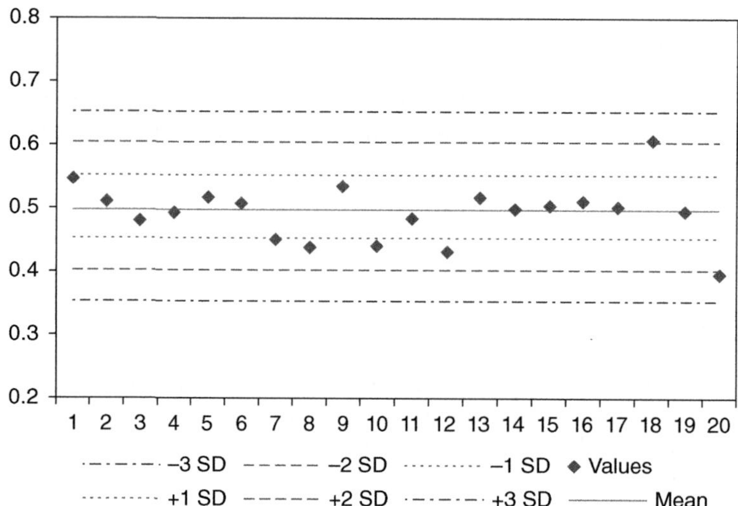

Fig. 7.2. Statistical control chart for 20 repeated samples.

Factors affecting sensitivity in antibody assay estimates include:

- number of animals in study;
- method used to determine disease or infection status;
- stage of disease;
- cut-off point selected;
- anti-species conjugate type;
- non-specific inhibitors;
- incomplete antibody; and
- suppression of immunoglobulin production.

7.5.2 Specificity

The diagnostic *specificity* of a test is the proportion of animals without the disease of interest that test negative (i.e. proportion of true negatives). Specificity is also defined as the conditional probability that a test will correctly identify those animals that are not infected (Pr T–|D–).

This compares with the laboratory definition of analytical specificity, which is the ability of the test to react only when the particular material is present and not react to the presence of other compounds.

Factors affecting specificity in antibody assay estimates include:

- number of animals in study;
- method used to determine disease or infection status;
- cut-off point selected;
- anti-species conjugate type;
- non-specific inhibitors;
- group cross-reactions; and
- non-specific agglutinins.

Table 7.2. Calculation of sensitivity and specificity estimates from results of testing on animals of known disease status.

	State of nature		
Test result	Diseased (D+)	Not diseased (D−)	Total
Positive (T+)	a	b	a + b = T+
Negative (T−)	c	d	c + d = T−
Total	a + c = D+	b + d = D−	n = a + b + c + d

a = true positives; b = false positives; c = false negatives; d = true negatives

Test characteristics	
Sensitivity (Se)	= a/(a+c)
Specificity (Sp)	= d/(b+d)
Infection probabilities	
Probability of having disease (Prevalence)	= (a+c)/n
Probability of not having disease (1−Prevalence)	= (b+d)/n

7.5.3 Estimating sensitivity and specificity from animals of known disease status

In order to estimate the test attributes of sensitivity and specificity, one must conduct the test on specimens from a number of animals for which the status of infection or disease is known. Often, experimental infections are used to determine these parameters, although field samples collected from known diseased and non-diseased animals (if a gold standard is available) are much better. Results from such a study can then be tabulated in a 2 × 2 table from which the sensitivity (Se) and specificity (Sp) can be calculated as shown in Table 7.2.

In probability notation, sensitivity is expressed as P(T+|D+) and specificity as P(T−|D−). Sensitivity and specificity are generally considered 'fixed' values, although for some diseases the amount of the agent and stage of disease may affect test sensitivity. Specificity can also vary with geographical region or other factors because of differences in cross-reacting agents.

Because of the difficulty in confidently identifying animals of known disease or infection status, it is often difficult to estimate sensitivity and specificity for a new test. Numerous methods have been developed to try and overcome these limitations and are discussed in more detail in the later section on evaluating diagnostic tests.

7.5.4 Sensitivity and specificity example

Table 7.3. Test Se and Sp with numbers for a theoretical test procedure.

	True disease status		
Test result	D+	D−	Total
Positive (T+)	33	2	35
Negative (T−)	4	141	145
Total	37	143	180

Estimated sensitivity and specificity are:

Se = 33/37 = 89.2% (95% binomial CI: 74.6–97.0%)

Sp = 141/143 = 98.6% (95% binomial CI: 95.0–99.8%)

7.5.5 Confidence intervals for Se and Sp

Confidence intervals should always be calculated when estimating sensitivity and specificity and can be easily calculated using computer software such as EpiTools (http://epitools.ausvet.com.au). Provision of confidence intervals allows users to evaluate the reliability of the estimates; wide confidence intervals because of a small sample size mean that the estimates are not very reliable and should be used with caution.

The precision of the estimates will improve (confidence interval width decreases) as the sample size increases. Ideally, there should be several hundred infected and non-infected animals for these calculations. For some diseases, sensitivity and specificity may be difficult or costly to determine but, wherever possible, such characteristics should be known for any test that is used in a national eradication programme or for official health status certification, so that test results can be interpreted with confidence.

7.5.6 Relationship between Se and Sp

For tests where the raw result is presented as a value on a continuous scale, such as an ELISA, there is an inverse relationship between Se and Sp as shown in Fig. 7.3.

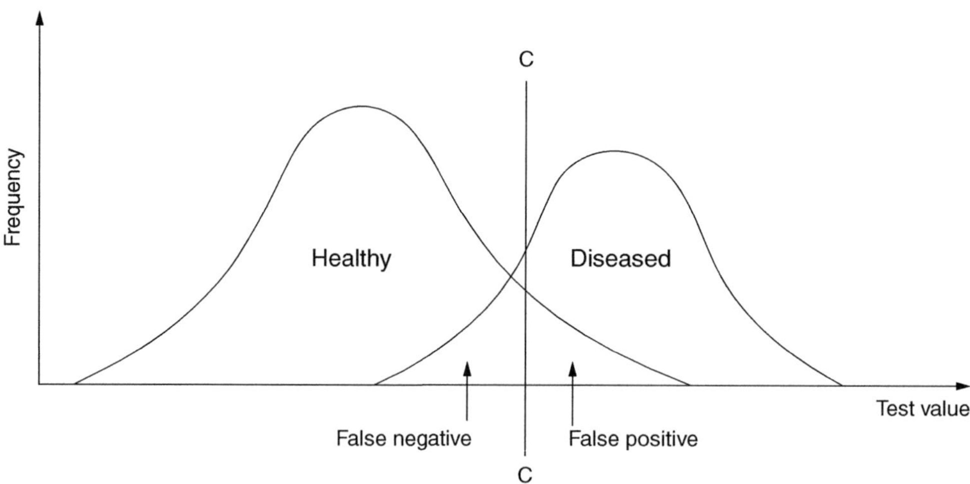

Fig. 7.3. Frequency distribution of test results measured on a continuous scale for healthy and diseased groups of animals with a theoretical cut-off point (C–C) separating reactors from non-reactors.

The frequency distribution of test results in a healthy population (D–) usually overlaps with the frequency distribution of test results in the diseased population (D+). Animals to the right of the cut-point (C–C) are classified as test positive and animals to the left are classified as test negative. If fewer false positives are required, C–C is moved to the right: specificity increases and sensitivity decreases. However, if fewer false negatives are required, C–C is moved to the left: sensitivity increases and specificity decreases.

Selection of the appropriate cut-off value will depend on a number of issues including the relative cost of false positives and false negatives, the stage of an eradication programme, if any, and the availability of other tests. An important consequence of imperfect specificity (i.e. <100%) is that if a large number of animals are tested from a population free of the disease in question, there is a significant chance of false-positive results occurring.

For example, if 100 independent samples were tested from a disease-free population, using a test with 99% specificity, the probability of at least one positive test result occurring is 63%. For a sample of only ten animals there is a 10% probability of one or more false positives, assuming a test specificity of 99%.

Because of this, cut-off values for screening tests are usually set to ensure a higher specificity, at the expense of reduced sensitivity.

7.6 Test Interpretation at the Individual Animal Level – Predictive Values

Sensitivity and specificity are important test characteristics that help us understand how well a test performs. However, both sensitivity and specificity depend on infection status of the animal, something we rarely know when we use the test. When interpreting test results, we are more interested in how well we can rely on the test result. Is a positive result indicative of an infected animal and, conversely, is a negative result truly indicative of an uninfected animal?

Predictive values are the conditional probabilities that answer these two related questions:

- What is the probability that a test-positive animal is truly infected (the positive predictive value or PPV)?
- What is the probability that a test-negative animal is truly not infected (the negative predictive value or NPV)?

Using probability notation, the predictive value of positive test results (PPV) is the P(D+|T+); for negative test results (NPV) it is the P(D–|T–). Formulae for calculating predictive values are based on Bayes' theorem of conditional probability and are presented here.

$$\text{Positive predictive value} = \frac{\mathrm{P} \times \mathrm{Se}}{\mathrm{P} \times \mathrm{Se} + (1 - \mathrm{P}) \times (1 - \mathrm{Sp})}$$

$$\text{Negative predictive value} = \frac{(1 - \mathrm{P}) \times \mathrm{Sp}}{(1 - \mathrm{P}) \times \mathrm{Sp} + \mathrm{P} \times (1 - \mathrm{Se})}$$

where Se = sensitivity, Sp = specificity and P = pre-test probability of disease (sometimes estimated true prevalence in the population).

The positive predictive value of a test (PPV) is the probability that a test-positive individual is truly infected.

The negative predictive value of a test (NPV) is the probability that a test-negative individual is truly uninfected.

In the above formulae, pre-test probability of disease (P) is a critical parameter for the calculations. In many cases, such as for a screening test in apparently health animals, the estimated true prevalence in the population can be used, as this is effectively an estimate of the probability of any selected individual being infected. However, in other situations, such as where the test is being used to confirm a diagnosed disease in a sick animal, prevalence in the broader population is not a good estimate. In this situation the clinician will assess the history and clinical signs of the animal and may decide that the pre-test probability of infection is considerably higher than the background prevalence (i.e. the animal is more likely to have the disease than if it was not showing the clinical signs observed).

For example, the estimated prevalence of heartworm disease in the population may be say 5%, based on practice records and local experience. However, the same records and experience may suggest that if a mature dog presents with specific signs of heart failure the likelihood of heartworm infection is much higher, perhaps 70%. If that is the case it is the latter value that should be used in calculating PPV and NPV.

7.6.1 Factors affecting predictive values

Predictive values are functions of the pre-test probability of infection and the test characteristics of sensitivity and specificity. As the pre-test probability declines so does the positive predictive value. The converse is true for negative predictive value. If the sensitivity and specificity of a diagnostic test are known for a particular target population, then predictive value graphs can be drawn for the range of all possible pre-test probabilities of disease from 0 to 1 (100%) (see Fig. 7.4).

When a disease is present in the population or region at low prevalence, PPV will be low and most positives will be false positives, unless test specificity is close to 100%.

For example, assuming a test with sensitivity of 99% and specificity of 95% and a pre-test probability of infection in the population (prevalence) of 1%, PPV is only 17% (more than 80% of reactors to the test will be false positives).

Of the two test properties, it can be shown that specificity exerts a greater influence on PPV than sensitivity. On the other hand, sensitivity exerts a greater influence on NPV.

7.6.2 Improving positive and negative predictive values

Some strategies that can be used to improve the predictive value of a positive test result:

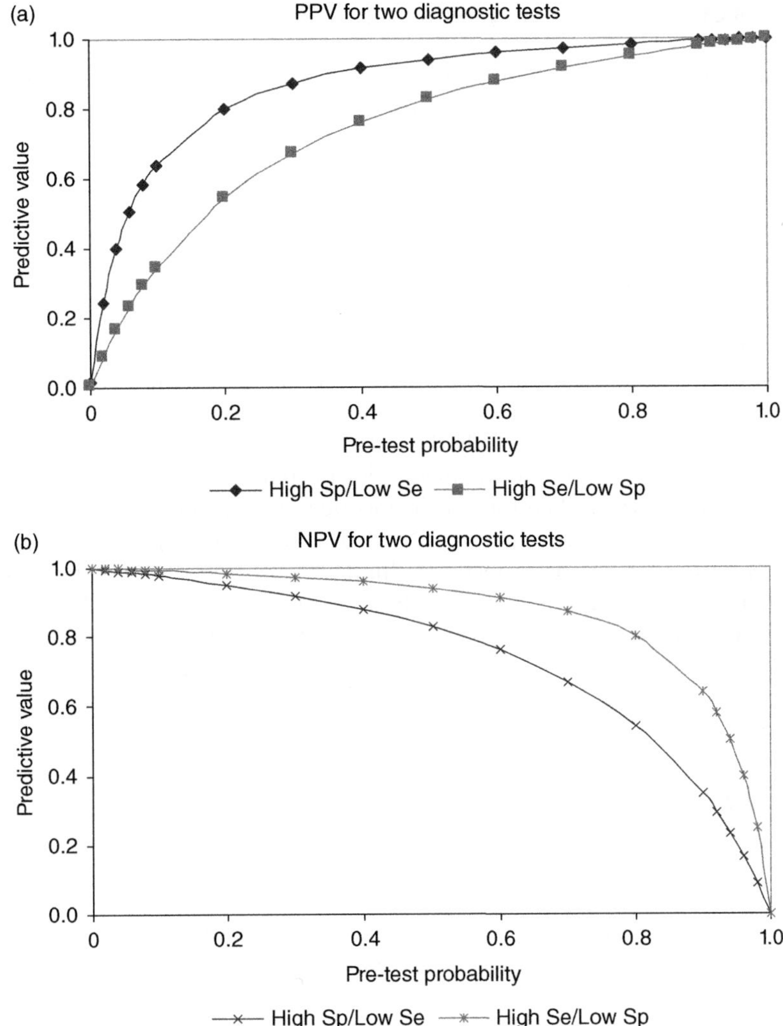

Fig. 7.4. Relationship between pre-test probability of disease and predictive values for two tests. Test 1 has Se = 80% and Sp = 95% while test 2 has Se = 95% and Sp = 80%. (a) Positive predictive values are better for test 1 because of its higher specificity. As pre-test probability approaches 0, PPV falls rapidly unless specificity is virtually 100%. (b) Negative predictive values are better for test 2 because of its higher sensitivity. As pre-test probability approaches 0, NPV approaches 1.

- Test high-risk groups – those with clinical signs rather than normal animals.
- Use a test cut-off value to provide a higher specificity, or use another test with a higher specificity than the original test.
- Use multiple tests in series (see below).

Some strategies that can be used to improve the negative value of a positive test result:

- Use a test cut-off value to provide a higher sensitivity, or use another test with a higher sensitivity than the original test.
- Use multiple tests in parallel (see below).

7.6.3 Rules of thumb for using tests at the individual level

With an understanding of the principles of predictive values, the following rules of thumb for using tests in the diagnostic process at the individual animal level can be recommended (modified from Baldock, 1988).

1. Decide on the pre-test probability of disease or non-disease after clinical work-up, but before performing any diagnostic tests. Revise probability estimates in the light of new information.
2. Consider what action will be taken for both a positive and negative test outcome. If the planned actions are the same regardless of test outcome, then performance of the test may not be justified.
3. If the objective is to confirm a likely diagnosis (the rule-in situation), then choose a test that has high specificity (>95%) and at least moderate sensitivity (>75%). If a positive result is returned, then it is highly likely the individual has the disease in question (PPVs are high for tests with high specificity, unless prior probability of infection is very low). If a negative result is returned, then further diagnostic work-up is required.
4. If the objective is to confirm that an individual is free from a particular disease (the rule-out situation), then choose a test with high sensitivity (>95%) and at least moderate specificity (>75%). If a negative result is returned, then it is highly likely the individual is free from the disease in question. If a positive result is returned, then further testing is required with more specific tests to ascertain whether or not it is a true or false positive.

7.7 Multiple Testing

Two or more tests can be used either sequentially or simultaneously and results interpreted in series or parallel.

In parallel interpretation, an animal is considered positive if it reacts positively to either or both tests; this increases sensitivity but tends to decrease the specificity of the combined tests.

In series interpretation, an animal must be positive on both tests to be considered positive; this increases specificity at the expense of sensitivity.

In general, the greater the number of tests involved, the greater the increase in sensitivity or specificity, depending on the method of interpretation that is used.

7.7.1 Sensitivity and specificity for multiple tests

Overall values for sensitivity for interpretation of tests in series or parallel, assuming conditional independence of the tests, can be calculated from the following scenario tree (Fig. 7.5), as shown using the following example.

For this example the two tests are assumed to be independent and have the following characteristics:

Test 1: Se = 50%; Sp = 98.7%

Test 2: Se = 60%; Sp = 98.6%

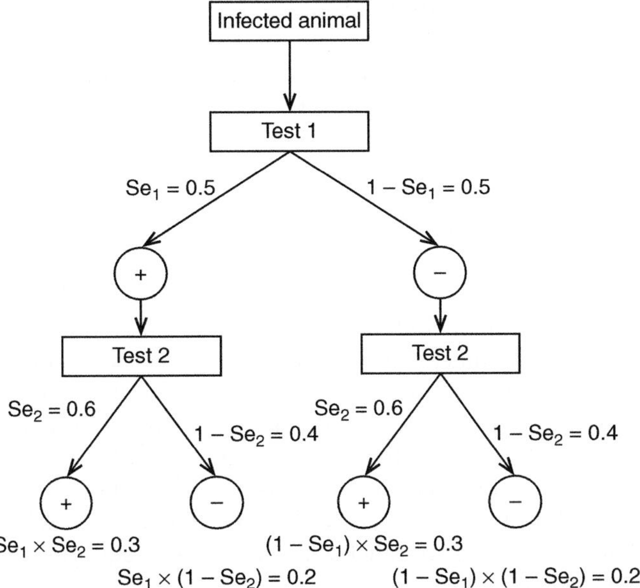

Fig. 7.5. Scenario tree for calculating overall sensitivity for two tests interpreted in series or parallel.

What are the theoretical sensitivities and specificities of the two tests used in parallel or series?

For sensitivity (Fig. 7.5), we assume an animal is infected and that it is tested with both Test 1 and Test 2. For Test 1, the probability of a positive test result (given that the animal is infected) is $Se_1 = 0.5$ and the corresponding probability that it will give a negative result is $1 - Se_1$, also = 0.5 for this example. For Test 2, the probability of a positive test result (given that the animal is infected) is $Se_2 = 0.6$ and the corresponding probability that it will give a negative result is $1 - Se_2 = 0.4$.

For series interpretation, both tests must be positive for it to be considered a positive result. From the scenario tree this is the result for the first limb on the left, which has probability $P(+/+) = Se_1 \times Se_2 = 0.5 \times 0.6 = 0.3$. Thus, the formula for sensitivity for series interpretation is $Se_{series} = Se_1 \times Se_2$ and for this example is 0.3 or 30%.

For parallel interpretation, the result is considered positive if either of the individual test results is positive. Alternatively, for a result to be considered negative both test results must be negative. Again this can be determined from the scenario tree, where the limb on the right represents both tests having a negative result and the probability of both negative results is $P(-/-) = (1 - Se_1) \times (1 - Se_2)$. Therefore the probability of an overall positive result for parallel interpretation is $Se_{parallel} = 1 - (1 - Se_1) \times (1 - Se_2) = 0.8$ (80%) for this example.

Similar logic can be applied to the example of an uninfected animal to derive formulae for specificity for series and parallel interpretation as shown below:

$Sp_{parallel} = Sp_1 \times Sp_2 = 0.973$ or 97.3% for this example; and

$Sp_{series} = 1 - (1 - Sp_1) \times (1 - Sp_2) = 0.999$ or 99.9% for our example.

7.7.2 Conditional independence of tests

An important assumption of series and parallel interpretation of tests is that the tests being considered are conditionally independent. This is also an important assumption of many non-gold-standard methods for estimating test sensitivity and specificity. Conditional independence means that test sensitivity (specificity) remains the same regardless of the result of the comparison test, depending on the infection status of the individual. If the assumption of conditional independence is violated then combined sensitivity (or specificity) will be biased. The conditional term relates to the fact that the independence (or lack of independence) is conditional on the disease status of the animal. Therefore sensitivities may be conditionally independent (or not) in diseased animals, while specificities may be conditionally independent (or not) in non-diseased animals.

If tests are not independent (are correlated), the overall sensitivity or specificity improvements may not be as good as the theoretical estimates, because two tests will tend to give similar results on samples from the same animal.

For example, let us assume that the two tests described above were applied to 200 infected and 7800 uninfected animals with the following results. What are the actual sensitivities and specificities for parallel and series interpretations and how do they compare to the theoretical values?

Table 7.4. Observed test results for 8000 animals.

Test 1	Test 2	Infected	Uninfected
+	–	30	70
–	+	50	80
+	+	70	30
–	–	50	7620
	Total	200	7800

Observed sensitivities and specificities of the two tests used in parallel or series are:

$Se_{series} = 70/200 = 35\%$ $Se_{parallel} = 150/200 = 75\%$

$Sp_{series} = 7770/7800 = 99.6\%$ $Sp_{parallel} = 7620/7800 = 97.7\%$

Sensitivity in series is slightly higher than was predicted previously (35% instead of 30%), and sensitivity of parallel testing has increased less than predicted (75% compared to 80%).

The apparent difference between calculated and observed values for combined sensitivities suggests that these tests are in fact correlated. Infected animals that are positive to Test 1 are also more likely to be positive in Test 2, as shown by the substantial difference in sensitivity of Test 2 in animals positive to Test 1 (70/100 or 70%) compared to those negative to Test 1 (30/100 or 30%).

The differences in observed and predicted specificities are much smaller and in this case probably due to random variation.

Lack of conditional independence of tests is particularly likely if two tests are measuring the same (or similar) outcome.

For example, ELISA and AGID are two serological tests for Johne's disease in sheep. Both tests measure antibody levels in serum. Therefore, in an infected animal, the ELISA is more likely to be positive in AGID-positive animals than in AGID-negative animals, so that the sensitivities of the two tests are correlated (not independent).

This is illustrated in Table 7.5, where the sensitivities of both tests vary markedly, depending on the result of the other test. In contrast, serological tests such as ELISA and AGID are likely to be less correlated with agent-detection tests, such as faecal culture.

Table 7.5. Comparison of test results for ELISA and AGID for Johne's disease in 224 histologically positive sheep.

	ELISA		
AGID	+	–	Total
+	34	21	55
–	13	156	169
Total	47	177	224

All 224 sheep are infected, so we can calculate sensitivities of both ELISA and AGID as follows:

ELISA Se overall	47/224 = 21.0%	AGID Se overall	55/224 = 24.6%
ELISA Se in AGID +	34/55 = 61.8%	AGID Se in ELISA +	34/47 = 72.3%
ELISA Se in AGID –	13/169 = 7.7%	AGID Se in ELISA –	21/177 = 11.9%

7.7.3 Application of series and parallel testing

Series testing is commonly used to improve the specificity, and hence the positive predictive value, of a testing regimen (at the expense of reduced sensitivity). For example, in large-scale screening programmes, such as for disease control or eradication, a relatively cheap, high-throughput test with only modest specificity may be used for initial screening. Any positives to the initial screening test are then tested using a highly specific (and usually more expensive) confirmatory test to minimize the overall number of false positives at the end of the testing process. For an animal to be considered positive it must be positive to both the initial screening test and the confirmatory follow-up test.

A good example of series testing is in eradication programmes for bovine tuberculosis, where the initial screening test is often either a caudal fold or comparative cervical intradermal tuberculin test, which is followed up in any positives by a range of possible tests including additional skin tests, a gamma interferon immunological test or even euthanasia and lymph node culture, depending on circumstances.

In the above situation it is important to realize that even though the follow-up test is only applied to those that are positive on the first test, this is still an example of series interpretation. Because an animal must test positive to both tests for a positive overall result, the result of the second test in animals negative to the first test is irrelevant, so that the test does not actually need to be done. Referring back to Fig. 7.5, it is apparent that deleting everything on the negative branch for Test 1 would have no effect on the final calculation of sensitivity for series test interpretation. This is an important consideration in control or eradication programmes, where testing costs are usually a major budget constraint and significant savings can be made by using a cheap, high-throughput screening test followed by a more expensive but highly specific follow-up test.

Parallel testing is less commonly used, but is primarily directed at improving overall sensitivity and hence negative predictive value of the testing regimen. Parallel testing is mainly applied where minimizing false negatives is imperative, for example in public health programmes or for zoonoses, where the consequences of failing to detect a case can be extremely serious. In contrast to series testing, every sample must be tested with both tests for parallel testing to be effective, so that testing costs can be quite high.

For example, in some countries testing for highly pathogenic avian influenza virus may rely on using a combination of virus isolation and PCR for detection of virus, with birds that are positive to either test being considered infected.

7.8 Measuring Agreement Between Tests

For many new tests, the true disease state of the animals in which it is being tested is not known and an investigator may only be able to measure how well a newly developed test agrees with an existing test. Unfortunately, sensitivity and specificity are often not available for the original test either. In this case, the new test can be compared with the existing test to see if it produces similar results.

For the same specimens submitted to each of the two tests, the investigator records the appropriate frequency data into the four cells of a 2×2 table, *a* (both tests positive), *b* (Test 1 positive and Test 2 negative), *c* (Test 1 negative and Test 2 positive) and *d* (both tests negative). The value kappa (k), a measure of relative agreement beyond chance, can then be calculated using software such as EpiTools or using formulae in standard epidemiology texts.

Kappa has many similarities to a correlation coefficient and is interpreted along similar lines. It can have values between –1 and +1. Suggested criteria for evaluating agreement are (Everitt, 1989, cited by Thrushfield, 1995):

Table 7.6. Interpretation of kappa statistic.

kappa	Evaluation
>0.8–1	Excellent agreement
>0.6–0.8	Substantial agreement
>0.4–0.6	Moderate agreement
>0.2–0.4	Fair agreement
>0–0.2	Slight agreement
0	Poor agreement
<0	Disagreement

Care must be taken in interpreting kappa – if two tests agree well, they could be equally good or equally bad. However, it may be possible to justify use of a newly developed test if it agrees well with a standard test and if it is cheaper to run in the laboratory.

Conversely, if two tests disagree, one test is likely to be better than the other although there may no way to tell which is better. The exception to this is where both tests have close to 100% specificity (i.e. no or few false positives). In this case the test with the larger number of positive results is likely to be more sensitive. McNemar's chi-squared test for paired data can also be used to test for significant differences between the discordant cells (*b* and *c*).

7.8.1 Examples of agreement between tests

Table 7.7. Comparison of results of two tests.

	Test 2 results		
Test 1 results	+	–	Total
+	121	36	157
–	34	931	965
Total	155	967	1122

Kappa = 0.74, indicating substantial agreement between the tests, but this result in isolation does not indicate which test is more sensitive or specific, or if either of the tests are any good. For this example, McNemar's chi-squared = 0.01, with df = 1 and P = 0.91, indicating that there is no significant difference in the discordant results between the tests, so the two tests have a similar (but unknown) performance.

As another example, a comparison of two herd-tests for Johne's disease in sheep yields the following results (from Sergeant *et al.*, 2002):

Table 7.8. Comparison of results of two tests for ovine Johne's disease.

	Test 2 results		
Test 1 results	+	–	Total
+	58	37	95
–	5	196	201
Total	63	233	296

How well do the two tests agree, and can you determine which test is better?

For these tests, kappa is 0.64, suggesting moderate–substantial agreement. However, McNemar's chi-squared is 22.88, with df = 1 and P <0.001. This means that the discordant cells (37 and 5) are significantly different. From the data available it is not possible to say which test is better – the additional positives on Test 1 could be either true or false positives, depending on test specificity.

In this case, Test 1 was pooled faecal culture (specificity assumed to be 100%) and Test 2 was the agar gel-diffusion test with follow-up of positives by autopsy and histopathology (specificity also assumed to be 100%). How does this change the assessment of the two tests?

Considering that both tests have specificity equal (or very close) to 100%, there are likely to be very few false positives. Therefore it appears that the sensitivity of Test 1 (pooled faecal culture) is considerably higher than that for Test 2 (serology), since Test 1 detected a greater number of positives overall.

7.8.2 Proportional agreement of positive and negative results

In some circumstances, particularly where the marginal totals of the 2×2 table are not balanced, kappa is not always a good measure of the true level of agreement between two tests (Feinstein and Cicchetti, 1990). For example, in the first example above, kappa was only 0.74, compared to an overall proportion of agreement of 0.94. In these situations, the proportions of positive and negative agreement have been proposed as useful alternatives to kappa (Cicchetti and Feinstein, 1990). For this example, the proportion of positive agreement was 0.78, compared to 0.96 for the proportion of negative agreement, suggesting that the main area of disagreement between the tests is in positive results and that agreement among negatives is very high.

7.9 Estimation of True Prevalence from Apparent Prevalence

When we apply a test in a population, we often get some positive results. The proportion of positive results observed is the apparent prevalence (sometimes also called seroprevalence). However, depending on test performance, apparent prevalence may not be a good indicator of the true level of disease in the population (the true prevalence). However, if we can estimate the sensitivity and specificity of the test, we can also estimate the true prevalence from the apparent (test-positive) prevalence (AP) using the formula (Rogan and Gladen, 1978):

$$\text{True prevalence} = \frac{\text{AP} + \text{Sp} - 1}{\text{Se} + \text{Sp} - 1}$$

All values are expressed as proportions (between 0 and 1) rather than percentages for these calculations. Confidence limits can be calculated for the estimate using a variety of methods implemented in EpiTools. When true prevalence is 0, apparent prevalence = 1 – Sp, the false-positive test rate.

Examples

Assume you have conducted a survey with a test whose sensitivity is 90% (0.9) and specificity is 95% (0.95) and you find a reactor rate (apparent prevalence) of 15% (0.15). By using the formula, you can estimate the true prevalence to be 11.8% (0.118).

Suppose you have conducted a survey of white spot disease in a shrimp farm, using a test with sensitivity of 80% (0.8) and specificity of 100% (1.0). You have tested 150 shrimp, and 6 shrimp tested positive. What is the estimated true prevalence?

The apparent prevalence is 6/150 = 0.04 or 4% (Wilson 95% CI: 1.8–8.5%)

Therefore, true prevalence = (0.04 + 1 – 1)/(0.8 + 1 – 1) = 0.04/0.8 = 0.05 or 5% (95% CI: 1.1 – 8.9%)

What happens if you assume that sensitivity and specificity are both 90%?

If Se = 0.9 and Sp = 0.9:

true prevalence = (0.04 + 0.9 – 1)/(0.9 + 0.9 –1) = –0.06/0.8 = 0.0625

The above example illustrates one potential problem with the Rogan and Gladen formula, which is that in some circumstances negative estimates can be produced. However, a negative (<0) prevalence is clearly impossible, so for this scenario the assumptions about sensitivity and specificity must be incorrect. For example, if specificity was 90% (0.9) and you tested 150 animals, you would expect to have 0.1*150 or on average about 15 false-positive results (even in an uninfected population). Therefore if only four positives were recorded, the specificity of the test must be much higher than 90% (a minimum estimate would be to assume all of the positives are false positives, so that specificity = 1 – apparent prevalence = 1 – 4% or 96%).

Because prevalence estimates are proportions we should also calculate and present confidence intervals for the estimate.

7.10 Group (Aggregate) Level Test Interpretation

The previous discussion describes the testing of individual animals. However, in epidemiological investigations, the study unit can often comprise a group of animals such as a herd of cattle, a flock of sheep, or a cage or pond of fish. For example, it is common practice to determine herd or flock status for some diseases based on the results of testing of a sample of animals, rather than testing the whole herd or flock.

In this situation, it is important to realize that testing for disease at the group or aggregate level incorporates a number of factors additional to those relevant to testing at the individual animal level. Thus, tests which may be highly sensitive and specific at the individual animal level can still result in misclassification of a high proportion of groups where only a small number of animals in each group are tested.

At the individual animal level, diagnostic test performance is determined by its sensitivity and specificity. The corresponding group-level measures are herd sensitivity and herd specificity. Herd sensitivity and herd specificity are affected by animal-level sensitivity and specificity, as well as the number of animals tested, the prevalence of disease in the group and the number of individual animal positive results (1, 2, 3, etc.) used to classify the group as positive. Just as we do for individuals, we also want high sensitivity and high specificity in our group-level interpretation.

Herd sensitivity (SeH) is the probability that an infected herd will give a positive result to a particular testing protocol, given that it is infected at a prevalence equal to or greater than the specified design prevalence.

Herd specificity (SpH) is the probability that an uninfected herd will give a negative result to a particular testing protocol (HSP).

7.10.1 Calculating herd sensitivity and herd specificity

The herd-level sensitivity (SeH) and specificity (SpH) with a cut-off of 1 reactor to declare a herd infected can be calculated as (Martin *et al.*, 1992):

$$\text{SeH} = 1 - (1 - (\text{Prev} \times \text{Se} + (1 - \text{Prev}) \times (1 - \text{Sp})))^m \text{ and}$$

$$\text{SpH} = \text{Sp}^m$$

where Se and Sp are animal-level sensitivity and specificity, respectively, Prev is true disease prevalence and m is the number of animals tested. SeH is equivalent to the level of confidence of detecting infection in herds or flocks with the specified prevalence of infection. SeH and SpH can be easily calculated using EpiTools or other epidemiological calculators.

If test specificity is 100% (i.e. any reactors are followed up to confirm their status), calculation of SeH is simplified:

$$\text{SeH} = 1 - (1 - \text{Prev} \times \text{Se})^m$$

Example

For example, assuming that we have tested 100 animals in a herd with a test that has Se = 0.9 and Sp = 0.99, what is the herd sensitivity for an assumed prevalence of 5%?

$$\text{SeH} = 1 - (1 - (0.05*0.9 + (1 - 0.05)*(1 - 0.99)))^{100}$$

$$= 0.996 \text{ or } 99.6\%$$

This means that if disease is present at a prevalence of 5% or more, there is a 99.6% chance that one or more animals in the sample will test positively.

For this scenario, herd specificity is:

$$\text{SpH} = 0.99^{100} = 0.37 \text{ or } 37\%$$

This means that there is a 37% chance that an uninfected herd will also have one or more animals test positively.

What happens if we assume that the prevalence of infection is 2% instead of 5%? Herd sensitivity:

$$\text{SeH} = 1 - (1 - (0.02*0.9 + (1 - 0.02)*(1 - 0.99)))^{100}$$

$$= 0.94 \text{ or } 94\%$$

SeH decreases as prevalence decreases.

Herd specificity:

$$\text{SpH} = 0.99^{100}$$

$$= 0.37 \text{ or } 37\%$$

SpH is unaffected by prevalence because, by definition, SpH applies only to herds with zero prevalence (uninfected).

In the above example, increasing the cut-point number of reactors for a positive result from 1 to 2 (i.e. if 0 or 1 animals test positive the group is considered 'uninfected' while if 2 or more test positive it is infected) results in an increase in SpH to 74% but a reduction in SeH to 77% (these calculations can be done using EpiTools: http://epitools.ausvet.com.au).

The formulae above assume that sample size is small relative to population size (or that the population is large). Similar formulae are also available for small populations or where the sample size is large relative to population size.

7.10.2 Risk of infection in test-negative animals

The only way to be 100% confident that no animals comprising a particular group are infected with a particular agent is to test every animal in the group with a diagnostic test that has perfect sensitivity and specificity. However, if only a low proportion of individual animals in the group are infected and only a small number are tested there can be quite a high chance that infected groups will be misclassified as uninfected. Table 7.9 shows the number of infected animals that may be present but undetected in a population of 100,000, despite a sample testing negative using a test with perfect sensitivity and specificity at the individual animal level.

The situation is further complicated where the test procedure being used has poor sensitivity, which is the case for many tests in regular use.

The probability of introducing infection in a group of tested-negative animals is the same as the probability that one or more animals in the group are infected but test negative. This probability can be calculated as:

$$\text{Probability} = 1 - \text{NPVm}$$

$$= 1 - ((1 - \text{Prev}) \times \text{Sp}/((1 - \text{Prev}) \times \text{Sp} + \text{Prev} \times (1 - \text{Se})))m$$

where NPV is the negative predictive value of the test in the population of origin, Se and Sp are animal-level sensitivity and specificity, respectively, Prev is true disease prevalence and m is the number of animals tested. As sample size increases the probability that the group will all test negative decreases, so that the overall risk associated with a group can be reduced by increasing the sample size. However, if all animals do test negatively the probability that one or more are actually infected increases (assuming that they are from an infected population), as shown in Fig. 7.6.

Table 7.9. Number of diseased or infected animals that could remain in a group of 100,000 after a small number are tested and found to be negative using a test that has perfect sensitivity and specificity at the individual animal level for 95% and 99% confidence levels.

No. of animals in sample tested from group of 100,000 and found negative	Confidence level 95%	Confidence level 99%
100	2,950	4,499
500	596	915
1,000	298	458
10,000	29	44

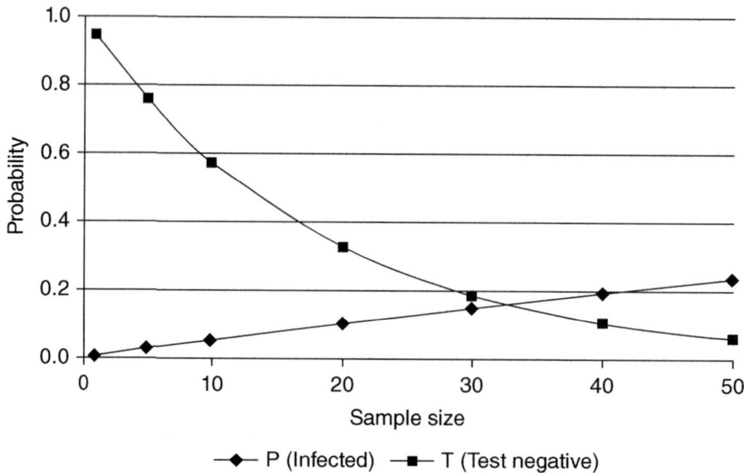

Fig. 7.6. Effect of sample size on the probability that a group of test-negative animals will include one or more infected (but test-negative) animals, and the probability that this will occur, for an assumed Se = 0.9, Sp = 0.99 and true prevalence = 0.05 (5%) in the herd/flock of origin.

For example, from Fig. 7.6: if 20 animals are selected from a herd or flock with a true prevalence of 0.05 (5%) and are tested using a test with Se = 0.9 and Sp = 0.99, and all 20 have a negative result, the probability that there are one or more infected animals in the group is about 0.1 (10%). In addition, the probability that all 20 animals will have a negative test result is about 0.33 (33%).

In simple language, there is a 1 in 3 chance that all animals test negative and also a 1 in 10 chance that there is one or more infected animals in the group, even if they have all tested negative.

Increasing sample size from 20 to 40 reduces the probability that all will test negatively from 33% to about 10%, but for those that are all negative, increases the probability that one or more are infected from 10% to 20% (1 in 5).

7.10.3 Demonstrate freedom or detecting disease?

As already discussed, it is impossible to prove that a population is free from a particular disease without testing every individual with a perfect test. However, demonstrating freedom from disease in a population is essentially the same as sampling to provide a high level of confidence of detecting disease at specified (design) prevalence. If we do not detect disease, then we can state that we have the appropriate level of confidence that (if the disease is present) it is at prevalence lower than the design prevalence. Provided we have selected appropriate design prevalence, it can then be argued that if the disease were present it would more than likely be at a higher level than the design prevalence, and therefore we can be confident that the population is probably free of the disease.

The selection of appropriate design prevalence is obviously critical: if it is too low sample sizes will be excessive, while if it is too high the argument that it is an appropriate threshold for detection of disease is weaker. For infectious diseases it is common to use a value equal to or lower than values observes in endemic or outbreak situations.

7.10.4 Important factors to consider in group testing

When testing a group of animals for the presence of disease, there are a number of important points to keep in mind:

- Individual and group-level test characteristics (sensitivity and specificity) are not equivalent.
- The number of animals to be tested in the group (sample size) is relatively independent of group size except for small groups (<~1000) or where sample size is more than about 10% of the group size. Alternative methods are available for small populations or where sample size is large relative to group size.
- The number of animals required to be tested in the group depends much more on individual animal specificity than it does on sensitivity.
- The number of animals to be tested in the group is linearly and inversely related to the expected prevalence of infected animals in the group.
- As the required level of statistical confidence increases, so the required sample size increases. The usual level is 95%. If this is increased to 99%, there is an approximate increase of 50% in the required sample size. For a reduction from 95% to 90% confidence, there is a decrease in sample size by 25%.
- As the sample size increases, group-level sensitivity increases.
- As the number of animals used to classify the group as positive is increased, there is a corresponding increase in specificity.
- As group-level sensitivity increases, group-level specificity decreases.
- When specificity = 100% at the individual animal level, all uninfected groups are correctly classified (i.e. group-level specificity also equals 100%).

7.11 Estimating Test Sensitivity and Specificity

There are two broad approaches to estimating test sensitivities and specificities.

Gold-standard methods rely on the classification of individuals using a reference test (or tests) with perfect sensitivity and/or specificity to identify groups of diseased and non-diseased individuals in which the test can be evaluated. In contrast, non-gold-standard methods are used in situations where determination of the true infection status of each individual is not possible or economically feasible.

Regardless of the methods used for estimating sensitivity and specificity, a number of important principles must be considered when evaluating tests, as for any other epidemiological study (Greiner and Gardner, 2000):

- The study population from which the sample is drawn should be representative of the population in which the test is to be applied.
- The sample of individuals to which the test is applied must be selected in a manner to ensure that it is representative of the study population.
- The sample should include animals in all stages of the infection/disease process.
- The sample size must be sufficient to provide adequate precision (confidence limits) about the estimate.
- Testing should be undertaken with blinding as to the true status of the individual and to other test results.

7.11.1 Gold-standard methods

Gold-standard methods have the advantage of using a known disease status as the reference test. This allows for relatively simple calculations to estimate sensitivity and specificity of the test being evaluated, using a simple 2×2 cross-tabulation of the test against disease status.

However, for many conditions a gold-standard test either does not exist or is prohibitively expensive to use (e.g. may require slaughter and detailed examination and testing of multiple tissues for a definitive result). In such cases the best available test is often used as if it were a gold standard, resulting in biased estimates of sensitivity and specificity. Alternatively, it may only be possible to use a small sample size due to financial limitations or the nature of the disease, resulting in imprecise estimates.

For example, the gold-standard test for bovine spongiform encephalopathy (BSE) is the demonstration of typical histological lesions in the brain of affected animals. However, false-negative results on histology will occur in animals in an early stage of infection. Therefore, if a screening test is evaluated by comparison with histology, specificity will be underestimated because some infected animals could react to the screening test but be histologically negative, resulting in misclassification as false positives. In addition, any infected but histologically negative animals that are negative on the screening test will be misclassified as true negatives, resulting in over-estimation of the sensitivity.

If a disease is rare, or if the gold-standard test is complex and expensive to perform, sample sizes for estimation of sensitivity are likely to be small, leading to imprecise estimates of sensitivity. If a disease does not occur in a country it is impossible to estimate sensitivity in a sample that is representative of the population in which it is to be applied. Conversely, if a disease does not occur in a country or region, it is relatively easy to estimate test specificity, based on a representative sample of animals from the population, because if the population is free of disease all animals in the population must also be disease-free.

Sometimes a new test may appear to be more sensitive (or specific) than the existing gold-standard test (e.g. new DNA-based tests compared to conventional culture). In this situation, the new test will find more (or fewer) positives than the reference test and careful analysis is required to determine whether this is because it is more sensitive or less specific. Even then, it is often not possible to reliably estimate sensitivity or specificity because there is no fixed reference point, so it may only be possible to say that the new test is more sensitive (or specific) than the old test, without specifying a value.

Gold-standard methods for estimating sensitivity and specificity of diagnostic tests and their limitations are discussed in more detail by Greiner and Gardner (2000).

Estimating specificity in uninfected populations

One special case of a gold-standard comparison is for estimating test specificity in an uninfected population. In this case either historical information or other testing can be used to determine that a defined population is free of the disease of concern. This can be based on either a geographic region that is known to be free, or on intensive testing of a herd or herds over a period of time to provide a high level of confidence of freedom.

If the population is assumed to be free, by definition all animals in the population are uninfected. Therefore, if a sample of animals from the population is tested with the new test, any positives are assumed to be false positives and the test specificity is estimated as the proportion of samples that test negatively.

For example, to evaluate the specificity of a new test for foot-and-mouth disease (FMD) you could collect samples from an appropriate number of animals in a FMD-free country and use these as your reference panel.

Two drawbacks of this approach are: (i) you cannot estimate sensitivity in this sample, since none of the animals are infected; and (ii) that by using a defined (often geographically isolated) population there is a risk that specificity may be different in this population to what might be the case in the target population where the test is to be used.

7.11.2 Non-gold-standard methods

Non-gold-standard methods for test evaluation can often be used in situations where the traditional gold-standard approaches are not possible or feasible. These methods do not depend on determining the true infection status of each individual. Instead, they use statistical approaches to calculate the values of sensitivity and specificity that best fit the available data.

Although these methods do not rely on a gold standard for comparison, they do depend on a number of important assumptions. Violation of these assumptions could render the resulting estimates invalid. Non-gold-standard methods for estimating sensitivity and specificity of diagnostic tests have been described in more detail by Hui and Walter (1980), Staquet *et al.* (1981) and Enøe *et al.* (2000).

Available non-gold-standard methods include the following.

Maximum likelihood estimation

Maximum likelihood methods use standard statistical methods to estimate sensitivity and specificity of multiple tests from a comparison of the results of multiple tests applied to the same individuals in multiple populations with different prevalence levels (Hui and Walter, 1980; Enøe *et al.*, 2000; Pouillot *et al.*, 2002).

Key assumptions for this approach are:

- The tests are independent, conditional on disease status (the sensitivity (specificity) of one test is the same, regardless of the result of the other test, as discussed in more detail in the section on series and parallel interpretation of tests).
- Test sensitivity and specificity are constant across populations.
- The tests are compared in two or more populations with different prevalence between populations.
- There are at least as many populations as there are tests being evaluated.

Bayesian estimation

Bayesian methods have been developed that allow the estimation of sensitivity and specificity of one or two tests that are compared in single or multiple populations

(Joseph *et al.*, 1995; Enøe *et al.*, 2000; Johnson *et al.*, 2001; Branscum *et al.*, 2005). These methods allow incorporation of any prior knowledge on the likely sensitivity and specificity of the test(s) and of disease prevalence as probability distributions, expressing any uncertainty about the assumed prior values. Methods are also available for evaluation of correlated tests, but these require inclusion of additional tests and/or populations to ensure that the Bayesian model works properly (Georgiadis *et al.*, 2003).

Bayesian methods rely on the same assumptions as the maximum likelihood methods. In addition, Bayesian methods also assume that appropriate and reasonable distributions have been used for prior estimates for sensitivity and specificity of the tests being evaluated and prevalence in the population(s). For critical distributions where prior knowledge is lacking it may be appropriate to use an uninformative (uniform) prior distribution.

Maximum likelihood and Bayesian methods of test evaluation are also often called latent class analyses or methods. This is because the methods are specifically designed to determine the latent (unknown) values required to populate the series of 2×2 tables representing test outcome against (unknown) disease status in each of the populations being investigated.

Comparison with a known reference test

Sensitivity and specificity can also be estimated by comparison with a reference test of known sensitivity and/or specificity (Staquet *et al.*, 1981). These methods cover a variety of circumstances, depending on whether sensitivity or specificity or both are known for the reference test. Key assumptions are conditional independence of tests, and that the sensitivity and/or specificity of the reference test is known.

In the special situation where the reference test is known to be close to 100% specific (e.g. culture or PCR-based tests), the sensitivity of the new test can be estimated in those animals that test positive to the reference test:

$$\text{Se(new test)} = \frac{\text{Number positive in both tests}}{\text{Total number positive to the comparison test}}$$

However, the specificity of the new test cannot be reliably estimated in this way, and will generally be underestimated.

Estimation from routine testing data

Where a disease is rare, and truly infected animals can be eliminated from the data, it is possible to estimate test specificity from routine testing results, such as in a disease control programme (Seiler, 1979). In this situation, test-positives are routinely subject to follow-up, so that truly infected animals are identified and removed from the population. It is also possible to identify and exclude tests from known infected herds or flocks. Specificity can then be estimated as:

$$\text{Sp} = 1 - (\text{number of reactors/total number tested})$$

In fact, this is an underestimate of the true specificity, because there may be some unidentified but infected animals remaining in the data after exclusion of tests from known infected animals or herds/flocks.

For example, the flock specificity of pooled faecal culture for the detection of ovine Johne's disease was estimated from laboratory testing records in New South Wales (Sergeant *et al.*, 2002). In this analysis, there were 9 test-positive flocks out of 227 flocks eligible for inclusion in the analysis. After exclusion of results for seven known infected flocks, there were 2/220 flocks positive, resulting in an estimated minimum flock specificity of 99.1% (95% binomial CI: 96.9–99.9%). In fact one or both of these flocks could have been infected, and the true flock-specificity could be higher than the estimate of 99.1%.

Modelling approaches

Several novel approaches using modelling have also been used to estimate test sensitivity and/or specificity without having to rely on a comparison with either a gold standard or an alternative, independent test.

Mixture modelling

One approach to estimating test sensitivity and specificity in the absence of a gold standard is that of mixture population modelling. This approach is based on the assumption that the observed distribution of test results (for a test with a continuous outcome reading such as an ELISA) is actually a mixture of two frequency distributions, one for infected individuals and one for uninfected individuals. Usually it is assumed that the results for the two subpopulations are either normally or log-normally distributed. This combination of underlying distributions results in a bi-modal distribution in a mixed population of infected and uninfected individuals.

Using mixture population modelling methods, it is possible to determine the theoretical probability distributions for uninfected and infected subpopulations that best fit the observed data, and from these distributions to estimate sensitivity and specificity for any cut-point.

For example, this approach was used to estimate sensitivity and specificity for ELISA for *Toxoplasma gondii* infection in Dutch sheep (Opsteegh *et al.*, 2010). ELISA results from 1179 serum samples collected from sheep at slaughterhouses in the Netherlands were log transformed and normal distributions fitted to the infected and uninfected components. The resulting theoretical distributions allowed determination of a suitable cut-point with estimated sensitivity of 97.8% and specificity of 96.4%.

While this is a useful approach for estimating sensitivity and specificity in the absence of suitable comparative test data, it does depend on the assumptions that the test results follow the theoretical distributions calculated and that the sample tested is representative of the population at large. If the actual results deviate significantly from the theoretical distributions, or the sample is biased, estimates will also be biased.

Simulation modelling of longitudinal testing results

An alternative approach, using simulation modelling, has been used where no comparative test data were available, but results of repeated testing over time were available.

In this example, the sensitivity of an ELISA for bovine Johne's disease was estimated from repeated herd-testing results over a 10-year period using a simulation model. Age-specific data from up to seven annual tests in 542 dairy herds were used to estimate ELISA sensitivity at the first-round test. The total number of infected animals present at the first test was estimated from the number of reactors detected at that test, plus the estimated number of animals that failed to react at that test, but reacted (or would have reacted if they had not died or been previously culled) at a subsequent test, based on reactor rates at subsequent tests. Reactor rates were adjusted for an assumed ELISA specificity of 99.8% to ensure estimates were not biased by imperfect ELISA specificity (Jubb *et al.*, 2004). Age-specific estimates of ELISA sensitivity ranged from 1.2% in 2-year-old cattle to 30.8% in 10-year-old cattle, with an overall age-weighted average of 13.5%.

This approach depends on the assumption that most Johne's disease-infected animals become infected at a young age, and that all animals that subsequently reacted to the ELISA were in fact infected at the time of the first test. If adult infection occurred in these animals the estimated sensitivity could have substantially underestimated the true value.

References

Baldock, F.C. (1988) Clinical epidemiology – Interpretation of test results in heartworm diagnosis. *Post-Graduate Foundation in Veterinary Science Proceedings No 107 – Heartworm Symposium*. Post-Graduate Foundation in Veterinary Science, Sydney, pp. 29–32.

Branscum, A.J., Gardner, I.A. and Johnson, W.O. (2005) Estimation of diagnostic-test semnsitivity and specificity through Bayesian modelling. *Preventive Veterinary Medicine* 68, 145–163.

Cicchetti, D.V. and Feinstein, A.R. (1990) High agreement but low kappa: II. Resolving the paradoxes. *Journal of Clinical Epidemiology* 43, 551–558.

Enøe, C., Georgiadis, M.P. and Johnson, W.O. (2000) Estimation of sensitivity and specificity of diagnostic tests and disease prevalence when the true disease state is unknown. *Preventive Veterinary Medicine* 45, 61–81.

Everitt, R.S. (1989) *Statistical Methods for Medical Investigation*. Oxford University Press, New York.

Feinstein, A.R. and Cicchetti, D.V. (1990) High agreement but low kappa: I. The problems of two paradoxes. *Journal of Clinical Epidemiology* 43, 543–549.

Georgiadis, M.P., Johnson, W.O., Singh, R. and Gardner, I.A. (2003) Correlation-adjusted estimation of sensitivity and specificity of two diagnostic tests. *Applied Statistics* 52, 63–76.

Greiner, M. and Gardner, I.A. (2000) Epidemiologic issues in the validation of veterinary diagnostic tests. *Preventive Veterinary Medicine* 45, 3–22.

Hui, S.L. and Walter, S.D. (1980) Estimating the error rates of diagnostic tests. *Biometrics* 36, 167–171.

Johnson, W.O., Gastwirth, J.L. and Pearson, L.M. (2001) Screening without a 'gold standard': the Hui-Walter paradigm revisited. *American Journal of Epidemiology* 153, 921–924.

Joseph, L., Gyorkos, T.W. and Coupal, L. (1995) Bayesian estimation of disease prevalence and the parameters of diagnostic tests in the absence of a gold standard. *American Journal of Epidemiology* 141, 263–272.

Jubb, T.F., Sergeant, E.S.G., Callinan, A.P.L. and Galvin, J.W. (2004) Estimate of sensitivity of an ELISA used to detect Johne's disease in Victorian dairy herds. *Australian Veterinary Journal* 82, 569–573.

Martin, S.W., Shoukri, M. and Thorburn, M.A. (1992) Evaluating the health status of herds based on tests applied to individuals. *Preventive Veterinary Medicine* 14, 33–43.

Opsteegh, M., Teunis, P., Mensink, M., Zuchner, L., Titilincu, A., Langelaar, M. and Van Der Giessen, J. (2010) Evaluation of ELISA test characteristics and estimation of *Toxoplasma gondii* seroprevalence in Dutch sheep using mixture models. *Preventive Veterinary Medicine* 36, 232–240.

Pouillot, R., Gerbier, G. and Gardner, I.A. (2002) 'TAGS', a program for the evaluation of test accuracy in the absence of a gold standard. *Preventive Veterinary Medicine* 53, 67–81.

Rogan, W.J. and Gladen, B. (1978) Estimating prevalence from the results of a screening test. *American Journal of Epidemiology* 107, 71–76.

Seiler, R.J. (1979) The non-diseased reactor: considerations on the interpretation of screening test results. *Veterinary Record* 105, 226–228.

Sergeant, E.S.G., Whittington, R.J. and More, S.J. (2002) Sensitivity and specificity of pooled faecal culture and serology as flock-screening tests for detection of ovine paratuberculosis in Australia. *Preventive Veterinary Medicine* 52, 199–211.

Staquet, M., Rozencweig, M., Lee, Y.J. and Muggia, F.M. (1981) Methodology for the assessment of new dichotomous diagnostic tests. *Journal of Chronic Diseases* 34, 599–610.

8 Sampling Populations

8.1 Introduction

Epidemiologists use population-based methods to investigate disease problems and to identify and evaluate interventions to control disease. It is thus vital that when selecting samples for study from a population that these samples are representative of the population of interest. If the sample is not representative of the population, the results will be biased and any inference based on the results of the study is likely to be flawed, leading to inappropriate decisions being made. In this chapter we discuss the various methods available for sampling populations and provide guidance on suitable methods to ensure that representative samples are obtained.

8.2 Why Do We Use Sampling in Epidemiological Studies?

When undertaking epidemiological studies it is usual to select a sample of the population for detailed study, rather than studying the population as a whole.

For example, sampling may be used to:

- estimate population parameters, such as average body weight or proportion with disease (prevalence);
- compare parameters between groups in a population (e.g. treatment/control or based on breed, age or some other risk factor); or
- demonstrate that a population is free of a disease or condition of interest.

We use sampling, rather than a census of the whole population, for a number of reasons. In particular, sampling is often a better option than a census because:

- It is usually much less costly.
- A properly constructed sample allows very precise and reliable estimates of population parameters (disease prevalence, mean body weight, etc.) to be generated.
- Sampling (if appropriate representative samples are taken) allows the calculation of confidence limits and the use of statistical tests to make inference about the parameter(s) of interest and to compare characteristics of different subpopulations (e.g. risk groups).

8.3 Populations and Samples

For the epidemiologist, the population is the patient. There may be a number of different populations that are of interest when investigating a particular disease condition. It is therefore essential to understand and define the population of interest. It is also important to note that different authors use slightly different terminology when referring to different populations. The terminology used here is based on that used by Thrushfield (2005).

8.3.1 Target or reference population

Before any epidemiological study is undertaken it is essential to understand where the results are intended to be applied. Are the results to be relevant to a single herd of animals, or a regional or national population, or are they restricted to a particular species, breed or sex of animals?

These considerations all affect the determination of the appropriate reference population for your study. The reference population should be clearly defined prior to beginning the investigation, so that it is clear to all involved how the results are expected to be applied. This also removes opportunities for ambiguity during analysis and interpretation of the results, as well as assisting in determining an appropriate study population from which to select your sample. The target or reference population is the population to which it is hoped to generalize or apply the results of the investigation.

For example, for a study of risk factors for foot-and-mouth disease infection in cattle in an endemic country the reference population might be all cattle (or cattle herds) in the country. Alternatively, if the study had broader application it might include all susceptible species, not just cattle.

8.3.2 Study population

The study or source population is the actual population from which eligible study subjects are drawn for the epidemiological investigation.

Ideally the study population should be the same as the target population. However, this is often not possible or practical, so the study population often comprises a subset of the reference population. The closer the study population is to the reference population, the less likely it is to be biased and therefore the more robust your results are likely to be, supporting a high level of confidence in any inference made. Conversely, the more differences there are between reference and study populations, the more likely that bias will be introduced and your study results may be invalid. It is therefore important to ensure that the study population selected is as much like the reference population as is possible.

Continuing the foot-and-mouth example, the study population might be all registered cattle herds in the country. This should be a reasonably good representation of the reference population, assuming that most cattle herds are registered, but might be very poor if only a small proportion of herds are registered. If the reference population is all cattle herds in the country, having only dairy herds as your study population might be a very poor choice of study population, particularly if the disease is likely to behave differently in dairy compared to non-dairy herds.

8.3.3 Study sample

The study sample comprises the units finally selected from the study population for inclusion in your study. The study sample is the group of animals or herds on which

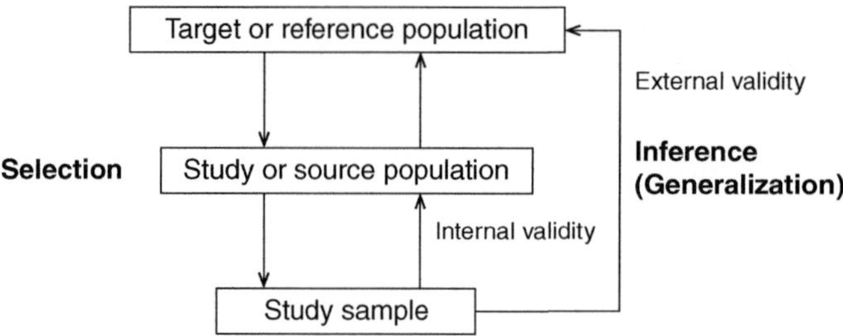

Fig. 8.1. The relationship of the reference population to the sample that is studied.

you will undertake your observations and measurements. For inference about the reference population to be valid, not only must the study population be similar in nature to the reference population, the study sample must also be similar to the study population (in this case we say that it should be representative of the study population). Obviously, for the sample to be representative of the study population it must have similar characteristics to the population and should be selected in such a way as to ensure that this is the case. This is achieved by using probability-based sampling methods, as described in more detail later in this chapter.

The relationship between the reference population, source population and sample for study are shown in Fig. 8.1. The aim is to have a sample that is representative of the reference population to which generalizations are made. If the sample is not representative, then generalizations will suffer error due to bias (selection bias). Representativeness can fail at either of two levels: (i) the study population may not be representative of the reference population (not externally valid); or (ii) the sample selected may not be representative of the study population (not internally valid). Failure at either of these levels will result in selection bias and study results that are flawed.

8.3.4 Population at risk

The population at risk is a particular example of an epidemiological population used mainly in disease outbreak investigations, as discussed in Chapter 3. When undertaking further investigations and specific studies as part of the investigation, the population at risk is also likely to be the reference population for your study and probably also the study population from which your sample is selected for further study.

For example, when investigating a particular disease within a single farm, the at-risk population may be all the animals on that particular farm or it may be limited to a particular subset of animals on the farm, such as a particular age group. On the other hand, if an outbreak of classical swine fever were to occur in a previously disease-free country, the at-risk population would be regarded as the entire pig population in the country.

8.3.5 Sampling units

Sampling units are whatever it is that you are selecting and on which you are intending to undertake measurements or observations. In many cases, animals will be the primary sampling unit. However, depending on the type of study, farms or subgroups within farms could be the primary sampling unit. In multi-stage sampling (see below), sampling can occur at multiple levels, so various levels of sampling units can also occur. For example, primary sampling units may be farms and secondary sampling units are animals within farms. Occasionally, this may be extended to a third or even fourth level.

For our foot-and-mouth disease example, primary sampling units are likely to be farms or villages and secondary sampling units animals within selected farms or villages.

8.3.6 Sampling frames

A sampling frame is a list of all members of the population, from which the sample is chosen.

Many probability-based sampling methods require a sampling frame from which the chosen sample is selected. For some sampling methods, additional information about each unit in the sampling frame may also be required, such as for stratification by herd size, region or some other factor. As for sampling units, sampling frames may be applied at multiple levels. For example, for a two-stage survey of cattle herds you would require a sampling frame of all herds in the study population, and then you might also require a sampling frame for each selected herd.

An example of a sampling frame for the foot-and-mouth disease study would be the register of all cattle herds in the country. This would provide a list of all registered herds, ideally with additional information such as herd size and location if stratification was required.

8.4 Approaches to Sampling

There are many ways to select a sample from a population for a survey or other epidemiological study. The appropriate method will depend on the purpose of the study, characteristics of the population and what information you have about the population.

The desirable characteristics of a sample are that it:

- is representative of the study population, to allow inference back to that population;
- produces unbiased estimates (i.e. estimates are accurate); and
- produces estimates of known precision (i.e. estimates are reliable and allow calculation of confidence limits for the true value).

8.4.1 What is a representative sample?

A representative sample is a sample selected in such a way that estimates of population characteristics calculated from the sample are not biased.

Specifically, it is a sample that has similar characteristics to the population from which it is drawn, with regard to important characteristics, including the outcome of interest.

For example, if we are studying the prevalence of brucellosis in cattle in a region, a representative sample would have similar characteristics to the study population (all the cattle in the region) and should produce a prevalence estimate that is unbiased with respect to the true value. A method is therefore needed to select a sample of animals so that they are very likely to have the same characteristics as the study population.

8.4.2 Probability versus non-probability sampling

Two broad groups of sampling techniques exist: probability sampling and non-probability sampling:

Probability sampling is a sampling technique in which each member of the population has a known, non-zero probability of being selected in the sample.

Non-probability sampling is any sampling method where members of the population do *not* have a known, non-zero probability of being selected in the sample (i.e. anything that is not a probability sampling method).

Probability sampling methods, if applied correctly, are more likely to produce a representative, unbiased, sample of the study population. Conversely, non-probability sampling is less likely to produce a representative sample, and then only by accident.

8.5 Non-probability Sampling Methods

Several non-probability sampling techniques are sometimes used. These methods are unable to reliably select a representative sample, and therefore inference about the target population should not be relied upon because estimates will be biased. Use of these methods may invalidate the results of an epidemiological study, and they should therefore be avoided.

8.5.1 Convenience sampling

Convenience sampling is an approach where units are chosen for sampling because they are easy, quick or inexpensive to collect.

For example, the first ten animals to pass through a race or crush represents a convenience sample. They are easy to examine, and you do not have to process all animals to select your sample. The problem with convenience sampling is that it is rarely representative of the population. The bias may not always be obvious, but it is often present, and is impossible to correct for.

A commonly used convenience sample is to use known cooperative farmers, because you know they will be supportive and are unlikely to drop out of your study part way through. The disadvantage of this is that they are often more progressive and more likely to seek advice than other farmers, leading to potential bias in your results.

8.5.2 Purposive sampling

Purposive or judgemental sampling is where animals are deliberately selected in an effort to achieve a representative or balanced sample of the population.

Typical animals may be chosen from a group, or animals which are thought to represent the range of animals present. This may be done be selecting some small animals, some medium-sized and some large animals. While this may seem reasonable, experience has shown that purposive samples are virtually always biased.

8.5.3 Haphazard sampling

Haphazard sampling is where units are chosen with no fixed purpose or reason, in an attempt to imitate random sampling (see below).

The problem with haphazard sampling is that people are very poor at picking things randomly. Judgement invariably plays a role, and efforts are made to keep the sample representative in the eyes of the person who is doing the selecting. This results in a type of purposive sample, with the same problems of bias. Both purposive and haphazard sampling also offer opportunities for deliberate bias when applied by unscrupulous operators, because the operator actually controls the sample selection process, whereas in probability-based sampling, selection is determined by the process itself.

8.5.4 Summary

Non-probability sampling techniques are unable to reliably select a representative sample.

Consider the example of a purposive sample, carefully chosen to try to be representative of the population. If we know that there are a number of risk factors for a particular disease, we may choose to select some animals with the risk factor and some without. Better still, if the data are available, we would choose these animals in the same proportion as the presence of the risk factor in the population.

Consider a survey of the seroprevalence of antibodies to foot-and-mouth disease in livestock. Animals that have been recently vaccinated are likely to have antibodies. If we know from vaccination campaign records that 80% of the population has been recently vaccinated, then we may choose to have 80% of the sample made up of recently vaccinated animals. This still does not ensure that the sample will be representative, because there are other risk factors that we have not taken into account, for instance recent exposure to the virus in an outbreak. Even if the sample is selected in such a way to take into account all the risk factors that are known, we do not have perfect knowledge of any disease, and the final sample may still be unrepresentative of the population. The solution to this problem lies in probability sampling.

8.5.5 When might non-probability sampling methods be useful?

Non-probability sampling can be useful in situations where statistical inference about the reference population is not required, so that a representative sample is less important. For example, when sampling to demonstrate freedom from disease or to determine if a disease is present in a population, biasing sampling to include those animals most likely to be infected will increase your likelihood of detecting disease, if it is present. It is important to realize that if you use non-probability sampling in this way, calculations to determine the true level of confidence that the population is free (assuming all samples are negative) are far more complicated, or may not be possible at all.

It is also not possible to reliably estimate the prevalence of disease (assuming disease is detected) or compare estimates between subpopulations.

For example, one approach to determining if a sheep flock is infected with Johne's disease is to preferentially select emaciated sheep for serological testing and/or post-mortem, as these are the sheep most likely to be showing typical lesions and in which test sensitivity is likely to be highest. If any of the sheep are positive the flock is infected. Conversely, if a reasonable number of the sheep are examined and are all negative the flock is likely to be free of Johne's disease. However, the results are only indicative of presence or likely absence of disease, it is not possible to quantify confidence of freedom or estimate prevalence in this situation.

8.6 Probability Sampling Methods

Probability sampling is based on the concept of randomness and the use of random numbers. Random numbers are best explained by an example using dice. Most dice have six numbered sides, 1 to 6, and when a die is rolled each side has the same probability of ending on top. However, at each roll, we never know which number will come up. What we do know is that if we roll the dice again and again, on average, all numbers will appear equally often. Rolling dice is one way of generating random numbers (in this case, between 1 and 6). Decimal dice exist, with ten sides numbered 0 to 9. In addition to a variety of other mechanical means of choosing random numbers there are two more convenient methods. Many statistical texts include tables of random numbers, which have been generated by some mechanical means. Alternatively, computer-generated pseudo-random numbers are available in many statistical programs. These pseudo-random numbers are not truly random as they come from a predictable sequence generated by a mathematical formula. Given the formula it is possible to predict the next number in the sequence. However, these numbers are usually indistinguishable from random numbers and are perfectly adequate for most random sampling situations.

There are a number of specific probability-based sampling methods, all of which use the principle of random numbers to generate a representative sample of the population.

8.6.1 Simple random sampling

Simple random sampling is a sampling technique where individuals are selected using random numbers or some other random selection technique, so that each member of the population has the same probability of being selected. It is the simplest form of probability sampling.

To select a simple random sample of ten animals from a herd of 100, ten random numbers are generated between 1 and 100 (either with dice, random number tables, selecting from pieces of paper in a bucket, using computer-generated random numbers, etc.). A list of animals (or sampling frame) is created and those corresponding to the chosen numbers are then selected (see Fig. 8.2). Alternatively, if a list of animals is not available, animals can be processed through a crush or race in order and animals corresponding to the chosen numbers are selected as they pass through.

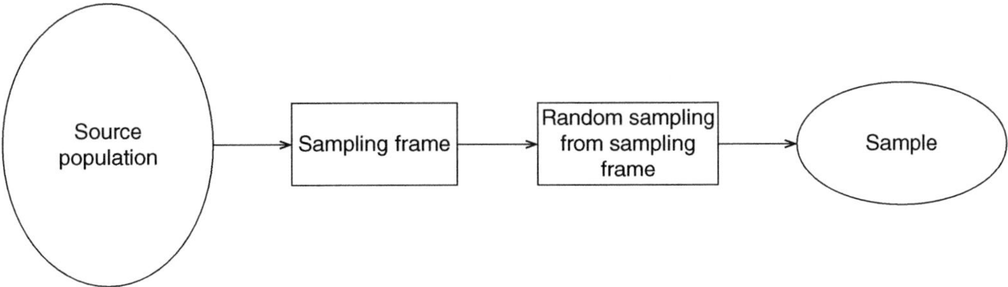

Fig. 8.2. Diagrammatic representation of simple random sampling.

To be able to do simple random sampling you must know the size of the population and either have a sampling frame of all sampling units (farms, animals, etc.) or be able to process the population in some ordered way.

8.6.2 Systematic random sampling

Systematic random sampling is where the selection procedure is according to some simple systematic rule, such as every *n*th animal in order. The first animal must be selected at random.

Systematic sampling is often more practical than simple random sampling, particularly where a sampling frame is not readily available. Consider a flock of 600 sheep. If we wish to examine samples from 30 sheep for parasites, simple random sampling would require that each sheep is first identified and assigned a number between 1 and 600. If the animals are not already identified, this process may be time consuming or impractical. Alternatively, we could select the required 30 random numbers between 1 and 600 and then count animals through a race. However, this would result in irregular intervals between sampling and could easily lead to mistakes. An alternative and simpler approach is to use systematic sampling.

Using systematic sampling, prior identification of the animals is not necessary and the interval between selected animals is fixed. The sheep are held in one pen and allowed to pass, one by one, through a race to another pen. Every 20th animal is then selected as it passes through, giving a total sample of 30 animals. In this case, 20 is known as the sampling interval. It is calculated as N/n, or the population size divided by the desired sample size (see Fig. 8.3).

Systematic sampling is only a form of probability sampling if the first animal chosen is selected at random. In our example, a number between 1 and 20 would be chosen at random, say 15. The 15th animal passing through the race would be the first animal chosen, and then every 20th animal (35, 55, 75, etc.). If, however, the first animal is chosen deliberately (not at random) there is no element of chance, and the technique becomes a form of non-probability sampling.

Under most circumstances, systematic random sampling will produce a sample with very similar properties to simple random sampling, and the same formulae may be used to analyse the sample data. There is a danger, however, if the population has some sort of cyclic variation that matches or nearly matches the sampling interval.

Fortunately, such clear cyclic ordering in animal surveys is very unusual, and so is rarely a problem.

For example, if we are sampling cows through a dairy, where the sampling interval was the same as the number of stalls in the dairy – in this case animals at the same position would be sampled each time, with an obvious potential for bias. Another example may be if we were sampling temperature records where our sampling interval worked out at being every 24 h. In this case we would be sampling records taken at the same time every day, which would not be representative of the temperature fluctuations experienced throughout the day.

For systematic sampling, we need to know the approximate population size and to be able to process the population in an ordered fashion to select our desired sample.

8.6.3 Stratified random sampling

Stratified random sampling is where the population is divided into a number of separate, mutually exclusive subgroups (or strata) according to some important characteristic, and representative sampling is undertaken from each group (stratum; see Fig. 8.4). Stratification of the population is usually based on some readily available characteristic of the population, often one that is likely to be associated with the outcome of interest (e.g. geographic location, herd size, etc.). For stratified sampling, not only do we need a sampling frame of primary units to select from, we also require information about what stratum each unit belongs to.

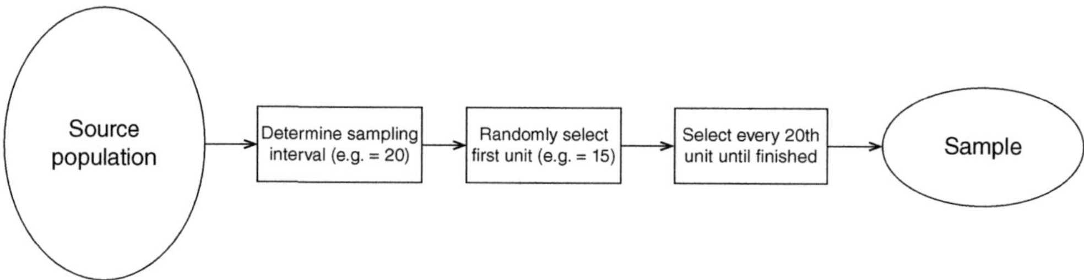

Fig. 8.3. Diagrammatic representation of systematic random sampling.

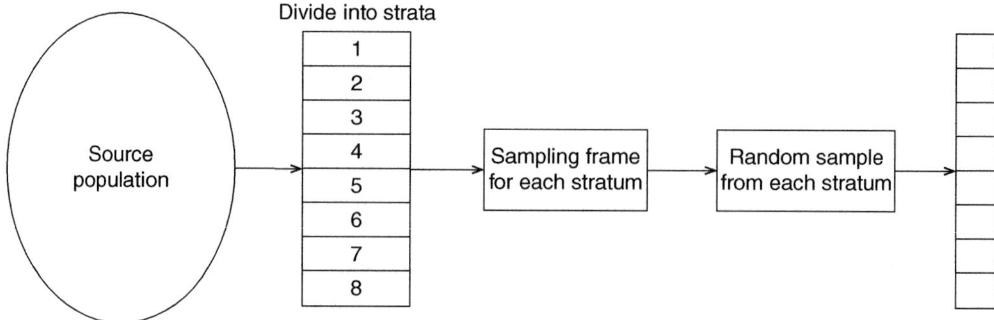

Fig. 8.4. Diagrammatic representation of stratified random sampling.

Why use stratified sampling?

There are three main reasons for using stratification.

1. It enables us to calculate estimates not only for the whole population, but for each stratum as well. For a national survey, stratification by province may provide a much more useful picture of the distribution of the disease, rather than just an overall estimate.
2. The second reason for using stratification is that it may produce more precise results. Imagine a survey of the prevalence of insect-borne blood parasites in cattle, in a country with several different climatic zones – hot and humid, hot and dry, cool and wet. The insect vectors for the disease are likely to be much more common in the hot and humid part of the country than in the other two zones. A national survey will find a lot of variability in the prevalence from one area to another. Stratification by climatic zone means, essentially, three separate surveys are conducted, one in each zone. In the hot humid zone, a uniformly high prevalence is likely to be found, while a low prevalence is likely in the other two zones. In each survey, the variability is much less. When the results of the three surveys are combined, the overall precision is greater. Alternatively, because of the expected increase in precision, the required sample size for the survey can be reduced, reducing costs.
3. From a practical perspective, stratification ensures that all strata, particularly those with relatively low numbers, are adequately represented in your sample. Stratification on a geographic basis also ensures that sampling is spread across all parts of the region or country, helping to share the workload.

Selecting your strata

To achieve improved precision from stratification, the aim is to have the animals within each stratum as homogeneous as possible with respect to the characteristic in question, and for the strata to be as different from each other as possible (low within-stratum variability, and high between-stratum variability). Before a survey we rarely know enough about the distribution of the characteristic in the population to ensure this, but we may know that the characteristic is linked to some risk factor (in our example, climatic zone). Stratifying on the risk factor will therefore help to improve the precision of the survey.

Depending on the purpose of the study, sample size within strata may be a fixed size, or may be proportional to the number of sampling units in the stratum. Generally, proportional sampling is simpler and results in an unbiased estimate, whereas for fixed size sampling the estimate must be weighted according to stratum sizes and calculation of variance is more complicated (see, for example, Cochran (1977) for more details).

8.6.4 Multi-stage random sampling

In simple random sampling, all animals need to be first identified. In systematic sampling, they need to be lined up in some sort of sequence for sampling. When surveying very large populations (e.g. national-level surveys) both simple random and systematic sampling are impractical, if not impossible. For example, it is not feasible to create a list containing each of the tens of millions of chickens in a country to allow simple random sampling.

Multi-stage sampling addresses this problem by utilizing our knowledge about the structure of the population and the fact that animal populations are often clustered into groups, based on farms or herds. Multi-stage sampling involves sampling of animals in several stages – first at the farm level and then animals within farms (see Fig. 8.5). While a list of all chickens would be impossible to compile, a list of all chicken farms in the country may be easily obtained from registration or other records.

First, groups of animals are selected (chicken farms) and then individual animals are chosen from the selected farms. This example uses two-stage sampling, the farm and the individual animal. The first-stage units (farms) are called the primary sampling units. The last-stage units (animals) are called the listing units (in this example they are also secondary sampling units). More stages can be included if necessary: a four-stage sample might involve random selection of districts at the first stage, villages at the second, livestock owners at the third and individual animals at the fourth.

Stratification may also be used in conjunction with multi-stage, usually at the first stage, if desired. In most cases, sampling at each stage will be either simple random or stratified random. However, in some cases, probability proportional to size sampling may be used for the first stage of a multi-stage sampling process (see below).

8.6.5 Cluster sampling

Cluster sampling is a form of multi-stage sampling where all animals are examined in the final stage (see Fig. 8.6). The key difference between cluster and multi-stage sampling

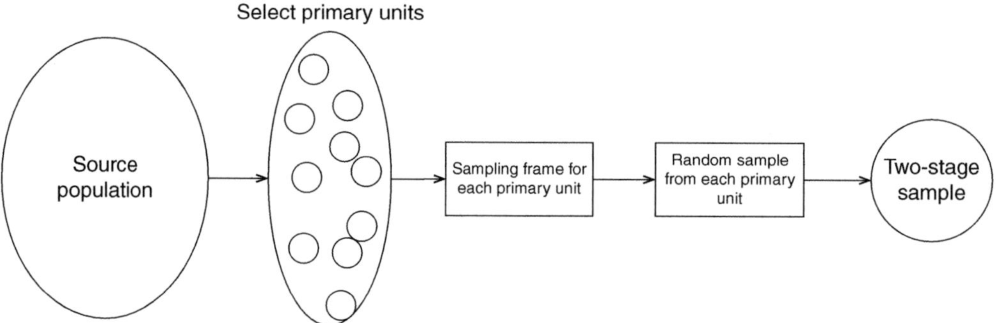

Fig. 8.5. Diagrammatic representation of multi-stage random sampling.

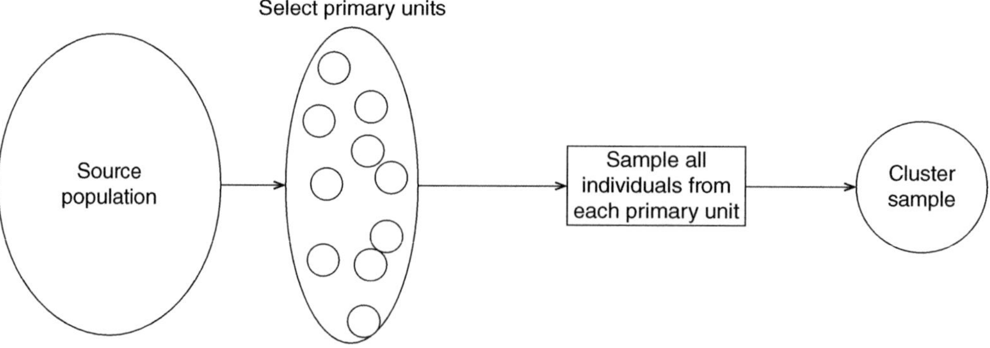

Fig. 8.6. Diagrammatic representation of cluster sampling.

is that for multi-stage sampling the sample is chosen by simple random sampling at all stages, whereas for cluster sampling a census is undertaken at the final stage. Stratification may also be used in conjunction with multi-stage or cluster sampling.

Multi-stage and cluster samples have two distinct advantages:

- They are easier to plan, as a complete list of all animals is not needed, only primary sampling units.
- They are more practical for the field-work team, as fewer sites need to be visited.

The disadvantages are that the results may not be as precise as with simple random sampling, and the formulae for analysis of the data are more complex.

8.6.6 Probability proportional to size sampling

So far we have considered variations on simple random sampling, where at each stage units have an equal probability of being selected. An alternative approach that can be used in some circumstances is probability proportional to size (PPS) sampling. PPS sampling is an alternative to simple random sampling that can be used at the first stage of a multi-stage sampling process.

PPS sampling is a multi-stage sampling method where the probability of selection for primary sampling units is proportional to their size. Sampling is weighted so that larger units (e.g. farms or villages) are more likely to be selected than smaller ones.

For example, consider the example of two-stage sampling to determine animal-level prevalence of disease. In this situation the first stage would be villages (or farms), while the second stage would be animals within villages/farms.

With simple random sampling, each village/farm would have an equal probability of being selected, whereas with PPS sampling, the probability of selection is proportional to the number of animals in each village/farm, so that villages with a higher livestock population have a higher probability of being selected than villages with fewer animals. This weighting towards larger villages takes account of the fact that more of the livestock population is located in the larger villages.

Therefore, PPS sampling requires the development of a sampling frame that includes livestock numbers for every village or farm in the area of interest. Conceptually, every animal in every village is numbered sequentially. The total number of animals in all villages is calculated, and a random number chosen, between one and this total. This number represents one animal in one village. The village in which that animal is located is thus also selected. This process continues until the required number of villages has been selected.

The main advantage of PPS sampling is that a fixed number of animals can then be selected within each village/farm and the resulting prevalence estimate is an unbiased estimate. Alternatively, if simple random sampling is used at the first stage, a fixed percentage of animals must be selected rather than a fixed number. PPS sampling also has the advantage that estimates are more precise for a given sample size (or sample sizes are smaller for a given precision of the estimate).

8.7 Sample Selection Techniques

In addition to selecting an appropriate random sampling method, there are some important practical sampling issues that must be considered when planning your sample collection.

8.7.1 Sampling frames

Simple random sampling requires a list of all members of the population, from which the sample is chosen. This list is known as the sampling frame. Similarly for multi-stage sampling, a sampling frame is required of the primary sampling units. Then for each primary sampling unit selected, a frame is required for the secondary sampling units contained in those primary units.

An ideal sampling frame for simple random sampling is a list that:

- includes every member of the population to be sampled (may be herds, villages or individual animals depending on level of sampling);
- does not include duplicates (every member listed only once);
- allows each member to be uniquely identified; and
- may contain additional information to be used for stratification or other sampling procedures (e.g. herd size, location, etc.).

For multi-stage sampling, the sampling frame at each stage must contain all the sampling units for that stage. At each stage, the sampling frame must be made up of units (herds, farms, villages) which uniquely contain every animal in the population (i.e. every animal appears in one of the units, and no animal appears in more than one).

In some circumstances, sampling frames may already exist. For instance, in the first stage of a two-stage national livestock survey, farms or villages may be used as the primary sampling unit. Government agencies will often hold comprehensive lists of farms or villages, which can be used as the primary sampling frame. These lists uniquely identify each farm by a registration number or village by name or number. Furthermore, they may hold valuable information for stratification, such as population size or location.

In many cases, however, no sampling frame is available, at least when planning the survey. In the second stage of our national survey, animals are the sampling unit. However, lists of all the animals in each farm or village in the country often do not exist (if they did we would not need to do two-stage sampling). The advantage of multi-stage sampling is that a sampling frame need only be created for those farms or villages selected, at the time that the samples are being collected, rather than every farm or village in the country. This can be done once you arrive at the farm or village to do the sampling or at the time of first making contact to arrange for sampling. At its simplest, a sampling frame of animals on a farm or village might be a sequential list of numbers starting at 1 and finishing at the number of animals present.

8.7.2 Sampling from a sampling frame

Once a sampling frame has been obtained or compiled, selection of units from it by simple random sampling is relatively straightforward. Consider a sampling frame of all villages in a country, listed one per line.

The first step is to number each line sequentially, from one to the total number of villages. Then random numbers are selected using a random number table or a computer, for example using EpiTools. Once the numbers are produced, each village on the list with the corresponding number is selected. Alternatively, EpiTools has a sampling program that uses sample size, sampling method and the sampling frame as inputs and generates a list of units to be sampled from the sampling frame, according to the user's specifications (http://epitools.ausvet.com.au/content.php?page=RandomSampling1).

8.7.3 Using random number tables

Although less commonly used now, random number tables provide a useful alternative to computer-generated random numbers, particularly in remote areas or other situations were computers may not be available. A random number table is simply a long list of randomly generated numbers, often listed in groups for ease of use. An abbreviated example of a random number table is shown below (Table 8.1), and a larger table of numbers is provided at the end of this chapter.

To use a random number table:

1. Choose a starting point for selecting your numbers. This can be anywhere in the table.
2. Choose a direction in which to progress through the table. This can be across by row, or down by column.
3. Calculate the range for your random numbers. What are the minimum and maximum allowable values?
4. Determine which digits to use from each group of numbers. This is determined by the size of the maximum number. For example if the sampling frame has elements numbered from 1 to 155, there are three digits in 155, so we need to use three digits from each group.
5. Decide on a strategy for using the numbers. For example, to improve efficiency we can use digits sequentially, regardless of groupings, or use two sets of numbers per group. Alternatively, for simplicity we might decide to only use one set of numbers per group (either first three or last three). Unused digits are ignored.
6. Proceed through the table according to selected direction, selecting numbers in the required range. Any number within your specified range is included, whereas any number outside the range is ignored. Continue searching until you have selected the required number.

For example, using the random numbers displayed in Table 8.1, we will select a sample of eight cattle from a population of 67 animals. We are assuming that you have constructed (or been provided) a sampling frame (list) of the 67 animals. For our sampling, we will start at the first column and third row (38481) and proceed across the rows. Because our sampling frame has only 67 animals in it, we only need to use two digits for each selection, and any numbers above 67 will be discarded. We also have decided that we will use the last two digits in each group. Following this approach, the first number (81) is greater than 67 and is discarded. The next three numbers (33, 43 and 42) are all

Table 8.1. Selection of numbers from a larger table of random numbers.

12856	93934	21797	56965	98947	45449	71469	90442	72779	86059
93916	47769	09132	72408	85773	88010	08745	35974	02562	48871
384~~**81**~~	419**33**	840**43**	515**42**	727~~**97**~~	341**45**	436**37**	239**31**	881**08**	541**20**
43770	59583	48269	09949	27091	72653	36310	64371	02933	32629
54282	98046	74715	37210	14501	80673	53026	80482	31827	95457
67146	90175	79848	05494	65282	39244	01903	60065	04783	79789

between 1 and 67 and are accepted. The next (97) is again discarded. The next five (45, 37, 31, 8 and 20) are all between 1 and 67 and are accepted, giving us our full sample size of eight. If more numbers were needed we would start again at the beginning of the next row.

8.7.4 Sampling animals without a sampling frame

In many cases a sampling frame is not readily available, particularly of animals at a village or farm level. Despite this, it is often possible to construct a sampling frame from available information. For example, a village may have multiple owners, each with a variable number of animals but for which there is no consolidated list. Similarly, a pig farmer may have many pens of pigs with a small number of pigs in each pen.

In such a situation, one way of constructing a sampling frame is simply to obtain or construct a list comprising each owner (or pen of pigs) with the corresponding number of animals for each. This may require some work and cooperation with the village head man and villagers, or the pig-farm owner. Once we have a list of owners (or pens) and numbers of animals we can generate a list of all animals in the population by adding a row to the list for each animal, identified by owner. EpiTools can generate this list for you from the list of owners and numbers of animals or it can be done in a spreadsheet or on paper. Consider an example where we might have 20 owners in a village and a total cattle population of 80 animals spread among those owners. Our sampling frame would end up as a list with 80 rows, so that if the first owner had five animals these would be in the first five rows, the next owner with nine animals would be rows 6 to 14, etc., a portion of which is shown below in Table 8.2.

We now have a sampling frame from which we can select our simple random sample. Once we have selected our sample, let us assume we select ten random numbers between 1 and 80, which come out as 17, 18, 22, 26, 36, 38, 63, 66, 71, 80. The first six of these are in the table above and represent animals 3 and 4 from owner 3, animals 4 and 8 from owner 4 and animals 6 and 8 from owner 6. We have now selected our random sample, at least on paper. The next step is to identify and select the animals identified in our sample.

This can also be a challenge, particularly if the individual animals are not easily identified individually. However, this challenge is usually not insurmountable and with a bit of care the random nature of the sample can be preserved. The key here is to ensure that you (as the person with the sample list) do not influence the process of identifying the animals. The simplest way of achieving this is to first identify the relevant owner from your list (or pen of pigs for the pig-farm example). You then get the farmer to point out each of his animals and count them out aloud. As each number on your sample list for that farmer is reached you identify that animal for sampling. Proceed in this manner until all selected animals for that farmer have been identified. To preserve randomness, it is important that during this process the person doing the counting does not know the numbers of the animals required.

8.7.5 Geographic sampling

In some situations random sampling is still possible, even when no sampling frame is available. Spatial sampling techniques (such as random geographic coordinate sampling)

Table 8.2. Example of a sampling frame.

ID	Owner	Animal
1	1	1
2	1	2
3	1	3
4	1	4
5	1	5
6	2	1
7	2	2
8	2	3
9	2	4
10	2	5
11	2	6
12	2	7
13	2	8
14	2	9
15	3	1
16	3	2
17	3	3
18	3	4
19	4	1
20	4	2
21	4	3
22	4	4
23	4	5
24	4	6
25	4	7
26	4	8
27	5	1
28	5	2
29	5	3
30	5	4
31	6	1
32	6	2
33	6	3
34	6	4
35	6	5
36	6	6
37	6	7
38	6	8
39	7	1
40	7	2

rely on the spatial distribution of the population to draw a random sample. Random geographic coordinate sampling is one approach that allows selection of a random sample of farms or villages in the absence of a sampling frame. Procedures for selecting and analysing random geographic samples can be quite complex and are described in detail elsewhere (Cameron, 1999).

8.7.6 Sampling with or without replacement

Probability sampling methods usually assume independence among sampling units and that the probability of a unit being sampled is constant, at least within strata. This implies sampling with replacement (i.e. sampled units are 'replaced' in the study population and can be sampled again). In practise, we rarely use true sampling with replacement and once a unit is selected it is not eligible to be sampled again. In most cases, particularly where population size is large relative to sample size, the impact of non-replacement is trivial. However, particularly in small populations or with large sample sizes the effect can be important. In such cases, it is important to either ensure that sampling with replacement is used, or that the methods used for sample size calculation take the non-replacement into account.

8.8 Sample Size Calculations

Before undertaking any sampling from a population for whatever purpose, it must be decided how many study units will be examined. This applies whether the study units are individual animals, farms, ponds, villages, etc. Also, the outcome to be measured must be known, as this will affect the method of estimation of the sample size.

Formulae exist for the calculation of sample size, and some computer programs implement these formulae to make the task easier. For example, sample size calculators for a range of circumstances are available at the EpiTools website (http://epitools.ausvet.com.au).

For any sample size calculation, some prior knowledge (or assumptions) is required. For example, when estimating a proportion (e.g. prevalence) using simple random sampling, the parameters needed to calculate the sample size are:

- the expected proportion (e.g. a prevalence of 70%);
- the level of confidence required (e.g. 95%);
- the precision (the allowable error in the estimate – equal to half the width of the desired confidence interval) required (e.g. ±5%); and
- the size of the population (e.g. 500 animals).

The first of these is likely to be the hardest to calculate, as this is what the investigation is designed to find out. Usually this has to be estimated from experience, or published figures from similar environments. If unsure, it is wise to err towards 50% (i.e. overestimate for low proportions, underestimate for high proportions) as this will produce a larger sample size, and better precision if your estimate is inaccurate.

Unfortunately, despite the most carefully worked sample size calculation, the actual sample size will often be as much determined by financial considerations as by science. If the budget is limited it may be more useful to decide what sample size is affordable, and then to determine if this sample size will produce information that is precise enough to answer the question properly. Common sample size calculations for epidemiological studies are discussed below.

8.8.1 Some terminology

Several new concepts and terms are introduced in this section. Readers are referred to Chapter 11, which provides a more detailed introduction to statistical principles and in particular to Section 11.10 on statistical error and statistical power.

A number of input parameters have to be defined for estimation of required sample size.

Statistical power is the probability of rejecting the null hypothesis when the null hypothesis is false. For sample size estimates a required power of 80% or 0.8 is commonly used, but alternative values may be chosen depending on the purpose of the study. Statistical power is equal to 1–beta, where beta is a measure of type II statistical error.

The confidence level is often required for sample size estimation and is generally defined as 1–alpha, where alpha is the statistical threshold of significance. Values of 90%, 95% or 99% are commonly used for the confidence level. The confidence level has the following interpretation. If a study aiming to estimate a proportion with 95% confidence were to be repeated an infinite number of times and a confidence interval was calculated for each sample, then 95% of those intervals would be expected to include the true population value.

When calculating sample size to estimate a population parameter, such as a population mean or proportion, one of the inputs required is the desired precision of the estimate, sometimes also called the acceptable error. This is usually presented as half the desired width of the confidence interval about the estimate.

8.8.2 Sample size for estimating a proportion

To estimate the proportion of individuals in a large population that have a characteristic of interest, the required sample size depends on the expected proportion, the precision (or allowable error) of the estimate (+/– %) and the level of confidence required in the estimate (commonly 95%). The required sample size can be calculated from the formula:

$$n = \mathrm{P} \times (1 - \mathrm{P}) \times (\mathrm{z} / \mathrm{e})^2$$

where P = expected proportion affected, e = allowable error (precision) of the estimate and z = the value from a standard normal distribution corresponding to the desired level of confidence (z = 1.96 for 95% confidence, 1.64 for 90% and 2.58 for 99%).

For example, assume that we want to know the proportion of sheep in a flock that are affected with footrot. Further, we want to estimate the true prevalence within +/– 5%, with 95% confidence and we assume that the proportion is likely to be about 20%. What is the sample size required?

From the formula, $n = 0.2 * (1 - 0.2) * (1.96 / 0.05)^2 = 0.2 * 0.8 * 39.2^2 = 246$

If we assume that the likely proportion is 50%, instead of 20%, the required sample size is 385.

The required sample size increases as the expected prevalence approaches 50%, as the desired level of confidence increases and as the allowable error decreases (estimate becomes more precise).

The above method assumes sampling with replacement or that the population is very large. For finite populations (or at least for relatively small populations – for example, if n is more than 5% of the population size), the sample size should be adjusted for the population size, as follows:

$$n_{\text{finite}} = (n \times N)/(n + N)$$

where n is the sample size for an infinite population and N is the population size.

In the above example, if we assume that there are only 1000 sheep in the flock, the required sample size drops to 198 for a prevalence of 20% and 278 for a prevalence of 50%.

8.8.3 Sample size for estimating a mean

To estimate the mean of a continuous variable (such as body weight), the required sample size depends on the assumed standard deviation for the variable, the allowable error of the estimate (+/– %) and the level of confidence required in the estimate (commonly 95%). The required sample size can be calculated from the formula:

$$n = z^2 \times s^2/e^2$$

where s = estimated standard deviation, e = allowable error precision of the estimate (measured in the same units as s) and z = the value from a standard normal distribution corresponding to the desired level of confidence (z = 1.96 for 95% confidence, 1.64 for 90% and 2.58 for 99%).

For example, assume that we want to know the average birth weight of calves. Further we want to estimate the true average within +/– 2 kg, with 95% confidence and the standard deviation of body weight is 5 kg. What is the sample size required?

From the formula, $n = 1.96^2 \times 5^2/2^2 = 3.84 * 25/4 = 24$

The required sample size increases as the expected standard deviation increases, as the desired level of confidence increases and as the allowable error decreases (estimate becomes more precise).

8.8.4 Sample size for comparison of two proportions or two means

Formulae are available for calculation of the sample sizes required for detection of significant differences between two population means or two population proportions.

A variety of methods for means or proportions, and which allow for differences in group size, are available in epidemiological calculators such as EpiTools (http://epitools.ausvet.com.au/content.php?page=SampleSize).

For comparing two proportions, sample size depends on the assumed values for the two proportions, the desired level of confidence, the power of the study and the desired ratio of the two sample sizes.

For example, suppose we want to carry out a survey of villages to compare the proportions of villages that experienced foot-and-mouth disease outbreaks during a 12-month period for two different provinces in a country. We think that one region had a higher prevalence (30% of villages), while the other had a lower prevalence (10%).

How many villages in each province do we need to visit, to have 95% confidence of detecting a significant difference with a power (1 – type II error) of 80%?

Using EpiTools, and assuming the same sample size for both regions, the required sample size is 72 villages for each province (144 in total) that would need to be sampled.

For comparing two means, sample size depends on the assumed difference between the means (or the assumed mean values), the estimated variance or standard deviations of the means, the desired level of confidence, the power of the study and the desired ratio of the two sample sizes.

For example, to compare the body weights of two groups of sheep where we would like to detect a difference of 2 kg with 95% confidence and 80% power, and assuming the body weights for the two groups are 48 and 50 kg, and the variance of the body weights is 5 kg, the required sample size is 20 per group (from EpiTools, and assuming equal group sizes and a two-tailed test).

8.8.5 Sample size for other purposes

Formulae, web-based tools and in some cases custom software are available for estimation of power and sample size requirements for a wide variety of study types and particular applications. Readers are encouraged to seek statistical advice for more detailed sample size estimates.

8.9 Random Number Table

12856	93934	21797	56965	98947	45449	71469	90442	72779	86059
93916	47769	09132	72408	85773	88010	08745	35974	02562	48871
38481	41933	84043	51542	72797	34145	43637	23931	88108	54120
43770	59583	48269	09949	27091	72653	36310	64371	02933	32629
54282	98046	74715	37210	14501	80673	53026	80482	31827	95457
67146	90175	79848	05494	65282	39244	01903	60065	04783	79789
10453	51747	13443	75009	26310	88892	59353	87097	60682	26322
67014	26549	80061	17302	93546	13876	39903	11597	35489	60192
18612	74655	14566	40014	35366	54253	41311	47110	51385	69066
29462	95644	41065	29669	61120	50223	37526	95068	91210	78897
71244	74020	81410	86862	52579	90019	33021	15029	09167	80397
54097	39541	53924	83483	36982	28966	65047	64275	91772	74937
81530	12331	99284	78071	17165	61383	60944	13618	44343	57035
58925	95623	88935	40573	26451	95147	96392	42901	51934	71081
39539	93819	24821	75184	92778	92986	86673	76737	22732	10490
98666	53413	28624	35818	30444	24610	07867	81424	92459	88301
90798	59552	19454	37808	29269	27567	25523	20221	20638	76094
64423	14601	64478	47615	30972	05802	51325	60907	28818	09316
23575	17006	62748	51490	15242	03282	51515	15322	50180	62030
53338	17493	84554	56128	17943	53272	08192	12864	47196	22014
74288	81287	88128	95338	88823	19352	49077	55923	80950	17870
27945	63600	29187	09838	54163	15946	52078	74939	41577	61534
54895	86295	49190	91844	83625	83873	76637	54611	01594	28812

Continued

Continued.

47679	55881	62618	43377	87739	15606	29020	42466	91614	32836
54013	62736	31765	71774	84032	03486	34924	50097	22891	31077
20784	65321	44037	52454	10231	74244	58917	22355	91850	22773
74627	98749	60999	30699	14915	84038	26241	03819	93615	23445
07036	11603	36911	56087	64838	50406	23308	49474	73281	85071
33583	11334	19388	43766	02486	70867	64228	42524	77679	94992
02176	94443	42411	08770	72092	22173	85381	44691	24223	76833
51498	37518	49619	73145	13958	09633	87586	35442	64323	38139
90379	91670	78226	54894	82413	40712	28655	49457	88703	03013
65127	34979	33702	68254	22477	43788	17307	51226	01760	81215
57020	55119	66573	77838	54208	53117	68243	21087	67509	70762
64926	27827	01319	41910	31815	82384	74502	74800	50157	40515
31764	47091	54805	05197	17745	16857	25268	10735	51825	50171
61257	31439	24684	95107	82964	66801	75563	68351	05528	70069
77325	41144	47995	12223	42843	08701	45184	65516	42226	74461
22726	60765	05154	78207	37205	68749	35848	03141	61870	16670
71988	17142	14850	35101	73250	31187	46146	16584	12096	28600
43012	74892	92762	87409	40137	97411	08959	13812	71240	04567
03144	81429	11198	83170	20674	67225	31782	36855	11230	69035
88380	99700	26451	59078	28358	30682	10149	48178	30055	30357
93093	44387	17938	76131	54733	32299	84888	24414	07673	33633
87935	95777	27955	48647	87835	30072	40736	86448	14056	14433
32230	02638	56942	87676	52855	80274	52455	06655	92140	15854
99062	39034	16860	95752	99695	72514	28914	03735	17234	90828
72009	89506	50885	29799	05551	09463	49269	95343	67718	47240
58977	40380	92496	61212	95904	58614	92000	21037	20037	61411
51860	54324	39827	57927	62456	38087	60725	86147	15772	86487
16877	82410	03204	95640	35431	82214	54859	05688	66478	67993
97407	00463	05384	66215	42976	72945	64542	95825	73600	98415
99120	15518	95584	31937	02373	63593	09363	80096	51874	47601
97402	53366	18418	02251	40511	19503	85178	69227	90000	10968
68691	14251	58122	14270	30444	86884	11028	82838	88738	74433
35241	44878	09850	27162	23295	76605	20171	39416	14368	30440
87199	93932	53610	59297	22178	64740	30449	76918	31183	16635
16443	19785	21061	96429	00591	16599	89155	51183	11601	03605
78721	56124	98055	39707	21010	27763	28910	17445	25738	70660
84584	17446	43401	74070	43955	84411	70816	44987	38902	29854
67666	80918	79380	29250	40298	84355	19160	38463	20005	56237
25788	29254	61624	76501	98753	39349	81548	24796	77671	29763
39673	91604	21904	77807	57838	95197	38223	66435	35654	03825
07633	31731	45261	86284	18631	09341	57058	05697	36222	93651
42923	25270	58238	44225	82520	06365	27620	54490	03004	62437
64597	46722	79943	33413	47003	13913	80781	25398	25282	39154
55013	05546	60813	16503	55638	76994	37800	37362	92625	30375
09966	53823	61848	16347	75326	42974	05395	92037	50957	60293
54853	93377	61009	85132	18959	70045	93599	22794	73699	95698
04450	94477	12167	67183	29492	02220	52641	68963	36848	51725
04937	13758	25043	71448	61006	76095	80217	34429	52739	75060
05859	85246	03695	25380	48757	28925	35843	73024	39864	94625

Continued

Continued.

38744	21252	64696	66715	25432	48137	34497	05880	43774	98023
21330	73927	06789	23732	60024	09203	71581	44115	65172	29160
94549	87410	95138	34373	36036	80860	89226	89768	10840	10499
36920	28279	16969	14671	12719	31915	82185	41680	91515	63166
82746	00686	72745	39783	02848	54543	00121	14690	49048	77040
35854	46187	66282	81947	41175	53647	39090	77867	07442	98757
45194	43620	78781	55616	63951	52926	85857	70911	07934	47310
19380	13632	42907	85457	75772	85479	09668	17185	72793	53133

References

Cameron, A.R. (1999) *Survey Toolbox – A Practical Manual and Software Package for Active Surveillance of Livestock Diseases in Developing Countries*. Australian Centre for International Agricultural Research, Canberra, Australia.

Cochran, W.G. (1977) *Sampling Techniques*. John Wiley & Sons, New York.

Thrushfield, M. (2005) *Veterinary Epidemiology*, 3rd edn, Blackwell Science, Oxford.

9 Data Collection and Management

9.1 Introduction

Epidemiological data are collected for many and varied reasons. However, the most important reason, one that should be common to all data collection, is that the data are needed to generate information for a specific purpose. In fact, the ultimate purpose is often to help make better decisions about disease control or prevention.

Data should only be collected if they are needed to answer a specific question or to assist in solving a particular problem. Collection of data for the sake of it, or in case they will be useful, is expensive and usually a waste of time and effort. Collection of data without a specific purpose can also be counter-productive, because people are likely to be less cooperative the next time you seek their assistance if the data collected previously have not been used productively.

9.1.1 Reasons for collecting epidemiological data

Some of the common reasons for collecting epidemiological data (adapted from Cameron, 1999) include to:

- identify if a disease is present in a country or region;
- determine the prevalence and distribution of a disease;
- determine the importance and impact of diseases;
- identify risk factors for a disease;
- identify and evaluate treatment or control options for a disease;
- set priorities for the use of resources for disease control programmes;
- assist in planning, implementing and monitoring disease control or eradication programmes;
- respond to disease outbreaks;
- meet international reporting responsibilities;
- demonstrate disease status to trading partners;
- monitor productivity and performance of livestock or aquatic animals;
- evaluate diagnostic tests and screening procedures for disease; and
- many others.

There are many types of variables which potentially can be used to record information. In this chapter, we explore the various types of data, sources of data, the methods used for collecting it and the best way to record it.

9.2 Variables, Data and Information

9.2.1 What is a variable?

A variable is a property or characteristic that can vary, either between animals, between groups or over time. In an epidemiological study, variables are the things that we measure or record about animals, groups and their environment. Examples of variables include:

- animal characteristics, such as disease state, breed, species, sex;
- things we can measure, such as weight, antibody titre, length, height;
- group characteristics, such as group size, location, group treatment; and
- environmental characteristics, such as soil type, water pH, rainfall.

9.2.2 What is data?

Data is a collection of facts about the animal or animals being studied. Where variables are the characteristics being measured or recorded, data are the actual values that are recorded – the values that variables take when measured in individuals or groups. For example, if a variable called disease is measured in a group of five cows the resulting data will be a series of five values, one for each cow, with each value being either diseased or not diseased.

9.2.3 What is information?

Data can be processed and analysed to generate information. Information is therefore not just the sum of the data available. Information can only be extracted from data if it is organized and analysed to provide meaning and allow interpretation.

For example, a database containing the results of a survey of villages for foot-and-mouth disease is just a collection of data. The information generated from these data might be that 20% of farms have had an outbreak in the last 12 months, but that farms in Region A are at three times the risk of an outbreak as farms in Region B.

9.3 Variable Types

There are two main types of variables, categorical variables and numerical variables, and several sub-types as shown in Fig. 9.1.

9.3.1 Categorical variables

A categorical variable is a qualitative property or characteristic of an individual or group. This type of variable is also known as a frequency variable. Categorical data can be cross-classified to create contingency tables for analysis and estimation of measures of association and the strength of association. The simplest form of contingency table is the 2×2 table, as shown in Table 9.1.

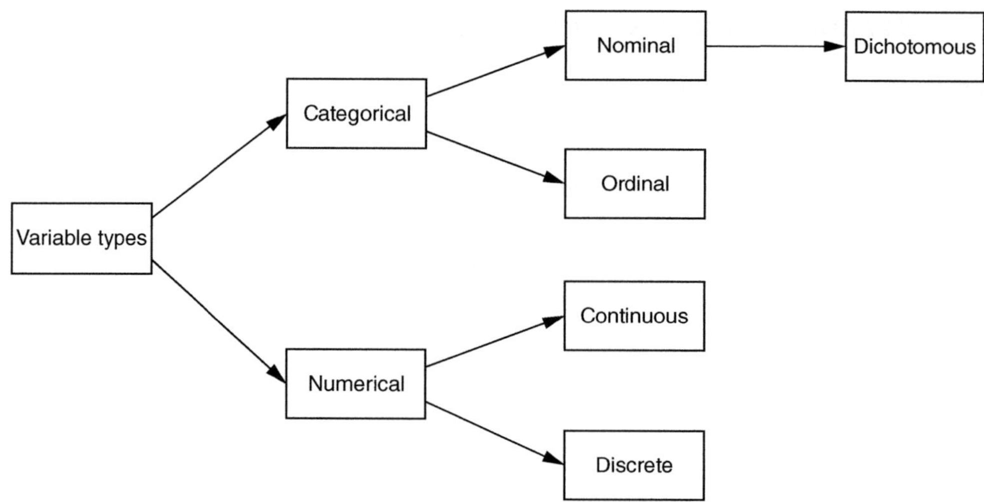

Fig. 9.1. Epidemiological variable types (adapted from Thrushfield, 2005).

Table 9.1. A 2×2 table of disease status against sex.

	Disease status		
Sex	Diseased	Not diseased	Total
Male	a	b	a+b
Female	c	d	c+d
Total	a+c	b+b	n=a+b+c+d

There are two main types of categorical variables, nominal and ordinal.

Nominal variables

Nominal variable categories are subjective, with no inherent order or ranking. Even though categories may have a number assigned to them to allow for ease of coding there is no relationship between the categories. Examples of nominal variables include animal characteristics, such as breed, sex and species.

Dichotomous variables are a specific type of nominal variable that can take only two values, often yes or no. Examples of dichotomous variables include disease states (diseased or not diseased) and exposure states (exposed or not exposed).

Ordinal variables

Ordinal variables are those that have categories represented by numerical values, and an inherent order. Examples of ordinal variables include age and score (such as lesion severity). Because ordinal data have an inherent order, an age = 3 cannot come before age = 1. Age can also be treated as a continuous variable (see below).

9.3.2 Numerical variables

Numerical variables are those that have values that are numbers, usually representing quantities. Values of numeric variables may be either continuous (measurements) or discrete (e.g. counts).

Continuous variables

Continuous variables are often measured with an instrument or assay, providing a measure that may take any value within the valid range. The precision of the measured value is only limited by the technology employed. Examples of continuous variables include age, weight, length and antibody concentration.

Epidemiologists sometimes convert continuous data to categorical data for analysis. This is done by converting to an ordinal variable based on classes or ordered groupings. For example, age of cattle could be grouped as ~<1 year, 1–5 years, 6–10 years and ~>10 years.

Discrete variables

Discrete variables are those that can have only values from a specified set of values. The possible values for discrete variables are often integer numbers (such as 1, 2, 5, 10, etc.) and represent counts. Examples of discrete variables include the number of animals on a farm, the number of quarters with mastitis, the number of cows that are lame. Age can also be treated as a discrete variable when measured in years (or months).

9.3.3 Variable states

Variables can exists in two states. These states are static and dynamic. A static state is a fixed characteristic that cannot change with time. A dynamic state is dependent on other factors. Examples of variable states are shown in Table 9.2.

9.3.4 Paired or unpaired data?

Data may be paired or unpaired (independent). Datasets are independent when the values in one set are not influenced by the values in the other set. Conversely, datasets are paired when values in one set are related to values in the other in some way. The most closely paired data are repeat measurements from the same individuals. However, data can also

Table 9.2. Examples of static and dynamic variables.

	Static (fixed)	Dynamic
Categorical variable	Breed	Disease status
Continuous variable	Adult height	Weight

be paired, for example, where animals are matched on age or production status, or where farms are matched on characteristics such as location and size. Data values for paired individuals are more likely to be similar than values for unpaired individuals, and therefore different analytical methods are used for paired data.

For example, if two randomly selected groups of animals are selected separately from a population and weighed, the weights for the two groups are independent. On the other hand, if one group is selected at random and individuals are identified and weighed on one occasion, and then the same individuals are selected and weighed again on a second occasion the two sets of weights are paired.

9.3.5 Dependent and independent variables

Variables can also be classified according to whether they are *dependent* or *independent variables* in an analysis. A dependent (*response*) variable is one that represents the outcome of interest in an epidemiological study, while an independent (*explanatory*) variable is one that represents any factor that is hypothesized as being associated with the dependent variable. For any particular study there are usually only a small number of dependent variables (often only one), but there may be many independent variables. For any individual analysis within a study there is usually only one dependent variable (often disease status) and one or more independent variables, depending on the type of analysis.

For example, disease state would be the outcome variable and age, breed, sex and a range of risk factors could all be independent variables in a study investigating possible risk factors for a particular disease.

9.4 Where Do Data Come From?

Data can be obtained from many different sources, depending on the type of data you require. Most of your categorical data will come from the field, for example, sex, species, age, class, disease status, etc. Often you will collect the data or they will have been collected by someone who is helping you. Continuous data, as well as coming from the field, can potentially come from other sources as well. Things such as antibody titre, hormone concentrations or parasite burdens could come from a lab, while data such as weight, growth and age will be obtained from the field.

9.4.1 Sources of data

There are many possible sources of epidemiological data. These sources vary greatly in the quality, accessibility, validity and usefulness of the data they can provide. This variability between data sources determines the value and potential uses for data from any particular source.

Common potential sources of epidemiological data include:

- epidemiological studies;
- government organizations (animal health, fisheries, statistics, local government);
- veterinary laboratories (government and private);

- veterinary practices;
- abattoirs, processing plants, etc.;
- serum banks;
- certification or assurance programmes;
- industry and service organizations;
- farmers; and
- others.

9.4.2 Validity of data

A critical issue for any epidemiological data is their validity. Validity of data is the degree to which the data accurately reflects the true situation in the population of interest. The validity of data can be affected by a range of important biases, particularly selection bias, misclassification bias and confounding. This is particularly the case when utilizing data that have been collected for some other purpose, such as many of the data sources listed above.

Therefore, before using such data, it is essential to consider the types and magnitudes of potential biases that may be present. Where possible, the impact of any biases should be controlled during analysis, and if this is not possible the likely magnitude and direction of the potential bias must be documented and considered in any decision making. If the potential biases are severe or unpredictable, it may be appropriate to discount the data and place little reliance on the resulting analysis when making decisions.

For example, an animal health authority is reviewing official policy on footrot in sheep, and is using a database of owner-notifications of disease on which to base its decisions. Because of owner resistance to notification, the notifications database could seriously underestimate the true prevalence of the disease, resulting in an inappropriate policy. In this situation it would be more appropriate to survey producers or to use some other method (such as sales of footrot-specific treatments) to determine the significance of the disease, instead of using the notifications database.

9.4.3 Strengths and weaknesses of data sources

Some of the main strengths and weaknesses of data sources are listed in Table 9.3.

9.4.4 Information from laboratory data

Laboratory information systems are often used as a source of epidemiological data for a variety of purposes, including:

- detection of new or emerging diseases;
- demonstration of freedom from some diseases;
- temporal or geographic trends in disease diagnosis; and
- identification of endemic disease cases for follow-up action.

However, laboratory data must also be used and interpreted with care due to the many inherent biases present in the data, including:

Table 9.3. Strengths and weaknesses of various data sources.

Source	Strengths	Weaknesses
Epidemiological studies	Usually good quality data Results may be applicable to the population of interest	Cost to run the study Delay in getting results Often only suitable for specific purpose Not always applicable to the population of interest
Government organizations	Readily available (usually) Cheap to obtain (being collected for other reasons)	May need to be extracted from paper files Not representative of population Usually limited in scope – often only diseases that are regulated May be confidentiality issues
Veterinary laboratories	Readily available (usually) Cheap to obtain (being collected for other reasons) Often computerized	May be severely biased – not representative of the population Limited to conditions requiring laboratory testing May be confidentiality issues
Veterinary practices	Useful for small animals or clinical conditions	Difficult to access Variable quality between practices Limited in scope
Abattoirs	Large throughput of animals Covers broad cross-section of farms	Limited to conditions with obvious gross pathology or requires additional testing Biased sample – healthy animals, mainly young or older animals Industrial and workplace health and safety issues with putting staff in abattoir Trace-back to farm of origin may be difficult unless effective animal identification and tracing systems are in place

- submissions are not representative of the population at risk;
- some species not represented or under-represented;
- affected by interests of laboratory staff and submitters;
- affected by changes and variations in technology used;
- reliable denominator information often not available;
- limited to diseases or conditions requiring a laboratory diagnosis;
- may be avoidance of testing for regulated diseases;
- only sick animals tested; and
- only healthy animals tested, for example for export testing.

9.5 Data Management and Information Systems

9.5.1 Managing data

Data can occur in many forms. The most common forms are:

- paper reports and files, such as in government agencies and laboratories;
- questionnaires or data-collection sheets;

- electronic format generated by automatic data-collection devices such as ELISA plate-readers, electronic scales, etc.; and
- electronic format in spreadsheets or databases.

Before data can be analysed and interpreted, they need to be organized into a format that can be easily analysed. For data that are on paper this means extracting the relevant data from the paper forms or files and entering them into a database or spreadsheet. For data that are already in electronic format, they must be organized and linked together ready for analysis. Even if data are not being analysed electronically, it is essential to organize the data so that all the data for each individual are collected together for the analysis.

Where data are being used from a number of different sources, it may be necessary to collate the data (either manually or electronically) to link related data elements together. For example, in Fig. 9.2, a single proposed analysis may include data from diverse sources such as:

- field data collection (questionnaire or data-collection form);
- automated data-collection equipment (electronic scales, GPS);
- laboratory testing records; and
- existing records from previous investigations.

These diverse data sources must be linked together either physically (by combining in a single data table, spreadsheet or database) or logically by including data in each separate data source that allows the data to be linked together for analysis (e.g. in a relational database).

In electronic (or paper) formats, data are usually arranged in a tabular format to facilitate analysis. In this format, each row in the table represents a record for an individual about which data have been collected and each column represents a field, which holds data for a specific variable about which data have been collected, for each record. Figure 9.3 is a typical table of data, showing four records each with five fields. Each row in the table contains data about one unit of interest (in this case the unit of interest is a farm, identified by FarmID), and each column (field) corresponds to one variable about which data has been collected for each individual. Field names correspond to the variables for which data were collected. Ideally, each record should have data in every field, but in many cases this does not happen, resulting in missing values.

A variety of software packages can be used to store and manage data, as discussed in more detail in the next section. For simple data, requiring only a single data table,

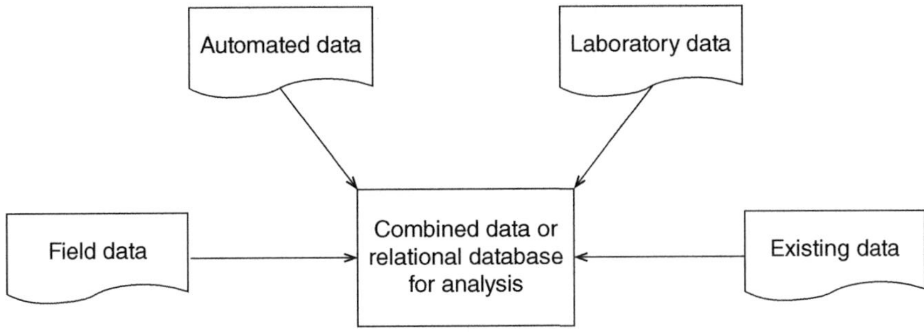

Fig. 9.2. Multiple data sources need to be combined or linked to enable analysis.

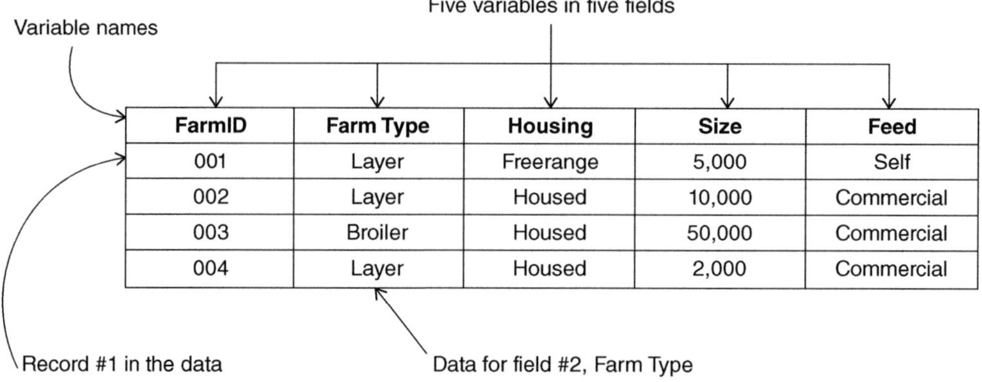

FarmID	Farm Type	Housing	Size	Feed
001	Layer	Freerange	5,000	Self
002	Layer	Housed	10,000	Commercial
003	Broiler	Housed	50,000	Commercial
004	Layer	Housed	2,000	Commercial

Fig. 9.3. Tabular organization of data into records and fields.

a spreadsheet or simple database is often sufficient. For more complex data, particularly where there are multiple related data sources and multiple records per unit of interest, a more complex relational database may be required.

9.5.2 Field types

We have already discussed the importance of different variable or data types. Once data are organized into records and fields in a spreadsheet or database, it is important to understand that there is also a range of field types that are used to record and format the data. The main field types are:

- Text – representing words or phrases. In some cases text fields might be limited to a specified length and only specified letters, words or phrases might be permitted. Text fields are useful for recording data for nominal variables, such as sex or breed, or for general comments.
- Integer numbers – whole numbers such as counts or ordinal variables where each category is recorded as a whole number.
- Real numbers – decimal numbers used for recording measurements such as age, weight or length.
- Date and time – special fields used for recording date and time data.
- Logical – special fields used to record dichotomous yes/no or true/false type data.

Use of these field types can help to reduce mistakes in data entry, and ensure that data are consistent and easily analysed. For example, coding a field for sex to only accept the values M and F ensures that other possible entries, such as male or female are prevented, simplifying analysis. On the other hand, it is also important that any field is able to accept any valid value that could occur in the data, so that in the sex example it would be important to include codes for desexed animals, if this is appropriate.

9.5.3 Computerized data management

Computers, hand-held tablets and smartphones are now ubiquitous and provide a variety of options for capturing and managing data. However, the data still need to be stored somewhere electronically, in a form that is amenable to analysis and interpretation. To do this requires some form of electronic data management system. Options to achieve this are discussed in this section.

The most important decision to make when establishing a data management system is probably not what type of computer to use, but the type of software to use. There is a vast array of software available for all imaginable purposes. As the purpose of computers is to manage data, all software may be thought of as data management software. However, some types of software are specialized for different types of data management functions.

The broad categories of software of primary interest for epidemiological studies are:

- word processors;
- statistical analysis tools;
- spreadsheets; and
- databases.

In order to highlight the different strength and weaknesses of the different software available, consider the data shown in Fig. 9.3. The data are arranged as a table, made up of rows and columns. These data can be represented in any of the four different types of programs.

Word processors are specialized for dealing with free-text data and their layout on the printed page. While they may serve important roles in a study, they are not suited to serious data management tasks. Despite this, some people insist on using word processors as the prime data storage software for study data. This may be in the form of free-text lists or tables.

Statistical programs sometimes have built-in database systems, but often rely on external data management software to prepare the data, and concentrate on their primary function of analysing data.

Spreadsheets and databases are both designed specifically to store data in an organized manner, suitable for manipulation and analysis. These should be the first choice for any significant data management task, and it is important to understand which of the two should be used in any given situation. Superficially, they often look similar, with data presented in a grid with columns and rows. However, their capabilities are very different. Spreadsheets and databases are discussed in more detail in the following sections.

Spreadsheets

The key characteristic of spreadsheets is that they are non-prescriptive arrays. This means that the grid of cells is simply a grid of cells, and any data type (number, text, date, logical, etc.) can be entered in any cell, at the whim of the user. The second most important characteristic is the ability to enter formulae in cells, referencing any other cell.

This lack of enforced structure results in a number of important advantages:

- Spreadsheets are very quick to set up for data entry. Simply type a heading in one cell, and you are ready to start entering data. If you are really impatient, you do not even need to type a heading.

- Data can be mixed in any way. If you want to have different datasets on the same page, there is nothing to stop you. If you want to divide the data into groups with headings, you can enter text cells in the middle of a group of numeric cells. Subtotals can be sprinkled where you will, at the bottom of columns or the end of rows.
- The ability to reference any cell or block of cells within a formula allows very flexible calculations. For instance, in ordered data, one record may have a relation to the previous record. Consider the example of data from a sentinel herd bled at regular intervals to check for the presence of seroconversion to a pathogen. If one is interested in calculating the time between bleeds, it requires a calculation involving values in the current row (date of current bleed) and the preceding row (date of previous bleed). Spreadsheets make this type of calculation very easy, by simply referencing the row above.

Other advantages of spreadsheets include very powerful in-built statistical functions (although these are often weighted towards financial applications), excellent graphics, and good import and export capabilities. Data entry is rapid, but there are limited or no data-checking capabilities. Spreadsheets are also extremely good at summarizing data in tabular form using the pivot table (or equivalent) function. This function can summarize counts, mean values and other summary values across many rows of data into a simple contingency table format, cross-classified by one or more variables of interest.

The flexibility, non-prescriptive layout and speed of set-up make them ideal for quick tasks involving relatively small amounts of data, or involving many complex calculations.

Examples of the type of tasks for which spreadsheets are ideal include:

- calculating budgets;
- creating epidemiological models (especially when combined with stochastic modelling plug-ins);
- summarizing data; and
- producing good-looking graphs from summary data.

The disadvantages of spreadsheets also stem from their flexibility and lack of prescriptive structure. The fact that an individual cell can contain any type of data means that it is possible to accidentally type a text value in the middle of a column of numbers. This can be easily missed, and may not show up obviously in the analysis. It is possible with modern spreadsheets to set up data-type controls for particular cells to partially overcome this limitation. More fundamental problems with the use of spreadsheets for large or complex datasets is their lack of relational ability (it is not possible to easily and reliably relate one set of data to another) and the limit on the number of rows that can be stored (particularly in older versions of some software). This is not a problem for many studies, but means that very large datasets cannot be managed with a spreadsheet. Note that some spreadsheets do not warn you when importing large datasets, and simply truncate the data.

Databases

Internally, spreadsheets store data as an array (actually a pointer-linked sparse array, which means that empty cells are not stored). This is a relatively complex data structure and provides spreadsheets with their power and flexibility. In contrast, data in a database are stored in a very simple column and row structure. The first record consists of the first field, followed by the second and so on, until the last field is followed by the first of the second record. Each data item in each field is stored as a specific data type (numeric data as binary numbers, dates as a date/time code, etc.). Where a cell has no data, the database still stores that cell, marked as empty.

The result of this internal data storage system is that databases are not nearly as flexible as spreadsheets. When a database is created, it is necessary to define the data type for each column or field. Once defined, no other data types can be stored there. So if a field is specified as an integer, for storing the number of dogs in a household, then it will not be possible to store a real number (with decimal places), text, a date, or a logical value in that field. Only integers are possible. The result is that during analysis, you can be guaranteed that all the data in that column will be valid. Unlike a spreadsheet, there is no risk of having a stray text value in the middle of a column of numbers, because it is simply not possible to store text in that column. This does not guarantee that the integer value entered is the correct value from the original data source, but it does guard against many possible errors.

This strict control of data types makes databases ideal for large datasets intended for statistical analysis. It makes it much easier to ensure the quality of the data. Because of this, modern databases also have a range of other features to improve data quality, including range checking and the ability to select categorical values from a defined list.

However, the greatest strength of databases (or at least relational databases) is that they can be designed to capture the complex data structures that occur in the real world. Consider the example of a study to determine risk factors for a disease of farmed poultry. One type of information that is required relates to the birds themselves and whether they have the disease or not. Others may relate to the shed or poultry house, the farm (e.g. management factors) and the region (e.g. factors common to many farms, such as weather). Further complexities may arise when changes over time are considered. For instance, one group of birds may be in one cage initially, where they are subject to a number of risk factors. Later, that group may be split and mixed with other groups.

One of the other significant advantages of databases is that they may contain very large amounts of data. Modern databases are generally only limited by the size of the storage available, with existing databases capable of easily managing tables with over 5,000,000,000 rows or up to multiple gigabytes in size.

Databases are very often the best way to manage data from studies, but they do have a number of drawbacks compared to spreadsheets. The most significant of these is the time and effort required to set up a database. In addition to defining the characteristics of each field in each table, there may be other set-up tasks, such as developing a data-entry interface and creating data-entry rules to maintain data quality. Database software also often has fewer built-in analytical functions than a spreadsheet, although neither type of software is capable of sophisticated statistical analysis without extensive programming. In most cases, when statistical analysis is required, dedicated statistical packages should be used, and most of these are able to import data from databases more easily than from spreadsheets.

Finally, modern database systems now run over the Internet, allowing for multi-user capability and remote access for data entry and reporting. Strict security

Table 9.4. Functionality of various computerized data management options.

Function	Word processor	Statistical analysis software	Spreadsheet	Database
Primary purpose	Text manipulation	Statistical data analysis (quantitative or categorical data)	Data storage and analysis (free-form)	Data storage and analysis (structured)
Secondary purpose		May have integrated database capability	Graphics capability	
Data entry	Yes	Maybe	Yes	Yes
Restrict input	No	Maybe	No (optional)	Yes
Linking	No	Maybe	Limited	Yes
Analysis	No	Yes	Yes	Limited
Access	Local	Local, may be able to access centralized database	Local	Remote

controls allow management of access to ensure only registered users can access the system (and only for specific actions for which they are approved). For example, a user approved for data entry may not be able to access reporting features, or users from different regions may be able to see detailed data for their region but only summarized data for other regions.

With the increasing availability of smartphones and tablets, users can enter data on their phone or other device and upload them automatically to the central database as soon as an Internet connection is available. Similarly, new approaches such as use of coded text messages (SMS) can be used to allow prompt and simple reporting to a central location.

As an example, national animal health information systems are now functional in many countries, with field staff at remote locations entering the data (reducing transcription errors associated with paper recording and use of data-entry clerks). District and regional staff can access reasonably low-level data to help manage diseases in their areas, while provincial and national staff can access summarized data to support national policy development and meet international reporting requirements.

Having a centralized database with remote access means that there is always only one version of the data, that it is updated automatically whenever a user submits data and it can be easily and securely backed up to ensure data security.

Summary

The functionality of the different computerized data management options are summarized and compared in Table 9.4.

9.6 Data Entry

Data entry refers to the process of transferring data from the form in which it was collected into an electronic form suitable for analysis. Data entry may be avoided when:

- a computer interface is used to collect the data (e.g. web-based survey forms);
- the data are generated and captured in an electronic form (electronic scales, data loggers);
- existing data are available in electronic format; or
- the data set is small enough or the analysis simple enough not to warrant computerized analysis.

In other situations, data-entry systems will need to be designed, balancing the objectives of speed, cost and accuracy. This discussion assumes that data are being entered into a database. Many of the same principles apply and the same tools are available when using spreadsheets for data entry and analysis.

9.6.1 Speed and simplicity

The process of data entry can be made faster and simpler by using a number of simple strategies.

On-screen layout

The order of questions and the layout of the form on the screen should match, as closely as possible, the paper layout of the data-collection form. This makes it much easier for the data-entry operator to identify the correct piece of information to be entered quickly.

No calculations

A great deal of concentration is required to enter data quickly and accurately. If there is a need to switch concentration to other activities during the process, this will interrupt the flow, slow down the task and possibly introduce errors. This can occur when data have to be transformed so that they are entered into the database in a different format to that on the data-collection form. This may involve coding (already discussed), or transforming units. For instance, if a respondent has recorded a value in gallons but the data-entry form requires the value in litres, the data-entry operator will have to do the conversion before they enter the data. This situation should be foreseen, and the calculation should be automatically performed by the database software. For instance, a field to record milk production may be followed by another to record the units. The automatic conversion can either take place during entry or during analysis, but either way removes the need for the data-entry operator to perform the calculation.

Keyboard versus mouse

Many form elements used for data entry can be completed simply by using a mouse. Many computer users find the mouse faster and easier to use than typing on a keyboard. However, experienced operators may often be faster at using the keyboard than using a mouse. Problems arise when the data-entry process calls for users to constantly switch between using the mouse and the keyboard. Try to design the interface so that one or the other is used, or, if both are required, that they are used in blocks without regular swaps between the two. Even graphical elements that are normally designed for the mouse can be used solely with the keyboard, for instance by using the tab, space, enter and arrow keys.

9.6.2 Accuracy – error checking and validation

Two approaches can be taken to data entry. The first is the use of a passive data-entry system, which accepts all data. Data checking and validation is then done as a second step by examining, and if necessary correcting, the data that have been input. The second, and more efficient approach, is the development of an active data-entry interface that assists with data checking while data entry is taking place. The advantage of this approach is that errors can be automatically detected while the data-collection form is still readily available. If errors are only identified when data entry is completed, the original form will need to be extracted from the file and the right value found – a time-consuming and inefficient task.

Active data-entry systems can analyse the data in a number of ways during data entry, and warn the user of problems. Examples of active data-entry checks include the following.

Range checks

For numeric values, there is often an expected permissible range. For instance, the number of quarters affected by mastitis will always between 0 and 4. The age of sheep is virtually always going to be between 0 and 20 years. The weight of a cat will usually be between 0 and 15 kg. The database can be instructed to either warn the user, or refuse to accept data, when a value outside these ranges is entered. Dates can also be subjected to range checking. For example, the date of examination should always be between the date of the beginning of the survey and the date of data entry.

Logic checks

While range checks examine only the data entered into a particular field, logic checks examine data in multiple fields, to determine if the data entered are logical. For instance, if the sex of animal is recorded as male, a record of mastitis would be invalid. These can be combined in powerful ways to cross-check multiple aspects of a record and avoid problems which may otherwise be difficult to detect.

Automation

The completion of a data-entry form can be automated in two ways. First, values can be entered into the fields automatically, without the need for the data-entry operator to type them. This can either be based on the previous record (if, for instance, sequential records often describe animals sharing many of the same characteristics), common default values, or common values based on examination of other fields in the record. The second way in which automation can improve the speed and accuracy of data entry is by automatically skipping certain fields that, based on the data previously entered, are not required.

Valid values

For categorical variables with a limited number of pre-determined responses, the database can be programmed to accept only valid values, or to prompt for confirmation if a value is not in the list of valid values.

9.6.3 Types of data-entry fields

There are a number of types of data-entry fields commonly available on computerized data entry systems, including databases, web-forms and spreadsheets, although other specialized data-entry fields exist in different software, but the most common are the following.

Text box

These are used for typing either numeric or text data from the keyboard. Specialized text boxes may be designed to accept only numeric data, or enforce a certain format (e.g. a specified number of decimal places). Others have mouse controls to increment or decrement the value. Another version is the multi-line text box, which is useful for including large blocks of text, or fields with variable numbers of lines, such as addresses.

Drop-down lists

These are especially useful for categorical data, and offer the main mechanism whereby categorical text-based data from a data-collection form can be automatically coded into numeric data by the computer. They are usually used with the mouse and, by clicking an item, an associated code can be entered into the database. Variations include list boxes (which permanently show all or part of the selection list, rather than just the one selected item) and lists from which more than one item may be selected (which may be useful for describing complex relationships).

Radio buttons

These are groups of buttons that allow only one item to be selected at a time. These are useful for shorter categorical questions, including dichotomous questions or questions with only a small number of mutually exclusive responses (e.g. Yes/No/Unknown responses).

Check box

These are single boxes that may have two states – checked (meaning yes or true) and unchecked (meaning no or false). These are commonly used for dichotomous data types. A variation on these is the three-state checkbox, which includes an intermediate half-shaded check, indicating unsure.

9.6.4 Missing values

Most datasets for epidemiological analysis are incomplete and contain missing data. There is a wide variety of reasons for this, but they are a fact of life and appropriate plans need to be put in place to deal with them.

The best approach is to take all possible steps to avoid missing data, and there are several strategies for this. Well-designed data-collection forms can make it much easier to avoid missing data, by providing alternative options in case none of the others seem suitable, asking only questions that have been tested and are answerable or willingly answered, and ensuring the questionnaire is short enough not to place an undue burden on the respondent. Where computerized data-collection systems are used, they can be programmed to enforce a response to each question.

For ongoing data collection, another good approach to minimize missing data is paying close attention to follow-up. When a person has failed to provide the required data, it is always a good idea to contact the person and ask for it. This has several benefits: they may be able to provide the missing data on the spot, or go and get it, avoiding the loss of that item of data; and they may also be more motivated to get the data next time it is requested, because they know that the data are important enough to somebody to make them get on the phone and ring. The realization that a person's individual contribution to a data-collection exercise is noticed and is considered valuable is often all that is required to ensure ongoing collection of high-quality data.

On the other hand, there have been cases where field staff conscientiously submit required data every month, until one month when an unforeseen illness or event results in no report being submitted for the month. If this is not noticed and there is no follow-up request for the field officer to submit the missing report, there is a good chance that the field officer will question the value of their efforts and they may simply stop submitting monthly data. This can result in a situation where head office staff lament the poor compliance rate while field staff comment on the lack of feedback and recognition of their efforts.

Even when the most diligent efforts are made, there will still be situations when data are unavoidably missing, and data entry and analysis procedures need to be able to cope with this.

In addition to planning to minimize missing data it is important to define what gets entered into the database when data are missing. In many cases, numeric fields may default to a value of 0 if nothing is entered. However, there is an important difference between a value of 0 (implying the presence of information) and a missing value. Some databases will permit the use of an empty field, or allow one to enter the 'null' or absent value. Others are less flexible and demand that some number be entered. In these cases, it is common to enter a special, out-of-range number or code to indicate a missing value, such as –999.

Whatever system is chosen, you should also have a clear understanding of how these values are treated during data analysis. This includes knowing exactly how different programs or software deal with different types of data when data are moved from one program to another during analysis. Some statistical programs allow you to specify a code for missing values, and these records are automatically omitted. In many other cases, it is necessary to explicitly exclude coded missing values from the analysis.

9.6.5 Duplicate-entry systems

While automated data-entry checking systems, good data-collection form design, avoiding transcription and follow-up all contribute to improving data quality, there is still a risk of errors occurring during data entry.

Duplicate data entry can reduce this risk and can produce a measure of error rate (errors per keystroke or per field). Duplicate data entry involves two (or more) data-entry operators entering the same data independently. The data is then compared, and any inconsistencies are checked against the original data-collection form to determine which is correct. This approach virtually eliminates error, due the low likelihood that both operators would make exactly the same mistake in the same record. If only a subset of data is double-entered, it can be examined to estimate the error rate. Clearly the problem with this approach is that it doubles the labour required for data entry. It is therefore often restricted to data of critical importance.

9.6.6 Multi-site data entry

When a large study involves data entry at more than one location, new problems may arise for data entry. Normally each record is coded or indexed using a sequential number within the database. If two or more databases are being compiled simultaneously, both will share the same index numbers for different records. When the data are merged, this may lead to problems with analysis. The best solution to this problem is to set up a centralized database that all users can access independently, so that duplication of records is prevented. If a centralized system with remote access is not possible, an alternative approach is to ensure that record identification includes not only the sequential index number but also an extra identifier unique to each data-entry location.

References

Cameron, A.R. (1999) *Survey Toolbox – A Practical Manual and Software Package for Active Surveillance of Livestock Diseases in Developing Countries*. Australian Centre for International Agricultural Research, Canberra, Australia.

Thrushfield, M. (2005) *Veterinary Epidemiology*, 3rd edn, Blackwell Science, Oxford.

10 Exploratory Data Analysis

10.1 Introduction

Exploratory data analysis (EDA) is the very first step in the process of analysing a dataset. The general aim of EDA is to summarize the data, identify and address oddities and in the process help identify a strategy for more elaborate or formal analyses. Although it is common to think of the analysis process as largely linear, it is more likely to be iterative with initial analyses identifying issues that need to be addressed or suggesting different coding systems and alternative analyses. Initial findings inform modifications and are then followed by further analyses and in some cases even collection of more data. At some stage a final analysis is completed and reported.

As a rule of thumb you should expect to spend more time on EDA than on your actual final analyses. EDA may be slow, iterative and involve analyses that are tried and discarded (blind ends). However, the reward is that once it is finished, the final and formal analysis may be completed quickly and smoothly.

Ideally EDA is done without any great assumptions about the data or about the type of statistical model that might be used on the data – the approach is to let the data reveal their own structure and secrets.

10.2 Goals of Exploratory Data Analysis

The main goal of EDA is to maximize insight into a dataset and into the underlying structure. Part of this involves assessment of:

- outlier values and how to manage these;
- which measures are outcomes of interest and which are explanatory factors;
- robustness of associations and conclusions from analyses;
- estimates for parameters;
- uncertainties for those estimates;
- which factors appear to be more or less important; and
- options for final statistical analyses.

Real insight and feel for a dataset involves more than just coming to grips with the list above and comes only as the analyst uses multiple approaches to explore different aspects of the data. It is particularly important to use graphical summaries in EDA – these will enhance insight into a dataset in ways that numerical summary measures are unable to do. Statistical analysis is a bit like detective work – there may not be a clear way forward. You examine the evidence, develop some theories or hunches and follow them. Your first hunch may not pay off and you should count on making several tries on your data. As a result it follows that tools used to explore the data must be flexible.

10.3 Backups and Records

Whenever you receive a dataset from a client or prepare to begin EDA on your own dataset, you should always start by making an original copy of the dataset and then use a working copy for all processing. In addition you should keep a log or record of all analyses and findings and in particular a detailed record of any changes that you make to the data file. These steps ensure that you can always go back to the original data if required and that you can identify and justify every step and decision that was made in the process.

Many statistical packages allow you to save some form of log file that can include details and often code for every analysis and processing step undertaken and even the output from every step. These files can be annotated with comments and can serve as a detailed record of all analyses. When combined with the original data file it is then possible to recreate every step in the analytical process.

10.4 Process of Exploratory Data Analysis

The overall process of EDA can be summarized as follows:

- processing data into a suitable form for analysis;
- checking data quality including assessment of missing data, implausible values, errors, outliers and variability;
- modifying data if necessary, including processes such as recoding, transformation, error correction, aggregation or other approaches;
- completing EDA using one or more of:
  - single variable (univariable) graphical displays;
  - single variable (univariable) non-graphical summaries;
  - multiple variable graphs assessing associations; and
  - multiple variable non-graphical measures of association.

10.4.1 Data structure

The first step is to understand the structure of the data and to consider the number and type of variables and number of observations in the dataset. Be wary of small sample sizes (less than 10 to 30 measurements) and also be wary of studies with more variables than observations.

Thought needs to be applied to the coding and use of categorical and ordinal variables.

Identify which variables are outcome variables (dependent) and which are predictors or explanatory variables (independent). If this is difficult, that is if you have a set of variables without a clear outcome variable, then certain techniques such as principal components analysis become more useful.

10.4.2 Processing data

It is also important to pay attention to variable coding and variable format. It is highly likely that you will be dealing with data in spreadsheets or database programs or both.

If an observation is missing, the simplest coding is to leave the cell blank or add a period '.'. In some cases it may be useful to distinguish missing cells (where the respondent did not answer) from observations that are not applicable and from observations with a zero value.

It is very important to understand the impact of missing values and coding on analyses. Zero values must be differentiated from missing values. Most statistics software packages will not tolerate text values (M for missing, NA for not applicable) being entered into a column of numeric values. If missing values are coded as some form of numeric value (e.g. –999), then the missing value codes must be defined in the software before analysis or they may be incorporated into any statistical processing.

Similar cautions can be applied to text coding for nominal variables and the use of numbers to represent categorical variables. For example, most statistical programs will treat integer codes as numbers (rather than categories) unless you specifically tell the program that they are to be treated as factors (categories).

For categorical data it is also important to think about which level might serve as a reference level in modelling. Some packages will default to using the lowest level (numeric) or first level in alphabetic order (for text variables). In some cases you may be able to change this in the modelling setup. Alternatively, you can prepare for this when coding data.

If data are entered via a key board then some form of verification and error checking should be performed. If you have paper forms or hard copies of data, then a simple method of checking is to randomly select sheets or questions and check values against entries in the spreadsheet or database. Record any errors that you find and the response or outcome for each error (e.g. excluded from the analysis, corrected, etc.).

10.4.3 How common and serious are spreadsheet errors?

Panko (1998, revised 2008) published a fascinating and revealing insight into spreadsheet errors. In summary:

- Between 20 and 40% of all spreadsheets are likely to contain errors.
- One study reported 90% of all spreadsheets with more than 150 rows of data, contained human-source errors (errors were not related to the program itself).
- A number of studies, covering over a thousand subjects and including both novices and experienced spreadsheet developers, found cell error rates ranging from about 1% to >20%, with most between about 5% and 10%.
- When Excel novices did formula-related tasks in Excel, 50% of the spreadsheets contained errors.
- When post-graduate students completed more complicated modelling in Excel with multiple worksheets, over 90% of worksheets had errors.
- When a researcher gave three spreadsheet development tasks to nine professional developers, all made at least one error and 63% of their spreadsheets contained errors. Yet all were very confident that their output was error free.

These error rates are consistent with normal human activity; for example, when people type they make undetected errors in about 0.5% of all actions. When more complex logical activities are performed the error rate rises to about 5%.

In general, people using spreadsheets for data management often build large and complicated spreadsheets that they intend to use to support important decisions and yet rarely appear to audit or check their spreadsheets for errors.

It is good practice to expect errors to occur even when specific measures are implemented to minimize errors. Some form of error checking should be undertaken for every dataset and every analysis. There is a variety of ways of doing this and a variety of software packages to assist you.

The following examples (accessed 15 April 2015) are auditing tools available for Microsoft Excel® for example:

- Power Utility Pak 2000: http://spreadsheetpage.com/index.php/products
- Spreadsheet Detective: http://www.spreadsheetdetective.com/
- Excel Auditor: http://www.bygsoftware.com/auditor/auditor.htm

There is also an excellent page of information on a University of Melbourne website with advice about using a spreadsheet to prepare data for analysis (http://www.scc.ms.unimelb.edu.au/dataprep.html (accessed 15 April 2015)).

10.5 Data Quality

The next step is to check data quality, including:

- Are there any suspicious, unlikely or impossible values?
- Are there any missing values and if so why, and what can be done about them?
- Have too many or too few significant digits been recorded?
- How were the data collected, how were variables measured, were the same instruments and precision used?
- In general, using data from several different sources increases the risk of inconsistencies. For example the same variable may have been measured at different locations but using different precision instruments at each location.

The three main types of data quality problem are errors, outliers and missing values.

An error is an incorrect value, either because it was recorded wrongly in the first place or copied/typed incorrectly. An outlier is an extreme observation that does not appear to be consistent with the rest of the data. Errors and outliers are often confused. An error may or may not be an outlier while an outlier may or may not be an error.

Checks for missing data should be relatively easy to do though you may need to develop a standard method of coding or entering missing values. It is valuable and important to find out why missing observations have occurred. There is a big difference between missing values lost through random events and situations where missing values are more likely to occur under certain circumstances. Then the probability that an observation may be missing may be dependent on the value of the observation or the value of the explanatory variables.

Credibility checks are a useful method for error detection. Performing a range test on each variable to compare the extremes against a pre-specified credible range for that variable is a quick and useful way to test for unexpected or unlikely values. For example, you may expect sheep body-weight to lie between 40 and 100 kg. If you find one value at 1000 kg, it is likely to represent a data-entry error. Sorting every variable in ascending and descending order is another simple way to check for extremely large or small values compared to the bulk of the measurements.

Bivariate and multivariate checks for consistency can also be done; for example, are age and date of birth consistent, are all cows considered for breeding actually post-calving? Another common method of checking data is to randomly select 5 to 20% of data cells and check them manually against paper records. This will give you estimates of error rates in data entry.

Graphical methods, such as frequency histograms for each variable, box plots and scatter plots are discussed in detail in a later section, but all help to understand data and appreciate gaps, extreme values, etc. There are also more formal procedures for detecting outliers (including significance tests). Some of these involve looking for large residuals after a model has been fitted, but these techniques do not pertain to the initial analysis phase.

When a suspect value (error) is identified, it is important to determine what to do. It may be possible to go back to original records and check the value for typing or recording error, inversions, etc. In many cases correction may not be possible and a decision may be made to exclude that value.

Extreme observations that could conceivably be correct are more difficult to handle. Tests for determining whether an outlier is significant provide little information as to whether it is actually an error or not. Expert advice may help and in some cases further data may help. Outright omission of an outlier is a drastic step, particularly if there is any evidence of a long tail in the distribution for that variable. Sometimes outliers are the most interesting observations.

A classic case is the early work on South Pole ozone depletion. Ozone measurements were made for many years in an automated fashion by satellite. Coded into the satellite was an automatic screening process that included outlier-rejection (i.e. for several years the satellite was measuring low ozone but those data points that exceeded thresholds were classified as outliers and then automatically deleted from the data prior to any further analysis). It was not until ground-based measurements were made and low ozone levels detected that someone then checked to see why the satellites had not observed the depletion – in fact they had but the data were thrown out! Outliers should always be assessed carefully because they may be an indication of underlying processes that are of genuine interest and value.

One alternative for managing outliers is to use robust methods of estimation that automatically down-weight extreme values towards the mean.

Chatfield (1995) suggests that for outliers with no evidence that they are errors, repeat the analysis with them in and with them out. If the conclusions are the same then the suspect values do not matter. If the conclusions differ substantially then the values do matter and additional effort should be expended to check them.

10.5.1 Precision

As part of assessment of data quality it is important to consider precision and the number of significant digits (Preece, 1981).

There are some rules of thumb on things such as how many digits to round to. Chatfield (1995) and others have said that in general data should be rounded to two variable digits where a variable digit is defined as one which varies over the full range from 0 to 9 in the data under consideration.

For example consider the following numbers:

181.633 182.796 189.132 186.239 191.151

The first digit, 1, is fixed while the second digit is either 8 or 9. The remaining four digits are variable digits (vary between 0 and 9). Therefore the numbers should be rounded to one decimal for summary statistics.

10.6 Descriptive Statistics

10.6.1 Qualitative data

For qualitative or categorical data, frequency tables are the most commonly used summary statistics. Simple tables are very useful for understanding coding and identifying miscoded variables (e.g. male animals may be recorded as male, M, m, Male, MALE) and simple tables of counts or proportions can help identify apparent patterns in the data for subsequent statistical evaluation.

Table 10.1 presents a two-way table of frequencies of AGID serology result against body condition score for 224 sheep infected with paratuberculosis. The table provides a summary of the coding levels used for the condition score variable, can be used to identify missing values (animals with no entry for condition score) and provides preliminary evidence of association between condition score and AGID result in that there is a decreasing trend in percentage of positive results as condition score increases.

10.6.2 Quantitative data

Summary statistics should be calculated for each numeric variable in the dataset and for subgroups based on outcome variables and any other variables of interest. Summary statistics for quantitative data include things such as mean, standard deviation (SD), median, minimum, maximum, correlation between each pair of variables, and other measures.

Table 10.1. Frequency of AGID serology results and body condition score for ovine paratuberculosis in 224 confirmed infected sheep.

	AGID result			
Condition score	Positive	(%)	Negative	Total
1	16	(94%)	1	17
2	16	(55%)	13	29
3	17	(14%)	103	120
4	6	(10%)	52	58
Total	55	(25%)	169	224

It is often useful to present summary statistics in a table and care should be taken to ensure the table conveys the information you want in a clear and uncluttered way. However, it is also important to remember that summaries can also sometimes mask underlying patterns and differences in the data.

Example

Consider the following four pairs of data which represent potential datasets for regression analyses (Table 10.2). Each pair consists of an outcome variable (Y) and an explanatory variable (X). Summary statistics and quantitative results of regression analyses are presented under the four pairs. The regression output (intercept, slope, correlation and residual standard deviation) is based on simple linear regression analysis ($Y = a + bX$).

The regression results for the four different pairs of data look very similar when the numeric output values are considered. However, when we look at scatter plots we get a completely different story, as shown in Fig. 10.1. In fact, as we can see from the scatter plots, the datasets are far from equivalent. The first set is linear, the second is quadratic, the third has an outlier and the fourth is clearly unusual with one influential extreme value.

This example simply reinforces the principle that quantitative analyses by themselves are incomplete numerical summaries that reduce the data to a few numbers and in the process important information may be filtered out. This can be misleading. Taking the time to do more extensive EDA that incorporates multiple assessments, both numeric and graphical, will usually result in a better final model (if and when a statistical model is completed).

Table 10.2. Comparison of four paired datasets.

Observation	X1	Y1	X2	Y2	X3	Y3	X4	Y4
1	10	8.04	10	9.14	10	7.46	8	6.58
2	8	6.95	8	8.14	8	6.77	8	5.76
3	13	7.58	13	8.74	13	12.74	8	7.71
4	9	8.81	9	8.77	9	7.11	8	8.84
5	11	8.33	11	9.26	11	7.81	8	8.47
6	14	9.96	14	8.1	14	8.84	8	7.04
7	6	7.24	6	6.13	6	6.08	8	5.25
8	4	4.26	4	3.1	4	5.39	19	12.5
9	12	10.84	12	9.13	12	8.15	8	5.56
10	7	4.82	7	7.26	7	6.42	8	7.91
11	5	5.68	5	4.74	5	5.73	8	6.89
Mean	9	7.50	9	7.50	9	7.5	9	7.5
SD	3.3	2.0	3.3	2.0	3.3	2.0	3.3	2.0
Intercept	3		3		3		3	
Slope	0.5		0.5		0.5		0.5	
Correlation	0.816		0.816		0.816		0.817	
Residual SD	1.237		1.237		1.236		1.236	

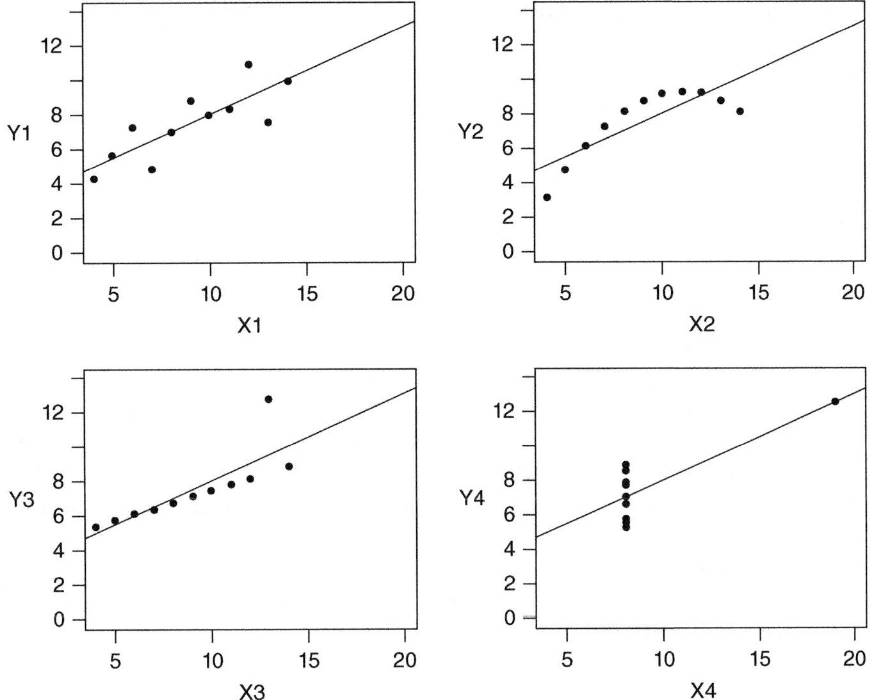

Fig. 10.1. Scatter plots comparing data from four datasets with similar summary statistics, from Table 10.2.

10.7 Quantitative Techniques

EDA should include both graphical and quantitative approaches. Often as part of the EDA approach it is useful to use some simpler quantitative techniques including both interval estimation and hypothesis testing.

A mean, for example, is a point estimate of the unknown population mean. Interval estimates (e.g. confidence intervals) expand on this by incorporating the uncertainty of the point estimate.

10.7.1 Mean

The mean of a sample is a measure of central tendency – a single number close to the centre of the distribution that represents all the data points in the sample. The arithmetic mean is the most commonly used form.

$$\bar{X} = \frac{\sum_{i=1}^{n} X_i}{n}$$

10.7.2 Alternatives to the mean

There are also a number of other alternatives as a measure of central tendency, either used in addition or instead of the arithmetic mean, including:

- Median: the middle value (half the values are higher and half lower).
- Mode: the most frequent value (the peak of the frequency distribution).
- Mid-mean: this is an arithmetic mean using only the data between the 25th and 75th percentiles.
- Trimmed mean: similar to the mid-mean except different percentile values are used. For example, a common choice is to trim off 5% of the points in both the upper and lower tails.
- Winsorized mean: similar to the trimmed mean but instead of trimming the points they are set to the lowest or highest value. For example all data below the 5th percentile are set equal to the value of the 5th percentile and all data greater than the 95th percentile are set equal to the 95th percentile. One of the main benefits of winsorizing is that it does not result in any loss of sample size compared to trimming.
- Mid-range: equal to (smallest + largest) / 2.
- Geometric mean: a mean usually calculated on a logarithmic or other transformed scale, useful for highly skewed data.

10.7.3 Measures of spread (variability)

There are two key components of data variability: how spread out are the data values near the centre and how spread out are the tails. The histogram is a useful graphical way of showing both these components.

Specific measures of variability include:

- Variance: for univariate data the variance is a common numerical measure of spread. Because it is roughly the arithmetic average of the squared distance from the mean, it has the effect of giving greater weight to values that are further from the mean. Although it is meant to be an overall measure of spread it can be greatly affected by tail behaviour.
- Standard deviation (SD): the square root of the variance. This is a measure of variability of individual observations.
- Standard error of the mean (SEM): this is a measure of variation of sample means around the true but unknown population mean.
- Range: the largest value minus the smallest value. The range does not capture the spread near the centre – it is based only on the two extreme values.
- Average absolute deviation: does not square the distance from the mean and so is less affected by extreme values than the variance and SD.
- Median absolute deviation: a variant of the average absolute deviation that is even less affected by extremes in the tail since they have less influence on estimation of a median than a mean.
- Interquartile range: 75th percentile value minus the 25th percentile value. This attempts to measure the variability of the points near the centre.

If data are non-normal, and in particular if there are long tails, then using alternative measures such as median absolute deviation or average absolute deviation of interquartile range can be more informative than conventional variance or SD.

10.7.4 Skewness

Skewness is a measure of symmetry or more precisely of lack of symmetry. A distribution is described as symmetric if it looks the same to the right and left of the centre point.

Skewed distributions may be called right (positively) or left (negatively) skewed depending on whether the tail is drawn out to the right or the left. The skewness for a normal distribution is zero and any symmetrical data set with a single central peak should have skewness close to zero. If a distribution is skewed the mean is dragged nearer to the tail than the median and mode. The ratio of skewness to its standard error can be used as a test of normality (i.e. you can reject normality if the ratio is less than –2 or greater than +2). A large positive value for skewness indicates a long right tail; an extreme negative value, a long left tail.

This interpretation of skewness is based on the fact that the ratio of the skewness to its standard error estimate is considered to have a standard normal distribution.

10.7.5 Kurtosis

Kurtosis is a measure of whether the data are peaked or flat relative to the normal distribution. Data with high kurtosis tend to have a distinct tall peak near the mean, decline rather rapidly and have heavy tails. Datasets with low kurtosis tend to have a flat top near the mean rather than a sharper peak. A uniform distribution is the extreme case of low kurtosis.

The ratio of kurtosis to its standard error can also be used as a test of normality (i.e. you can reject normality if the ratio is less than –2 or greater than +2). A large positive value for kurtosis indicates that the tails of the distribution are longer than those of a normal distribution; a negative value for kurtosis indicates shorter tails (becoming like those of a box-shaped uniform distribution).

10.7.6 Multivariable non-graphical techniques

The basis of multivariable EDA is cross-tabulation or some similar approach. Where one variable is continuous and one categorical, we can do summary statistics of the numeric variable for each level of the categorical variable (i.e. mean body weight for each of four treatment groups). Correlation matrices will also work for continuous variables. In epidemiology we might use a series of odds ratios or relative risk ratios. These are often referred to as screening tests.

10.8 Graphical Techniques

Graphs are an ideal way of displaying information about data (i.e. its shape of distribution, trend or direction of change over time or relationships). In the initial data analysis it is common to produce many different graphs in order to inspect the data in many different ways, although at the end of the process only a small number may be retained or displayed to others. The most useful univariate graphs are histograms and box plots. Scatter plots are very useful for exploring bivariate relationships between two numeric variables.

In general, special graphical effects, such as 3D bars or shadows, should be avoided or only used with care, since such effects often obscure the data. Even the use of a lot of colour can interfere with simple appreciation of graphical information.

A graph should communicate information with clarity and precision. It should not distort what the data are trying to say. It should make large datasets coherent in a small space and encourage the eye to compare different parts of the data.

Critical elements to consider in preparing graphs include:

- Keep graphs simple – do not try to put too much information on one graph.
- Clear, self-explanatory titles and units of measurement should be presented on the graph.
- All axes should be labelled.
- Scale on each axis needs to be chosen with some care to avoid distorting or suppressing information, as does the placement of tick marks.
- Use scale breaks for false origins. Scale breaks are breaks usually in the *y*-axis to allow graphs to show data that may be widely disparate in value. Alternatively, a false origin (lowest value) can be used.
- Mode of presentation should be chosen carefully, for example, size and shape of plotting symbol (asterisks, dots, etc.) and the method, if any, of connecting points.
- Consider trial and error to find what you want.

One expert on graphical presentation of data (Tufte, 1983, 1997), has defined a lie factor, which is:

$$\text{Lie factor} = \frac{\text{Apparent size of effect shown in graph}}{\text{Actual size of effect in the data}}$$

To avoid deception, the lie factor should be kept close to one.

Tufte's books contain many excellent examples of graphical presentation of data, including examples of poor and misleading presentations.

Most graphs are static and two-dimensional. In recent years there has been great interest in interactive and dynamic graphs. The essential feature here is that the analyst can interact with the graph on a computer screen so that the graph can change to display different information. Typically, interaction involves mouse clicking or hovering and actions include revealing values, showing labels, changing axes or scales, eliminating selected points and rotating a 3D graph.

Increasing visual and processing capabilities have changed the way some people are using and teaching statistics. Interactive graphical approaches offer an alternative approach to numerical analytical methods for some forms of analysis. In many cases these techniques complement and enhance traditional numerical based methods and in some cases offer insights that are simply impossible to achieve with numerical analyses.

10.8.1 Histograms

Histograms are the most commonly used graphical technique for showing the distribution of values for a quantitative variable. Histograms are produced by dividing the range into a set number of equally spaced intervals and plotting the count of values in each interval as a bar. Many statistical and graphics packages will produce histograms simply and automatically. Histograms are a useful method for assessing normality and compete with the probability plot for this purpose.

There are two broad decisions to make when producing a histogram:

1. How best to group the data into classes? Varying the number of intervals and the width of intervals can alter the appearance of the plot. If too many classes are used the graph may appear rough and strung out. With too few, it may look too smooth. The suggested approaches to try and overcome this are to use either 10–12 classes as a convenient standard, or to use the square root of the number of observations in your sample as a guide to the number of intervals. Most packages have default routines for producing histograms that will be adequate for most situations.
2. The second decision is whether frequencies (counts) or relative frequencies (proportions or percentages) appear on the vertical axis. There are no strict rules for this and it largely depends on preference and the purpose for which the graph is to be used.

Histograms may be described as symmetric, left or right skewed or showing multiple peaks, gaps, outliers, etc. Histograms are typically drawn with no spaces between the adjacent columns unless a class is empty. In a histogram, because classes are the same width, and height reflects the value, then the area of each column reflects the contribution by that class to the total. Within one interval, the rectangles make it appear that the data are spread uniformly throughout the interval though this is often not the case. Figure 10.2 shows a reasonably symmetrical histogram for body weights of 50 sheep, overlaid with a frequency polygon for the same data.

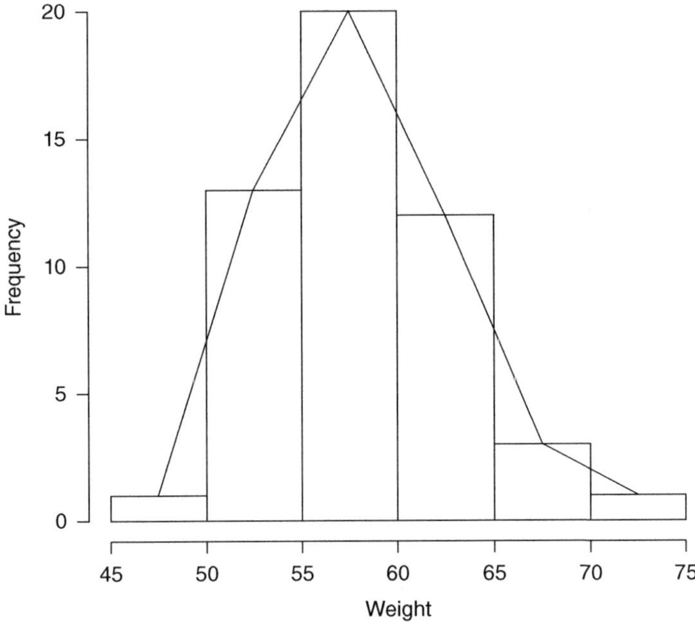

Fig. 10.2. Histogram and frequency polygon of 50 sheep weights.

If the histogram indicates a symmetric moderately tailed distribution then the recommended next step is to do a normal probability plot to confirm approximate normality.

If the histogram is bimodal then consider alternatives (e.g. a mixture of two distributions or some other pattern such as sinusoidal). Histograms can also be very useful for identifying outliers, as shown in Fig. 10.3.

10.8.2 Frequency polygon

Frequency polygons are similar to histograms, but instead of drawing bars to represent the frequency of each X-class we simply draw points where the mid-points of the tops of the bars would be. Connecting these points with lines produces a frequency polygon. The histogram in Fig. 10.2 also shows a frequency polygon and the same polygon is shown in Fig. 10.4 on its own. The polygon contains the same information as a histogram but in a slightly different form.

10.8.3 Stem-and-leaf plots

Stem-and-leaf plots are a simple and versatile way to view data. They are essentially modified histograms, where numerical values replace the bars. The initial digits (before the decimal point) of each value are listed on the left to form the stem and the first of the remaining digits are shown on the right, representing the leaves, as shown in Fig. 10.5. Stem-and-leaf plots allow patterns in the data to be appreciated quickly. The skewed nature of the data in Fig. 10.5 is quite easily apparent.

It may be possible to increase or decrease the level of detail shown by changing the scale of the stem, for example by decreasing each stem unit to 0.5 or increasing to 2.

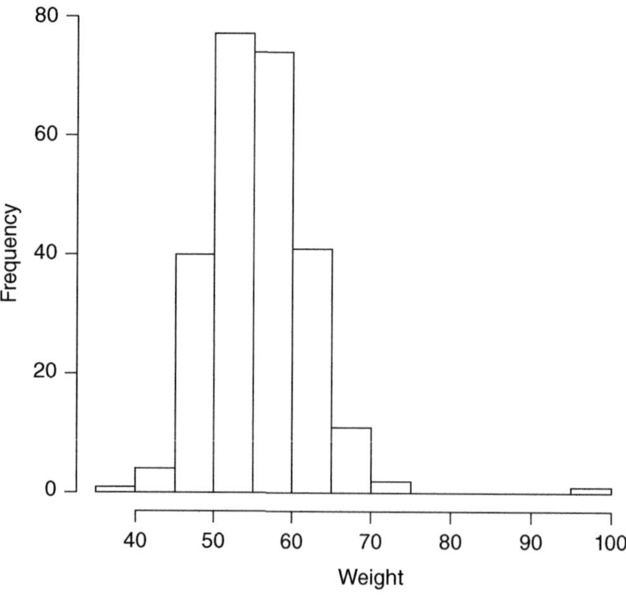

Fig. 10.3. Symmetrical histogram with a possible outlier.

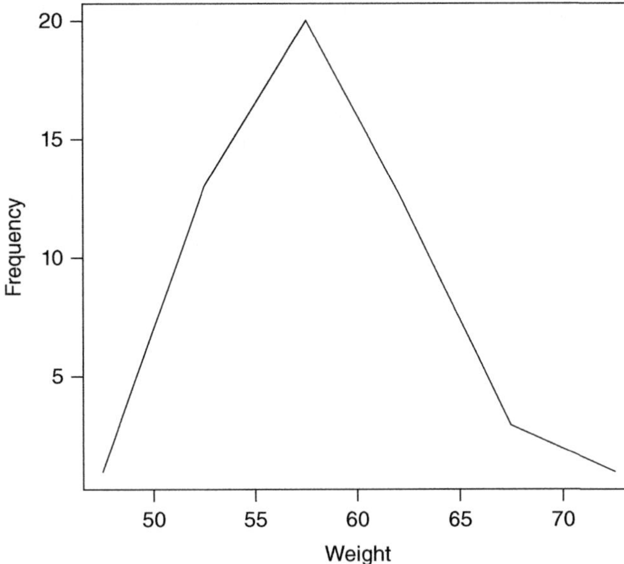

Fig. 10.4. Frequency polygon for body weights of 50 sheep.

```
The decimal point is at the |

3 | 9
4 | 59
5 | 47
6 | 013
7 | 012356778
8 | 01124556788
9 | 02
```

Fig. 10.5. Stem-and-leaf plot for sample data with values ranging from minimum of 3 to maximum of 10.

10.8.4 Box plots

Box plots (also known as box-and-whisker plots) are another way of displaying information about the spread of a single batch of numbers and extreme values. Box plots are usually constructed from a single quantitative variable, although it is also common to use a second (categorical) variable to divide the first variable into groups for comparison. Figure 10.6 shows the general layout of a box plot.

Box plots have three main features: the centre, spread and outliers. The following points describe common approaches to interpreting box plots:

- The bottom and top of the box are the 25th and 75th percentiles. The length of the box is therefore the interquartile range (IQR). The box represents 50% of the data points. A line is drawn through the box at the median (50th percentile).
- Upper adjacent values lie between the 75th percentile and less than or equal to the 75th percentile plus 1.5 times the IQR.
- The lower adjacent value is the smallest observation that is greater than or equal to the 25th percentile minus 1.5 times the IQR.

- Adjacent values are shown as T-shaped lines (whiskers) that extend from either end of the box.
- Values outside the upper and lower adjacent are called outer or outside values. Values less than three times the IQR from the 25th and 75th percentiles are called mild outliers. Those outside three IQRs are called severe outliers.

Figure 10.7 shows a series of box plots for ELISA ratio results for paratuberculosis in sheep, for four different groups of sheep. There is a clear difference in the distribution

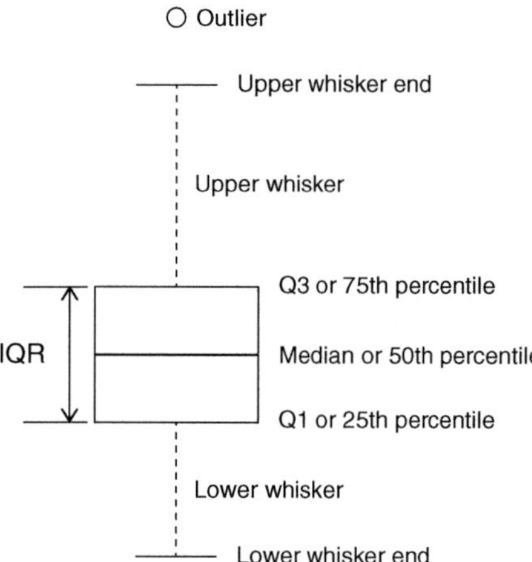

Fig. 10.6. Normal layout for a simple box plot.

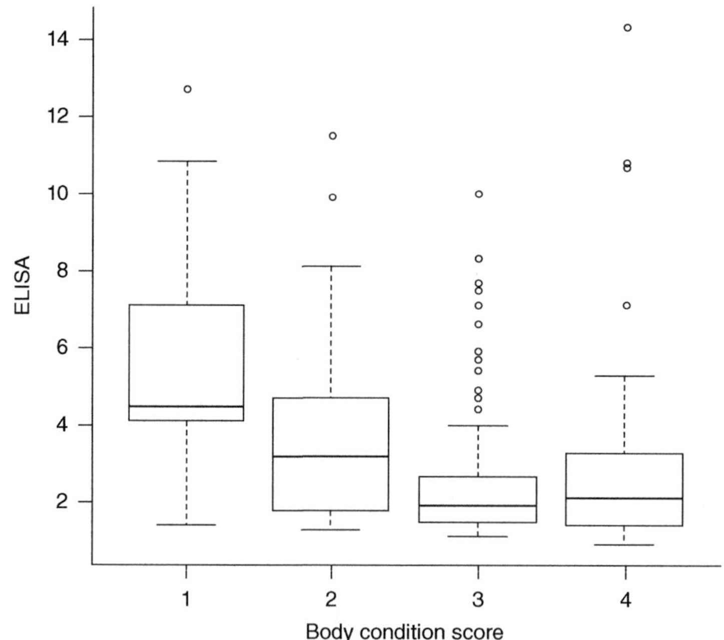

Fig. 10.7. Box plot of ELISA ratio values for 224 sheep infected with paratuberculosis, categorized into four groups, based on body condition score (1 = very thin, 4 = fat).

of results, with groups one and two having a higher median value and wider inter-quartile range compared to groups 3 and 4, which had more outliers.

10.8.5 Probability plot

There are numerous methods for testing whether data are normally distributed, both graphical and numerical (statistical). Graphical procedures are often preferred since they allow visual inspection, so that it is easy to see if the assumption is violated by just one or two outliers. The graphical appearance may also allow identification of the best transformation for the data if it obviously does not fit the chosen distribution (and subsequently allows checking of how well the new distribution fits). A normal probability plot is just one special case of the more general probability plot that can be used for this purpose. Most statistical packages have built-in routines for performing probability plots.

Quantile–quantile (Q–Q) plot or normal quantile plot

Q–Q or normal quantile plots are similar to probability plots. In fact some software packages call them both probability plots.

A Q–Q plot is a plot of the quantiles of the first dataset against the quantiles of a second dataset, usually a theoretical distribution. A quantile is simply a percentile expressed as a proportion (e.g. the 25th percentile is the same as the 0.25 quantile). The 0.3 quantile is the point at which 30% of the data fall below and 70% above that value. The Q–Q plot is a graphical way of determining if a dataset comes from a population with a common distribution.

Real data almost always show some departure from the theoretical normal model. It is important not to overreact against every little wiggle in the plot.

Most statistical software can now generate Q–Q or normal quantile plots automatically. Figure 10.8 shows a normal quantile plot for the data in Fig. 10.3. The diagonal line represents the line corresponding to the equivalent normal distribution.

The simple interpretation of probability plots is that if the points fall along a straight line, you can assume the data follow that probability distribution (for whatever distribution you are fitting). Outliers generally show up as extreme points at either end of the plot.

Sometimes points on the ends stray from the line and may appear to follow a pattern, for example, points at the top of the line my curve up or points at the bottom may curve down. This is caused by data with longer tails than expected. If the plot has a convex or concave curve to it the data are skewed to one side or the other (see Fig. 10.9).

Probability plots have a number of advantages. They are simple and rapid, work well for small and large sample sizes, can be used on single variables as well as inspecting the residuals from complex analyses (ANOVA, etc.). They can also be constructed for distributions other than the normal distribution. Probability plots also have disadvantages in that they are subjectively interpreted, and do not yield an objective assessment (no p-value).

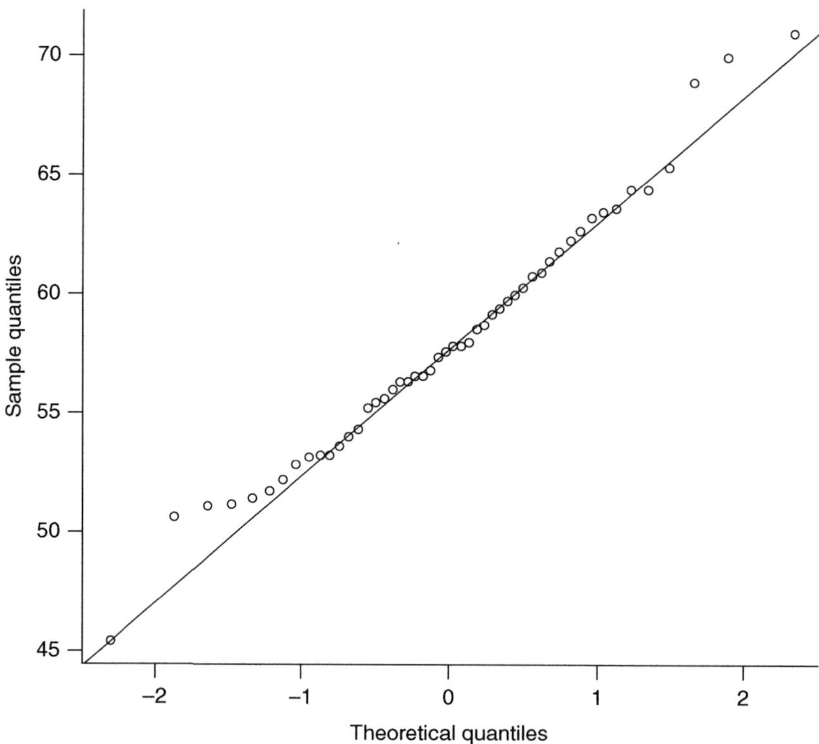

Fig. 10.8. Normal quantile plot for body-weight data for 50 sheep.

10.8.6 Bar charts and area charts

Bar charts are used to compare data values to one another, often frequency counts. Several variants exist, including vertical bar (column), horizontal bar, stacked bar, area chart, line chart and many more. Bar charts are generally easy to make and interpret. Figure 10.10 shows a bar chart for the distribution of body condition score (1–4) in 224 sheep from six flocks (1–6).

10.8.7 Error bar charts

Error bar plots can be used to graphically display tables of means and a defined interval represented by the bar. Bars may represent standard error, standard deviation or confidence interval. It is important to always add text to the legend to define what the bars represent. Figure 10.11 shows an error bar chart for the ELISA and condition score data for 224 sheep infected with paratuberculosis, shown previously in Figure 10.7.

10.8.8 Scatter plots

Scatter plots are a commonly used and powerful tool for investigating the relationship between two continuous variables – the values for one variable are plotted on the *y*-axis against the corresponding value for the other variable (on the *x* axis). All statistical

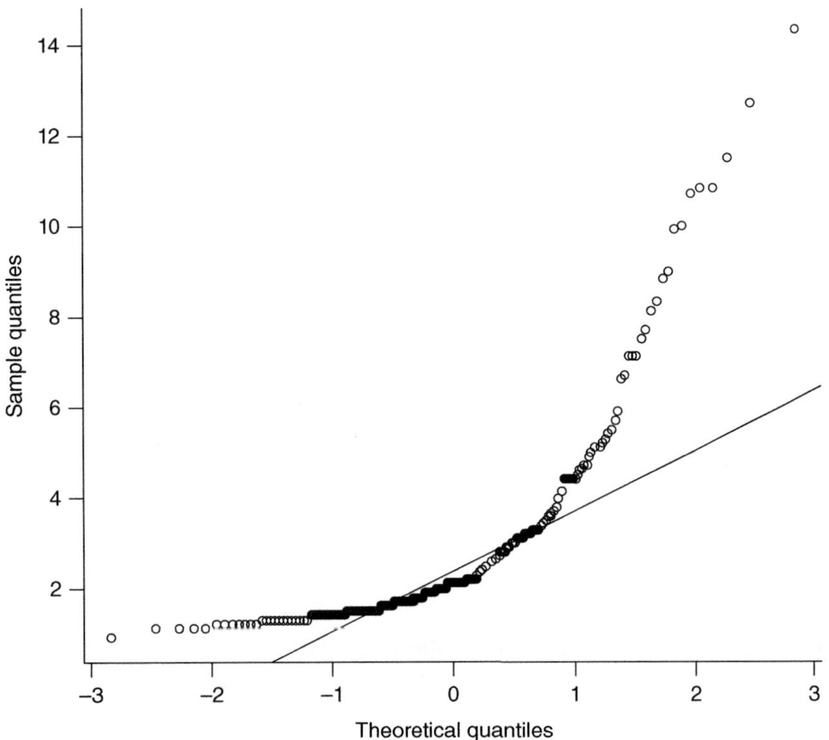

Fig. 10.9. Normal quantile plot for ELISA ratio values for 224 sheep infected with paratuberculosis.

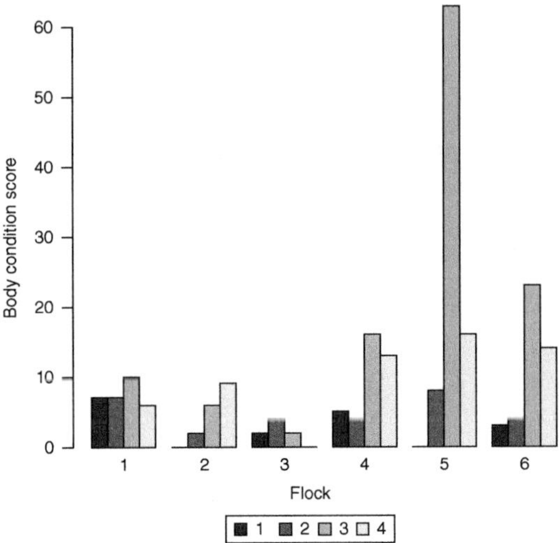

Fig. 10.10. Counts (frequency) of sheep classified by body condition score (1–4) and flock (1–6).

packages offer scatter plot capabilities. Figure 10.12 shows a scatter plot of simulated data for results of duplicate testing of 1000 serum samples using a test with a quantitative result such as an ELISA. For this example, the solid line is the line of identity – all points should lie on this line if the duplicate tests gave identical results.

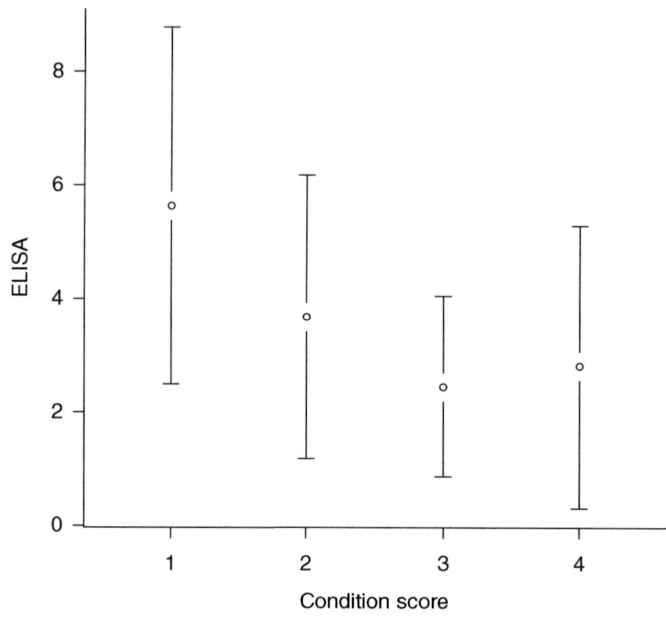

Fig. 10.11. Error bar chart (mean and standard deviation) for ELISA ratio values for 224 sheep infected with paratuberculosis, in four groups according to body condition score.

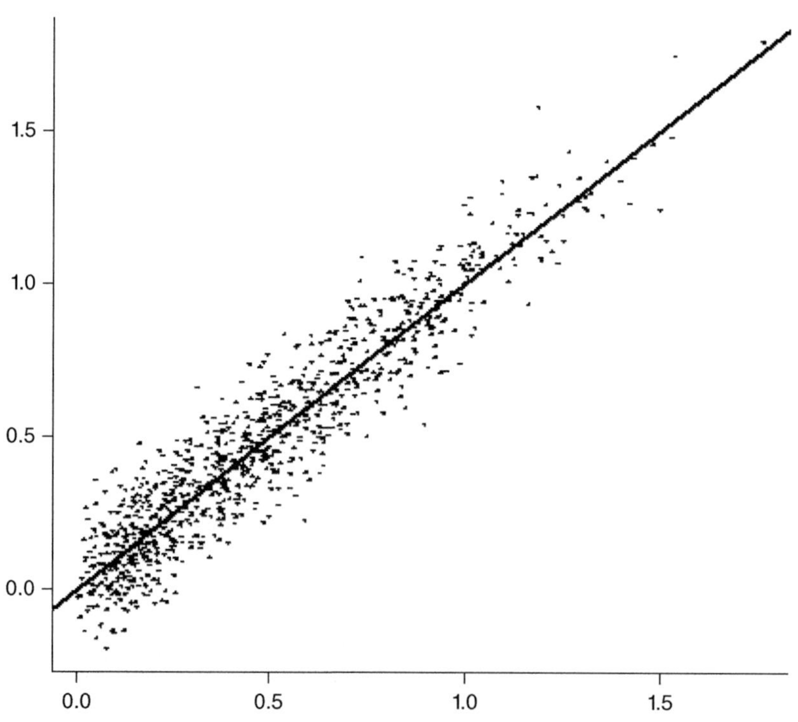

Fig. 10.12. Scatter plot of simulated duplicate testing results for 1000 serum samples.

10.8.9 Scatter plot matrix

A scatter plot matrix is a table (or matrix) of scatter plots for pairwise comparison of multiple continuous variables. Scatter plot matrices are very useful if you have a larger number of variables at the beginning of a regression analysis, for example. Given a set of variables, the scatter plot matrix contains all the pairwise scatter plots of the variables on a single page in a matrix format. If there are *k* variables the matrix will have *k* rows and *k* columns. Scatter plots provide rapid and cursory information about presence or absence of relationships between variables and nature of any such relationships. Figure 10.13 shows a scatter plot matrix for hypothetical data.

10.8.10 Time series plots

Whenever data represent measurements collected over time, it is useful to plot them against either time or the order in which the measurements were taken. This allows

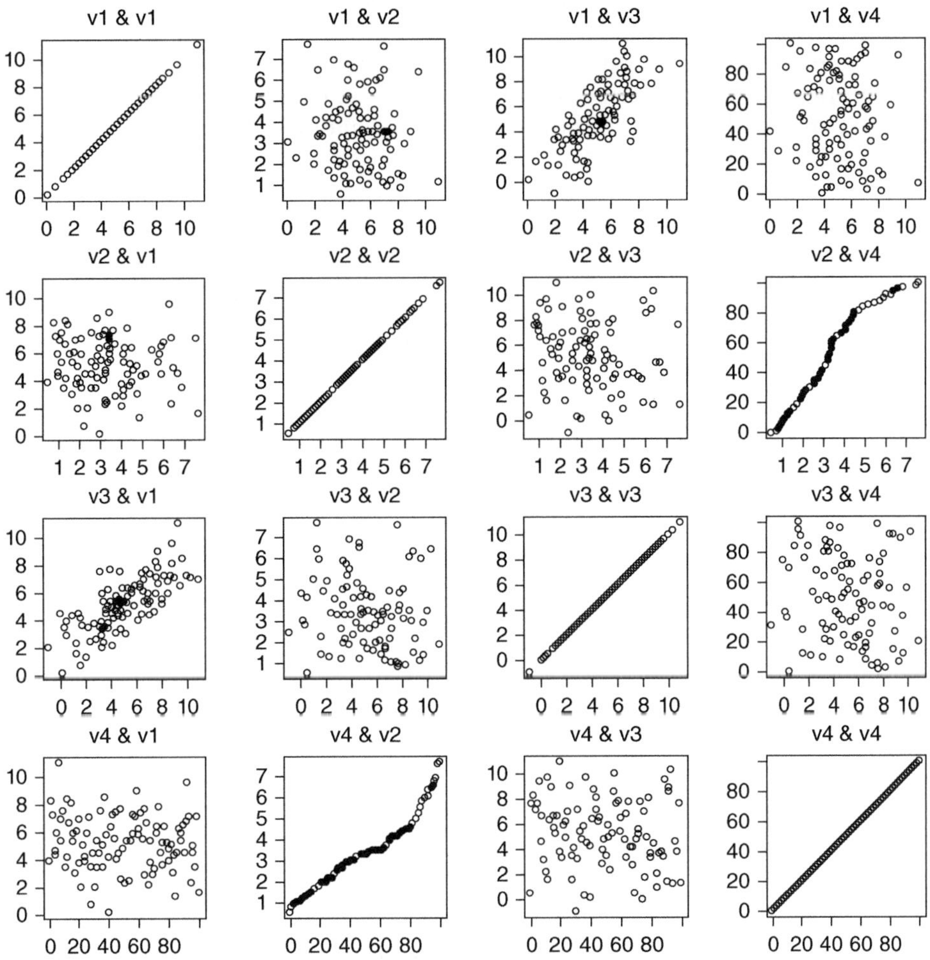

Fig. 10.13. Scatter plot matrix for hypothetical data for four variables, v1 to v4.

rapid identification of unexpected values or patterns in the data that might otherwise not be apparent.

Figure 10.14 shows 66 measurements of the passage time of light, made by Newcomb in 1882, in the order in which they were collected (Stigler, 1977). The plot shows several outliers in the data and quite an amount of random variation in the measurements overall. However, most measurements were broadly in the range of 25 to 40 units.

Many datasets are time series (measurements of the same variable taken at regular intervals over time). Government economic and social data and disease prevalence data are common examples. Weather and climatic data are also often presented in this way. Epidemic curves are another good example of time series data. Figure 2.1 is a good example of an epidemic curve, showing the number of cases of cholera in John Snow's cholera investigation in London in 1854.

Another example of simple time series data is that for control samples in diagnostic test applications (see Fig. 7.2 for example). A control sample (positive or negative) is usually run each time the test is performed and the resulting value can be plotted over time (or plate run) to investigate the performance of the test, as shown in Fig. 7.2.

There are a large number of methods for trying to simplify, smooth and generally extract meaning from time series plots. However, these methods are beyond the scope of this text and can be found in statistical and epidemiological texts.

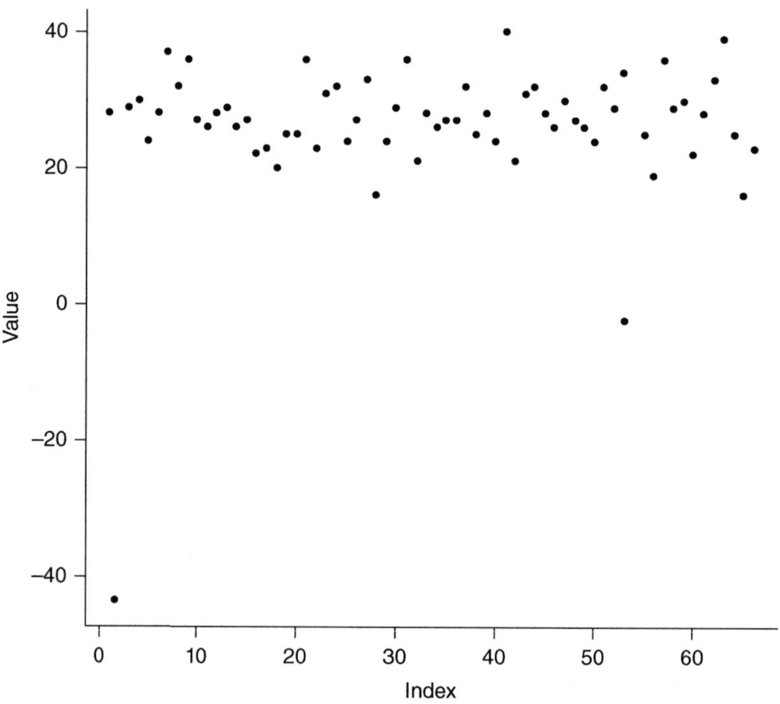

Fig. 10.14. Sixty-six measurements of the passage time of light made by Newcomb in 1882.

10.9 Statistical Tests of Normality

Several statistical tests are available to test data for normality and are available in most statistical packages. A significant result ($p < 0.05$) generally indicates a non-normal distribution while a non-significant result ($p > 0.05$) indicates that the data are consistent with a normal distribution.

The performance of statistical tests for normality is influenced by the size of the dataset. If the sample size is over 100 then you can be reasonably confident in the results. However, for smaller sample sizes visually inspecting plots (histograms and normal probability plots) and past experience will usually give as good an indication of whether the data are reasonably normal.

The two most common tests are briefly summarized here. There is a variety of other tests for normality.

10.9.1 Shapiro-Wilk test

The Shapiro-Wilk test is a useful test of normality in most situations. It is the ratio of two estimates of the variance of a normal distribution based on a random sample of n observations. It can be considered as roughly equivalent to measuring the straightness of the normal quantile–quantile plot and is commonly used for assessing normality of data.

10.9.2 Kolmogorov-Smirnov

The Kolmogorov-Smirnov test is an alternative test, based on the maximum difference between the observed distribution and expected cumulative-normal distribution. This test has relatively low power (unable to detect non-normality with small sample sizes) and the Shapiro-Wilk test is now generally the preferred test.

References

Chatfield, C. (1995) *Problem Solving: a statistician's guide*. Chapman & Hall, London.

Panko, R. (1998, revised 2008) What we know about spreadsheet errors. *Journal of End-user Computing* Special issue on Scaling up End User Development 10(2), 15–21. Available at: http://panko.shidler.hawaii.edu/SSR/Mypapers/whatknow.htm (Accessed 1 November 2014).

Preece, D.A. (1981) Distributions of final digits in data. *Journal of the Royal Statistical Society, Series D (The Statistician)* 30, 31–60.

Stigler, S.M. (1977) Do robust estimators work with real data? *The Annals of Statistics* 5(6), 1055–1098.

Tufte, E.R. (1983) *The Visual Display of Quantitative Information*. Graphics Press, Cheshire, Connecticut.

Tufte, E.R. (1997) *Visual and Statistical Thinking: displays of evidence for making decisions*. Graphics Press, Cheshire, Connecticut.

11 Introduction to Statistical Principles

11.1 Introduction

Research in animal health typically aims to make inferences about characteristics of a population in which we are interested. For example, we might be interested in the prevalence of a particular disease, or the mean value of a measurement such as body weight. We also want to know how accurate or precise our estimates of these values are. Alternatively, we might want to know if a particular treatment reduces the prevalence of disease, or increases body weight, or if a suspected risk factor increases the likelihood of disease occurrence and by how much.

It is usually impractical to attempt to address these questions by measuring every individual within a population of interest. Instead we enrol a sample of individuals from the target population, measure outcomes of interest on the sample and then use statistics to make inferences about the target population by estimating population characteristics with defined levels of precision. We can also estimate the likelihood that an observed difference between groups has occurred due to chance, or whether it is more likely to be due to the presence of a risk factor or treatment effect.

An understanding of statistical principles and analytical methods is therefore very important in achieving appropriate design and successful completion and publication for research projects and epidemiological studies. Areas of particular interest include generation of a statistical hypothesis that can be tested in the study, identification of treatment groups, sample size estimation, allocation of animals to groups, selection of outcomes to measure, choice of statistical tests and interpretation of findings.

An understanding of statistical principles is also essential for readers of scientific journal articles so they can critically evaluate and interpret the methods and results of such papers against relevant questions such as was the sample size sufficient to detect a real difference, was the analysis appropriate for the study design and the data, was the analysis undertaken correctly and are the results relevant to my practice.

Many professionals struggle with statistics. Difficulties may be exacerbated by the use of technical terminology or jargon with particular statistical meanings, a perception that statistical methods are a black box producing a binary answer (significant or non-significant), and lack of understanding of related principles derived from mathematic and probability theory.

This chapter is intended to provide an introduction to the theoretical principles that underpin statistics and review statistical concepts relevant to a wide variety of statistical methods. We use clear and non-complex terminology and aim to provide readers with sufficient familiarity with the core principles so they can identify issues, avoid common problems and determine when to seek further advice from individuals with statistical expertise.

11.2 What is 'Statistics'?

Statistics refers to 'the science of learning from data, and of measuring, controlling, and communicating uncertainty' (Davidian and Louis, 2012).

The term scientific method is used to describe an approach to research that begins with some form of hypothesis, which is then tested in an objective manner by collection of data that are analysed to determine whether the prior hypothesis is refuted or supported. If the observations differ greatly from the prior hypothesis, then the theory or hypothesis will need to be changed. This process of theory followed by observation followed by modification of the theory and further observation encapsulates the ongoing search for scientific truth.

Statistics underpins the scientific method and provides methods to support the design of research studies, collection and analysis of data and testing of hypotheses, as well as presentation and interpretation of results.

11.3 Sample versus Census

When undertaking a scientific investigation we generally want to make inferences about the target population of interest (e.g. the percentage of cattle in a village with antibodies to foot-and-mouth disease virus). However, we almost never take measurements on every single member of an entire population. Instead, we collect specimens or measurements from a sample of animals that are selected in some way from the target population. Even when we are dealing with a finite population, such as all cows on a farm or all dogs that attend a veterinary practice, we are still more likely to take a sample of the population, rather than a census.

In most cases we use sampling from the population because it is impractical to collect data on the entire population due to resource constraints (time, labour, money). It is also important to understand that the application of statistical methods makes it possible to obtain estimates of population values with perfectly acceptable precision by taking measurements from a sample and not attempting to measure the entire population.

Sampling from populations is a key mathematical concept that underpins statistics. However, a key aspect of sampling is that the sample must be representative of the population, in order to allow valid inference to be made from the sample estimates to the population values. See Chapter 8, Sampling Populations, for more information on selecting representative samples.

11.4 Probability Distributions and the Normal Curve

Figure 11.1 shows a histogram of 1000 data points created by taking random draws from a simulated distribution with a defined mean and standard deviation (SD). These 1000 data points are intended to represent actual measurements on a sample of 1000 subjects.

The smooth curve superimposed on the histogram is a (theoretical) normal curve derived from a mathematical formula using the same values for the mean and SD.

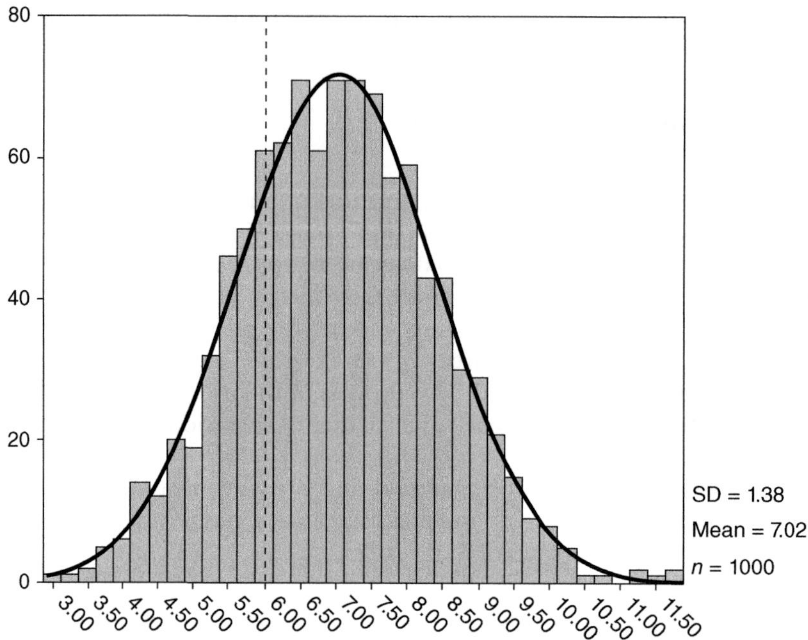

Fig. 11.1. Histogram of 1000 simulated measurements, with an overlaid normal curve with the same mean and standard deviation.

A vertical dotted line is drawn through a score of 6. From an examination of the 1000 data points, we find there are 243 data points with a value less than 6 (0.243 or 24.3% of the data points). Alternatively, we can use the mathematical model (the smooth line) to predict what proportion of data points would be expected to fall below 6, with a predicted value of 0.23 (very close to the observed number from the data points).

This sort of estimation from the mathematical model uses the area under the curve as an estimation of relative frequency. This is possible because the smooth curve is a probability density curve: the total area under the curve is equal to one (1) and the area under the curve between any defined set of values can be used as an estimate of the relative frequency (i.e. 23% of the area under the curve lies to the left of the dotted line).

Density curves are a way of using mathematical theory in combination with a sample of real-world observations to answer questions of interest such as those listed in Table 11.1.

The density curve used for the above examples is based on a normal distribution, but density curves can come in almost any shape. They simply represent idealized mathematical models for the distribution of a set of data. However, the normal probability distribution is commonly used in statistics because many continuous variables found in nature follow this distribution.

11.5 Standard Normal Distribution

A special form of normal distribution is the standard normal distribution, or z-distribution (Petrie and Watson, 2013). It has a mean = 0 and SD = 1. Any dataset that is

Table 11.1. Examples of the types of questions that can be answered from a normal density curve (see Fig. 11.2 for details).

Question	Answer	Figure
What proportions of data points are less than 6 and greater than 8 in the population represented by the sample of 1000 high-school scores above?	23.0% <6, 23.9% >8	11.2a
What is the threshold score separating the top 5% and bottom 5% of the population and the top and bottom 10% of the population?	Top 5% = 9.3	11.2b
	Bottom 5% = 4.3	11.2b
	Top 10% = 8.8	11.2c
	Bottom 10% = 5.3	11.2c
What proportion of data points lie within 1 SD from the mean?	68.3% between ±1 SD (5.64–8.4)	11.2d

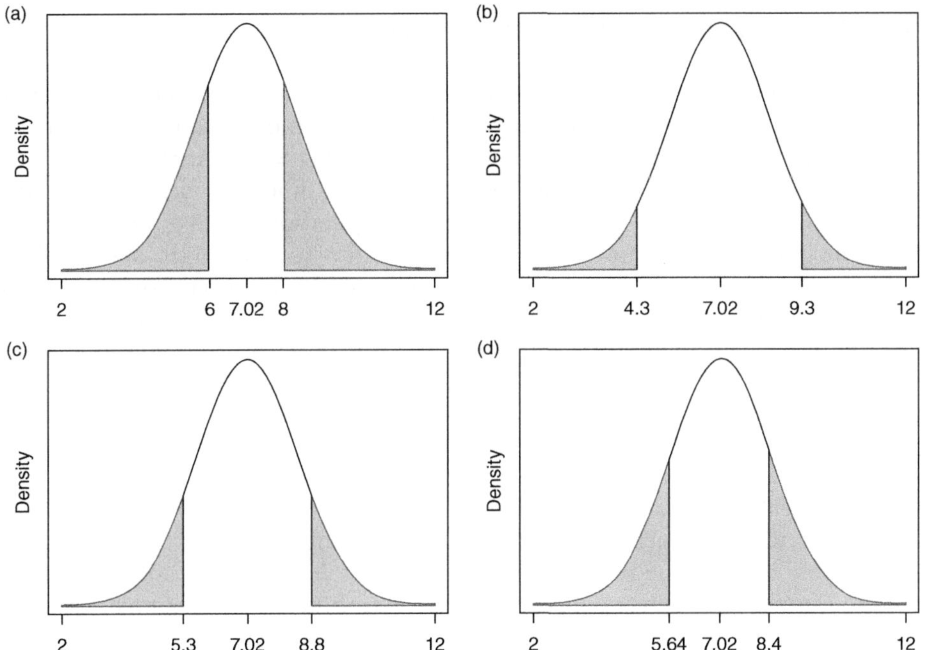

Fig. 11.2. Normal density curves for mean = 7.02 and standard deviation = 1.38, showing cut-points to answer the questions posed in Table 11.1: (a) percentages with scores <6 and >8; (b) cut-off scores for top and bottom 5%; (c) cut-off scores for top and bottom 10%; and (d) percentage within ±1 standard deviation of the mean.

normally distributed can be standardized or normalized (turned into a dataset with mean = 0 and SD = 1) by subtracting the mean from every point and then dividing every point by the SD. The benefit of doing this is that the units of the z-distribution are standard deviations. When combined with area under the curve estimations we can now estimate the proportion of the population that lie within 1, 2 or 3 standard deviations of the mean, for example.

Using the z-distribution we can see that 95% of the data points (or area under the curve) lie between −1.96 and +1.96 and 90% of the data points lie between −1.64 and

+1.64. These rules apply for any normally distributed dataset (i.e. 95% of the data lie between values that are 1.96 standard deviations either side of the mean).

We can now use this property of the z-distribution to identify the threshold scores for our data points from the 1000 observations (mean = 7.02, SD = 1.38). Given that 95% of the data points from a standard normal distribution lie within plus or minus 1.96*SD of the mean, the upper and lower limits of this range can be calculated in the original scale as:

Lower limit = 7.02 – 1.96*1.38 = 4.3

Upper limit = 7.02 + 1.96*1.38 = 9.7

11.6 Transition from Probability Towards Inference

11.6.1 Sampling distribution of a sample mean

Suppose we wished to measure serum cholesterol concentration in the entire population of dogs in Australia. Suppose further that the unknown and true population mean = μ (mu) and the unknown and true population SD = σ (sigma).

Note that it is common practice to use Greek symbols to denote population parameters (since we are not measuring the entire population we do not know the true value of the population parameters) and Roman letters to refer to the statistical outputs that we can estimate from measurements collected on a sample. For example, the standard deviation estimated from the sample data can be denoted using the Roman letter *s* and it is an estimate of the true but unknown population standard deviation, referred to by the Greek symbol sigma (σ). Similarly the variance of a sample is s^2 and it is an estimate of the population variance (σ^2).

We randomly select a sample of *n* observations and estimate a mean (mean_1). Then we obtain a separate and different sample of *n* observations and estimate a second mean (mean_2). It is highly likely that these two means will be similar but not identical, with the difference being due to chance or random error.

If we were to continue this process indefinitely, selecting all possible samples of size *n* and estimating the mean cholesterol concentration for each sample, we would end up with a dataset of values consisting entirely of the means from all of the samples. This is called the sampling distribution of mean cholesterol concentration in samples of size *n*.

11.6.2 The central limit theorem

The central limit theorem says that the sampling distribution of sample means computed for samples of size *n* has three important properties (Dawson-Saunders and Trapp, 1994; Petrie and Watson, 2013):

1. The mean of the sampling distribution (mean of all of the separate sample means) is identical to the population mean (μ).

2. The SD of the sampling distribution of sample means is equal to $\left(\sigma/\sqrt{n}\right)$. This quantity is known as the standard error of the mean (SEM) and can be estimated from

the sample SD and n. It reflects the variability of the sample means around the true population mean.
3. Provided that n is large enough, the shape of the sampling distribution is always approximately normal, no matter what the shape of the distribution of the underlying variable is. Even if the underlying distribution is skewed, for example, a sample size greater than about 30 is enough to make the sampling distribution normal in shape. This means that for a numerical variable, if the distribution of the population the sample is drawn from is normal (single peak and symmetrical), or if the sample size is reasonably large (>30), then the central limit theorem holds (i.e. the sampling distribution of means is normal).

We now have three different kinds of distribution, including:

- A population distribution with mean = μ and SD = σ.
- A distribution for each sample with mean = $\bar{x}$ and SD = s.
- A sampling distribution with mean = μ and SEM = $\left(\sigma/\sqrt{n}\right) \approx SD/\sqrt{n}$.

11.7 Application of the Central Limit Theorem

The sampling distribution and the central limit theorem provide the theoretical basis for the following assumptions:

- The mean of the sample is an unbiased estimate of the population mean.
- The SEM calculated from the sample mean, sample size and sample SD is a measure of the spread of all of the possible different sample means around our one estimate, if we were to repeat the sampling *ad infinitum* as per the sampling distribution.
- We can use the SEM to construct a confidence interval for the true population mean and for statistical hypothesis testing.

11.7.1 Confidence intervals

Assuming that our sample is randomly derived, then the sample mean is an unbiased estimator of the true but unknown population mean. The law of large numbers says that the sample mean must approach the population mean as the size of the sample increases. Given a specified sample size, how reliable might our estimate of the mean be?

Suppose we were able to select a random sample of 150 animals from the target population and we measure an outcome of interest in each animal (say body weight). Assume that the sampling strategy used was sufficient to be confident that the sample is representative of the population. Summary statistics for our sample are:

n = 150, mean = 80.7, SD = 9.2, SEM = 0.7512

It is reasonable to think that the sample mean may not be identical to the true but unknown mean of the population, but it should provide an unbiased estimate of the population mean.

In our discussion of the standard normal distribution, we found that 95% of the data points lie between the values –1.96 and +1.96. The SEM provides an estimate of the standard deviation of the distribution of sample means around the true but unknown population mean, so we can now use this value to estimate the 95% confidence interval for the true population mean, where:

- the lower 95% limit = 80.7 – 1.96*0.7512 = 80.7 – 1.47 = 79.2
- and the upper 95% limit = 80.7 + 1.47 = 82.2

The formal interpretation of this result is that if we took a large number of random samples, each with 150 subjects and estimated confidence intervals for each sample, 95% of those confidence intervals would include the true population mean (Motulsky, 2014).

The more commonly applied – and strictly speaking less correct – interpretation is that, based on this one sample, we are 95% confident that the mean of all animals in the population lies between 79.2 and 82.2.

It is worth noting that from our single sample of 150 measurements we can use either the SD or the SEM in conjunction with the z-distribution to estimate different intervals. An interval based on the sample SD is describing the spread of raw measurements around the sample mean. An interval based on the sample SEM is used to generate a confidence interval for the sample mean to provide an interval likely to include the true but unknown population mean.

11.8 Hypothesis Testing

Statistical significance testing involves the following steps (Motulsky, 2014):

1. State the null and alternative hypotheses.
2. Define a threshold value for declaring a p-value significant. This threshold value is commonly 0.05 and is termed the significance level or α.
3. Select an appropriate statistical test and calculate the p-value.
4. If the calculated p-value is less than the defined threshold the difference is defined as significant and the null hypothesis is rejected. If the calculated p-value is greater than α, the difference is said to be not significant and the null hypothesis is accepted.
5. If the null hypothesis is rejected then the alternative hypothesis is accepted by default.

The first step in statistical hypothesis testing is to formulate a null hypothesis, usually expressed as no effect or no difference. For example, we wish to see if treatment with additive A will cause an increase in body weight in animals of the same weight and gender and managed in the same way. We measure body weight in treated and control animals and express our null hypothesis as:

$$H_0: BW_{treated} = BW_{control}$$

We can also present the same null hypothesis in a slightly different way:

$$H_0: BW_{treated} - BW_{control} = 0$$

We then need to generate the alternative hypothesis that contradicts the null hypothesis such that the two hypotheses encompass all possible outcomes:

$$H_A: BW_{treated} \neq BW_{control}$$

or

$$H_A: BW_{treated} - BW_{control} \neq 0$$

Note that the alternative is the complement of the null hypothesis, so that together the null and alternate hypotheses cover all possible outcomes and consequently one of the two must be true. Under conventional statistical theory we then apply the statistical test to the null hypothesis.

11.8.1 Hypothesis testing logic

Hypothesis testing provides a means of assessing the likelihood that the null hypothesis is true. Generally, we do an experiment because we believe the treatment will have an effect (i.e. animals will grow faster, fewer vaccinated animals will die, infection rate will fall, etc.). However, statistical tests are based on evaluating the null hypothesis, and often the null hypothesis is phrased in the expectation that it will be disproved as a result of the study (e.g. treatment has no effect, vaccine does not alter disease rate, etc.).

Applying a statistical test will generate a test statistic. A t-test will produce a t-statistic, analysis of variance will produce an F-statistic, and so on. The test statistic is a random variable with a known distribution such as the normal distribution. This distribution can then be used to generate a probability, or p-value.

The p-value is the probability of getting an outcome as extreme as, or more extreme than the observed outcome, under the assumption that the null hypothesis is true. If the observed outcome is unlikely (p-value is low), then this is evidence against H_0 and in favour of H_A. The smaller the p-value, the stronger the evidence against H_0, based on the data.

In most cases we then compare the calculated p-value with a fixed value that we have pre-determined to represent a threshold. This threshold is called the significance level and is denoted by alpha (α). A common threshold value for alpha is 0.05 (5%).

Note that if we accept alpha of 0.05, then we accept that even if the null hypothesis were true, we could obtain an outcome as extreme or more extreme than the one actually observed up to 5% of the time. If the calculated p-value is less than the predefined alpha of 0.05, then we can say the test results are statistically significant at $\alpha = 0.05$.

For our previous example we used a two-sided test. However, hypothesis tests may also be one-sided, where:

$$H_0: A \leq B \quad \text{and} \quad H_A: A > B$$

or

$$H_0: A \geq B \quad \text{and} \quad H_A: A < B$$

In most cases a two-sided hypothesis test is preferable, unless there are compelling reasons to use a one-sided (often called a one-tailed) test. This is because we can rarely be absolutely certain that the treatment will act only in a certain direction. As much as we may believe that our treatment will reduce blood cholesterol levels or increase body weight, there is often a possibility that the actual effect could be in the unexpected direction. Therefore, it is essential to allow for differences in either direction. Also, a difference that would not be significant in a two-tailed test may be significant in a one-tailed test, leading to concerns that people may be trying to justify use of a one-tailed test in order to benefit from the increased power. This occurs because under a one-sided test the threshold value on the probability distribution occurs at α (0.05), instead of $\alpha/2$ (0.025) under a two-sided test (because α is split under both tails in the two-tailed test).

11.8.2 Test statistics

Almost all statistical tests involve the same general approach to estimation and interpretation of the test statistic.

The test statistic is based on two components: a numerator representing the effect size and a denominator representing a standard error term.

In a conventional t-test comparing two group means the effect size is the difference between the two means and the denominator is the standard error of the difference. In other tests, the numerator and denominator may be calculated in different ways but they will always represent broadly the effect size and standard error terms.

The larger the absolute value of the test statistic, the more likely the test will return a significant p-value. Increasing the effect size and/or reducing the standard error term will logically each contribute to making the test statistic larger.

Measures that will make the standard error term smaller include reducing the variability in measuring the outcomes (increasing precision) and increasing the sample size.

11.9 Choice of Statistical Tests

So far we have discussed significance tests in general terms. There are a large number of different statistical tests available, and the choice of which statistical test to use will depend on the nature of the data and the types of comparisons being made.

Test selection is determined by three main factors: the number and nature of explanatory variables, the nature of the outcome variable being analysed and whether or not the outcome variable can be considered to be normally distributed. There may also be variations depending on whether or not observations are paired or matched. Common types of statistical tests and the circumstances where they are used are summarized in Table 11.2 (Dawson-Saunders and Trapp, 1994; Petrie and Watson, 2013).

11.10 Statistical Error and Statistical Power

Conventional statistical tests often use a significance threshold of $\alpha = 0.05$, meaning that when the test returns a p-value less than 0.05 we interpret the result as being statistically significant.

If we use 5% significance tests repeatedly when H_0 is in fact true (and everything else behaves as it should), then 5% of the time the tests will return a significant p-value in error and the other 95% of the time the test should correctly return a non-significant p-value.

11.10.1 Statistical error

There are two types of statistical error, as summarized below and in Fig. 11.3 (Dawson-Saunders and Trapp, 1994; Petrie and Watson, 2013):

- Type I error or alpha error or α. Commonly accepted as $\alpha = 0.05$. This is the probability of rejecting H_0 when in fact H_0 is true. If we were to conduct repeated tests, we would expect to erroneously reject the null hypothesis 5% of the time.
- Type II error or beta error or β. This is the probability of failing to reject H_0 when in fact H_A is true. Commonly accepted as $\beta = 0.2$.

11.10.2 Statistical power

The probability of making a type II error is termed beta (β) and $(1 - \beta)$ is termed power (Petrie and Watson, 2013).

Table 11.2. Summary of statistical tests appropriate for different data types.

Test type	Categorical (counts) outcome	Continuous outcome
Simple tests (single explanatory variable)	Chi-square test Fisher's exact test Kruskal-Wallis Mann-Whitney U Mantel-Haenszel chi-square	t-test One-way analysis of variance
Multiple explanatory variables	Logistic regression Poisson regression	Multiple linear regression Analysis of variance Analysis of covariance Generalized linear models (GLMs)
Paired data	McNemar's test Wilcoxon signed ranks test Repeated measures logistic regression	Paired t-test Repeated measures ANOVA
Complex data	Mixed-effects logistic regression Multi-level models	Mixed-effects linear regression Multi-level models Survival analysis Spatial statistics

		Truth in the population	
		H_0 not true	H_0 true
Results of study	Reject H_0	Correct	Type I error (α)
	Accept H_0	Type II error (β)	Correct

Fig. 11.3. Types of statistical error.

Power is defined as the probability of obtaining a statistically significant result in a study given that there is a biologically real effect in the population being studied.

Power = $(1 - \beta)$

The probability of a type I error is defined by α and traditionally set at $p = 0.05$. Commonly used levels for α include 0.001, 0.01 and 0.05. As α is lowered, type I errors (mistakenly rejecting H_0 when the groups are actually not different) become less likely but type II errors (missing a real difference) become more likely.

Beta is commonly set within the range of 0.05 to 0.2. If $\beta = 0.1$, the analysis has a 10% chance of missing a real association or difference. Alternatively this can be described as a power of 90%, which implies that the analysis has a 90% chance of detecting an effect if an effect exists in the population.

There is always a trade-off between α and β. If you make α smaller to minimize the risk of a type I error, you increase the likelihood of a type II error (β becomes larger). Current practice is to devote huge attention to type I error and largely ignore type II error. Type I error is far less likely to occur because most experiments are designed such that the null hypothesis is highly likely to be false.

In recent decades there has been a growing awareness of the need to ensure reasonable statistical power in planning research studies. In fact along with 95% confidence intervals and 5% significance tests, 80% power is rapidly becoming another standard in statistical inference and funding bodies have begun to demand that power analyses and sample size determination be performed during project planning. This helps to ensure that studies are designed effectively and that if the effect being studied is in fact real, then there is a high likelihood of the study detecting it. As a result funding bodies can be more confident in effective use of money.

Power analysis can be very effectively used in the planning phase of a study to determine how many subjects/animals are required in order to be confident of achieving a statistical power of 0.8.

It may seem useful to try for more than 80% power but to do so usually makes it very difficult to also achieve $\alpha = 0.05$ (i.e. increases the risk of type I error) because of the conflict between the two sources of statistical error.

11.10.3 Power analysis

Many people only think of power analysis as a means to determining the optimal sample size requirements in the planning phase of a study. Although this application is arguably the most common (and perhaps most important), power analysis can be used to estimate any of the contributing parameters provided values can be provided for the other parameters. There are five parameters involved in power analysis and once values are set for any four, the remaining parameter can be estimated.

The five component parameters are:

- α;
- β (power = $1 - \beta$);
- effect size (ES);

- sample size; and
- precision/variation.

In order to estimate a value for any one of these variables, you need to be able to provide values for the others. For example, to estimate a sample size needed to detect a difference between two means, you will need to provide values for α, β, effect size and variability.

Defining β and χ

Type I error can only occur when the null hypothesis is true. Most of the time in experimental studies, the likelihood of the null hypothesis being true is actually small. As a result type I errors are probably rare and efforts to control type I error by making α more stringent are probably unwarranted. As a result it is suggested that α be set at 0.05 under most circumstances (more to fit with traditional expectations) and that under some experimental objectives it may well be preferable to make α larger rather than smaller (i.e. go to $\alpha = 0.1$ or $\alpha = 0.2$, etc.).

There are no specific rules regarding power $(1 - \beta)$ though power surely must be greater than 0.5. Traditional convention is to set desired power at 0.8 ($\beta = 0.2$). This means that in the scenario where the null hypothesis is false, the null hypothesis is four times more likely to be rejected (i.e. a correct outcome) than accepted erroneously (0.8 versus 0.2). It may well be desirable to have power >0.8, but in practical terms it is often prohibitively expensive in terms of sample size to achieve this.

There are occasions where you may choose alternative values for α and β. A classic example is in performing screening tests to screen a large number of candidate drugs to look for the next wonder drug. It is much more important to avoid making a type II error than a type I error. In this situation you may wish to maximize power (reduce β to as small a value as possible) and accept a much larger risk of type I error.

Effect size and variance estimation

Common ways to generate values of effect size and variance for use in power analyses include:

- from previously published studies of similar outcomes;
- from a pilot study; or
- from expert opinion.

Applications of power analysis

Power analysis serves the following functions.

1. Estimate sample size required to detect an estimated effect size having set α and β. Performed during the planning phase of an experiment. This is the most effective way to use power analysis – to run scenarios and inform sample size requirements before the project is begun. It is important to run a variety of scenarios (generally under different assumptions concerning effect size and variance) to get a feel for a sample size that will be robust and likely to deliver good power if there is a difference.

2. Post hoc power analyses (performed after completion of the study). This is a more controversial use of power analysis. Using the findings of the study as input parameter values for effect size and variability in estimating required sample size for a future study is legitimate since it is the same as the first application above.

Using the findings of a completed study to estimate achieved power is generally considered to be inappropriate. The findings will simply be consistent with the p-value derived from statistical tests and will not add any additional value.

11.10.4 Strategies to increase statistical power without increasing sample size

Using power analysis to calculate required sample size often results in an estimate that exceeds practicality and/or budget.

There are a range of strategies that can be considered as ways to try to maximize statistical power or to increase power for a given sample size.

1. Maximize the achieved or target effect size. It may not be possible to achieve a greater effect size.

2. Increase α (choose a less stringent significance threshold). This is often not possible but may be appropriate in selected situations such as screening tests.

3. Change an experimental hypothesis from two-tailed to one-tailed. This should only be considered in situations where there is clear and defensible justification for expecting a one-directional effect. Most of the time one-tailed tests are not justified and this should be avoided where possible.

4. Reduce the necessary confidence level. This is only reasonable under some conditions such as bioequivalence testing where 90% confidence levels are commonly applied instead of 95%.

5. Use continuous variables instead of dichotomous or categorical variables. If continuous variables can be measured with reasonable precision then use of parametric statistical tests may produce better statistical power than non-parametric tests.

6. Increase precision of data or reduce variation and standard error terms. It may be possible to use a more advanced measurement method or even to measure a different variable with more precision. Reducing data variation will also allow a smaller sample size for a given power.

7. Use paired or repeated measurements involving the same subjects. In some study designs it may be possible to alter the design slightly to involve paired measurements (before and after). This reduces data variation and hence required sample size.

8. Use unequal group sizes. In most circumstances using equal group sizes gives the greatest power for the total number of subjects. In some cases it may be easier or cheaper to increase the size of one group and not the other. Many case-control studies involve control groups that are considerably larger than the case groups.

9. Incorporate covariates and/or blocking variables. Under optimal conditions incorporating blocking variables can partition variation and effectively increase the effect size and reduce residual variation.

10. Ensure explanatory variables are not correlated with each other. Correlation between explanatory variables can reduce statistical power.

The strategies listed above are examples that may be used to maximize the chance of a study producing results which include statistically significant and meaningful results. Some involve making changes to study design and these must be considered with caution since they may actually alter the focus of the research objectives.

11.11 Conclusion

Statistical theory provides the fundamental basis for design and analysis of scientific studies. A basic understanding of statistics and the application of hypothesis testing is essential to ensure proper study design and the correct interpretation of results. Although statistics has its own jargon and can seem quite mystifying to the uninitiated, it has a logical basis in the practical application of mathematical and probability theory. The theory of sampling distributions and the central limit theorem are fundamental to all statistical applications and an understanding of these basic principles is essential for the appropriate application and interpretation of statistical tests in any scientific study.

A variety of interactive epidemiological calculators can be accessed via the AusVet website and used for performing simple statistical tests, power analyses and sample size estimations (Sergeant, 2013).

References

Davidian, M. and Louis, T.A. (2012) Why statistics? *Science* 336(6077), 12 doi: 10.1126/science.1218685.

Dawson-Saunders, B. and Trapp, R.G. (1994) *Basic Clinical Biostatistics*. Appleton and Lange, East Norwalk, Connecticut.

Motulsky, H. (2014) *Intuitive Biostatistics*, 3rd edn. Oxford University Press, New York.

Petrie, A. and Watson, P. (2013) *Statistics for Veterinary and Animal Science*, 3rd edn. Wiley and Blackwell, Oxford, UK.

Sergeant, E.S.G. (2013) Epitools epidemiological calculators. AusVet Animal Health Services. Available at: http://epitools.ausvet.com.au (accessed 7 November 2013).

12 Animal Health Surveillance

12.1 Introduction

Surveillance of animal health (and disease) is an important aspect of veterinary activity and also of information to assist in policy determination and decision making. Surveillance can take a wide variety of forms and produces many different outputs, all of which contribute to our knowledge and understanding of disease occurrence and distribution and factors affecting the health of livestock and other species.

At a fundamental level, surveillance information is critical for many of the decisions required to be made about disease control and prevention on a day-to-day basis.

For example, before embarking on a programme to control and perhaps eventually eradicate a disease, such as foot-and-mouth disease, from a country, it is essential to know things such as: how much of the disease is there; what impact is it having on animals and their owners and on the country as a whole; is the amount of disease increasing, decreasing or unchanging; where does it occur; are there areas where it does not occur or is less common, etc.

Similarly, once a control programme is initiated, decision makers need to know whether or not progress is being made and are goals being achieved. For example, is the number of infected herds decreasing, are free or low-prevalence areas remaining free and is the prevalence among animals decreasing.

The answers to these questions (and many others) are provided by surveillance.

This chapter provides a general introduction to the principles of animal health surveillance, while subsequent chapters provide specific guidance on planning and analysis of surveys for estimating prevalence of disease or demonstrating freedom from disease.

12.2 What is Population Health Surveillance?

In the broadest sense, population health surveillance is a mechanism applied to collect and interpret data on the health of animal populations, to describe accurately their health status and to support decision making. This concept is shown in Fig. 12.1, where stakeholders are the people whose livelihood depends on consistent and reliable animal productivity, government regulators with the responsibility for protection of trade and natural resources, and groups whose interest lies in environmental protection.

The terms population, monitoring and surveillance are defined in the OIE *Terrestrial Animal Health Code* (OIE, 2011).

Surveillance is the systematic ongoing collection, collation and analysis of information related to animal health and the timely dissemination of information to those who need to know so that action can be taken (OIE, 2011). Surveillance implies an active response to a defined outcome of the surveillance activities.

Monitoring is the intermittent performance and analysis of routine measurements and observations, aimed at detecting changes in the environment or health status of a population (OIE, 2011). Monitoring implies limited or no response to observations, regardless of the findings.

A population is a group of units sharing a common defined characteristic.

The term population health surveillance can be used in a wider sense to incorporate both surveillance and monitoring activities as well as the collection and interpretation of data about the structure of the animal populations of interest. Population health surveillance also is not limited to surveillance of disease, *per se*, but includes surveillance and monitoring of the health status of the population. Figure 12.2 shows the relationships among the components of a population health surveillance programme. This figure incorporates the OIE *Code* concepts of providing an effective

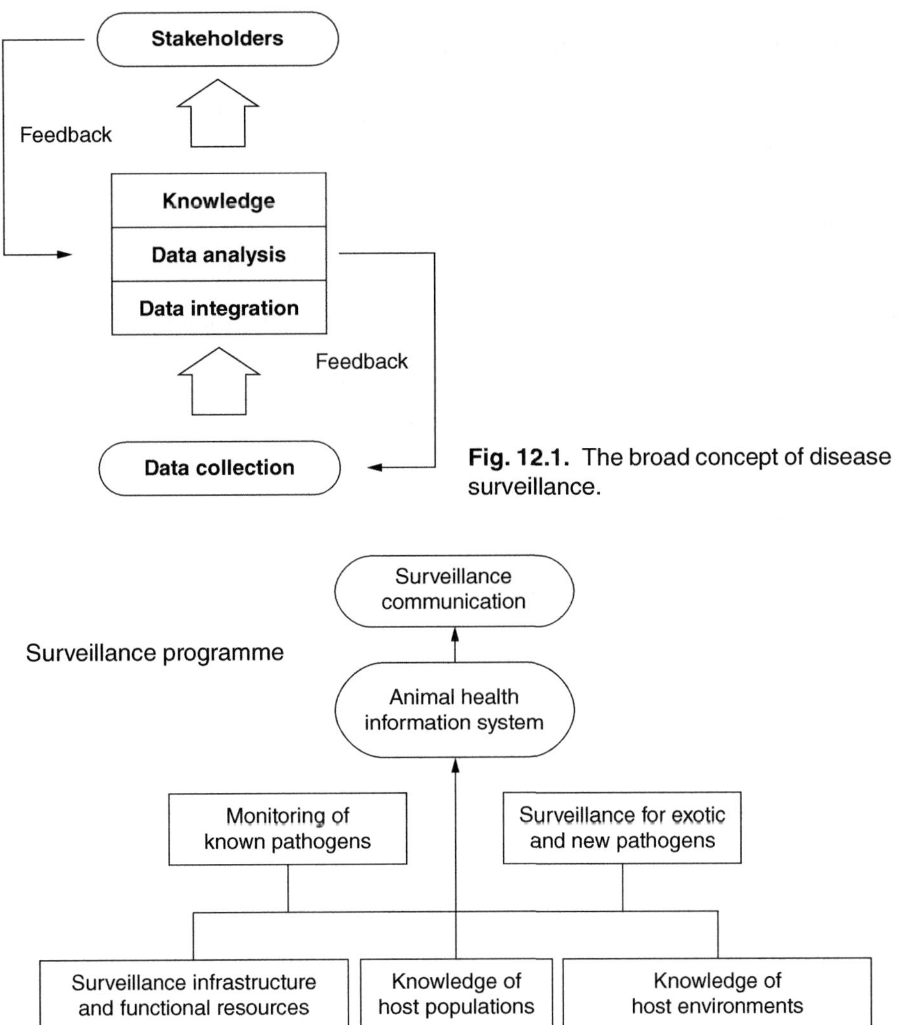

Fig. 12.1. The broad concept of disease surveillance.

Fig. 12.2. Relationships among different components of a population health surveillance programme incorporating OIE *Code* concepts.

surveillance infrastructure, as well as including a description of host population and environmental characteristics. In the rest of this chapter we will not distinguish between surveillance and monitoring, as the basic principles apply equally to both.

Figure 12.2 outlines the fact that surveillance requires supporting infrastructure and resources in the form of appropriately trained personnel, adequately equipped laboratories, legal support structures, transport and communication networks. Effective application of this infrastructure requires a good knowledge of susceptible/carrier host populations and their environments. Building on this foundation are the various surveillance and monitoring activities that lead to accurate knowledge of the whereabouts and problems caused by various pathogens. Last, but not least, all this information must be captured, analysed and communicated to relevant stakeholders to complete the objective of disease management.

12.2.1 Common features of surveillance

Surveillance comes in many different sizes and shapes. However, some of the common features include:

- systematic collection of relevant information;
- timeliness of data collection;
- ongoing, continuous data collection or periodic or on-off programmes depending on purpose;
- practicality, consistency and timeliness of methods rather than requiring absolute accuracy;
- analysis, interpretation and communication of the data;
- planned use of the data for decision making; and
- a focus on measuring level of diseases (or changes in level of disease) or on detection of disease incursion/occurrence.

12.3 Why Do We Carry Out Surveillance?

Surveillance is undertaken to obtain information about a disease or potential pathogen. This leads to the question: why do we need the information? In most cases, the information is required to help with decision making in relation to a particular disease or diseases. This could be high-level decisions by the government veterinary services, or lower-level decisions by farmers and their advisors.

The sort of decisions required includes such things as:

- Should we implement a control programme for this disease?
- Is an existing control programme working or does it need to be changed?
- Should we allow importation of animals or their products from another country (or farm)?
- How much is a particular disease costing farmers? Or the community?
- Should we impose controls on the movements of animals because of this disease?

Decision makers need relevant and good quality information derived from surveillance in order to make optimal decisions.

However, good decisions do not just depend on the technical data. In addition, decision makers must consider the political, economic and social aspects of the decision, so that the decision is a balance of these various factors.

In this context, the primary purpose of population health surveillance is to provide cost-effective information for assessing and managing risks associated with trade in animals and products (intra- and international), animal production efficiency and public health. The information thus generated can then be used to support rational decision making by government veterinary services.

This statement of purpose is consistent with the OIE *Code* and international perceptions of what disease surveillance is meant to achieve in animal production systems.

The specific aims of surveillance programmes may be many and varied, depending on the disease of interest, the overall purpose of the surveillance and the specific circumstances in the country or region where the surveillance is being undertaken.

Surveillance objectives can be categorized into one of four broad objectives based on whether the target diseases are present or not present in a country or region.

For diseases that are present in a country or region surveillance objectives include the following.

1. Accurate description of the distribution and occurrence of diseases relevant to disease control and domestic and international movement of animals and products.
2. Detection of cases of disease, usually as part of an ongoing control or eradication programme for protection of public health.

For diseases that are not present in a country or region, surveillance objectives include:

3. Rapid detection of new, emerging and exotic infectious diseases in animals.
4. Demonstration of freedom from diseases relevant to domestic and international movement of animals and products.

The above objectives are unambiguous for what surveillance is meant to achieve, whether the activity be undertaking a survey to describe the distribution and prevalence of an important disease, collecting information to ensure that disease zones are maintained, or assessing success of eradication or other disease control measures.

12.4 Some Terminology

A variety of names have been used to describe different types of surveillance, reflecting the many objectives for which surveillance is used. Terms such as passive surveillance, active surveillance, general surveillance, targeted surveillance and, more recently, scanning surveillance (Scudamore, 2002) are used, but it is not always clear what they mean. A brief explanation of each is given below. A more complete discussion on passive and active surveillance is contained in the text *Survey Toolbox for Livestock Diseases – A Practical Manual and Software Package* (Cameron, 1999). A comprehensive surveillance programme will comprise a combination of many approaches to the gathering of surveillance data.

12.4.1 Classification by how the data are collected

One common way of classifying a surveillance system is according to the way in which the data are collected, either passively or actively.

Passive surveillance

Passive surveillance is the secondary use of routinely collected data that was generated for some other purpose.

In other words, the collation of information on specific animal diseases is a by-product of more general disease investigation activities. These include the routine gathering of information on disease incidents, such as requests for assistance from farmers, reports from field officers and findings from tests performed on specimens submitted to diagnostic laboratories, or examined for research purposes. Passive surveillance is very useful for early detection of emerging diseases and often provides a general picture of the disease situation in a population. However, passive surveillance data is not adequate to quantify the level (prevalence/intensity) or geographic distribution of a disease, nor can this type of surveillance be used to reliably demonstrate absence of a particular disease from a given area.

Depending on the available data and the specific disease(s) of concern, passive surveillance may provide some indication of trends of disease over time or whether a disease occurs commonly or not.

Examples of passive surveillance activities include routine disease investigations and abattoir meat inspections.

Routine disease investigations are usually initiated when a farmer seeks assistance with a disease problem from either private veterinarians or government veterinary services for the diagnosis and treatment of a disease in his/her animals. Incidental to the diagnosis and treatment of the case is that surveillance data can be captured about the case as part of a broader passive surveillance programme. The surveillance data may be captured in any of several ways, including through collation of laboratory reports, reporting of investigations by government field officers, compulsory notification of specific disease by private veterinarians, or through veterinary practice sentinel networks.

Abattoir meat inspection is primarily undertaken to ensure quality of the meat and that it is fit for human consumption. However, during the inspection process specific disease conditions may be detected, resulting in condemnation of the affected carcass or part of the carcass. This data are recorded as the reason for condemnation but also provide surveillance data for the recorded disease conditions.

Active surveillance

Active surveillance is surveillance that is designed and initiated by the primary user of the data.

Active surveillance involves the active collection of data on the presence of a specific disease or pathogen within a defined animal population. In contrast to passive surveillance, the primary purpose of an active surveillance activity is for surveillance.

Active disease surveillance includes deliberate and comprehensive searching for evidence of disease in a specified population and, in some instances, provides the data required to demonstrate that the specified population is free of a specific disease. Active disease surveillance programmes may be non-specific, catch-all activities aimed at detecting any significant disease occurrences, or may target specific diseases or may monitor the progress of specific disease control or eradication efforts. In order to maximize the value of active surveillance, it should be based on survey techniques that provide representative samples of the population of interest. Appropriate analysis provides valid measures of infection estimates, such as prevalence.

Examples of active surveillance activities are provided here.

A serological survey to determine seroprevalence for bovine brucellosis represents an active surveillance activity that requires planning and selecting a representative sample of herds and animals, field visits to collect samples and laboratory testing of the samples, all at the cost of the government veterinary authorities. However, the results of a properly conducted survey will provide a precise estimate of the prevalence and distribution of brucellosis in the population of interest.

A survey of salmon farms to demonstrate population freedom from infectious salmon anaemia virus (ISAv) requires careful planning and implementation to ensure representative samples at both farm and fish levels and significant cost for laboratory sampling, but produces a quantitative estimate of the level of confidence that ISAv would be detected if present at a specified prevalence in the population.

Active surveillance activities have the advantage that they are planned and designed for a particular purpose, so that the quality of the resulting data is usually much better than for passive surveillance. In fact, a properly designed active surveillance programme should be able to support quantitative estimates of disease prevalence (with confidence intervals) and/or confidence of detecting disease if it is present. The downside of active surveillance is that it is usually considerably more expensive than passive surveillance. For passive surveillance the primary cost of data collection is borne by whoever initiates the activity (the farmer for on-farm disease investigation, the abattoir or inspection authorities for abattoir meat inspection). The government authorities may contribute to the cost through provision of laboratory services or by a payment for access to data, but these costs are relatively low. In contrast, the user of the data (usually the government veterinary services or the affected industry) for active surveillance is responsible for the entire cost of the activity. In some cases this can involve substantial cost for field activities to collect samples and for testing samples in the laboratory.

Distinctions between active and passive surveillance are not always clear. Passive surveillance is not always totally passive and active surveillance can include activities other than planned activities (e.g. investigation of disease outbreak reports). Consistent understanding of surveillance activities is further complicated by combinations of terms, such as targeted active surveillance when referring to surveys aimed at specific pathogens, or risk-based surveillance, referring to preferential sampling of subpopulations more likely to be infected.

12.4.2 Classification by disease focus

An alternative approach to classifying surveillance as active or passive, based on how the data are collected, is to classify surveillance according to the disease focus of the activity (Scudamore, 2002).

Targeted surveillance

Targeted surveillance is surveillance that is focused on a specific disease or pathogen. It collects information on a specific disease or condition so that its absence can be substantiated or its presence within a defined population can be measured.

In the above example of an active surveillance programme for bovine brucellosis, serum samples would be collected and tested using a serological test for brucellosis. The survey would provide no data on the occurrence of other diseases (foot-and-mouth disease, tuberculosis, etc.) because it is specifically targeted at brucellosis. To obtain information about other diseases, they would also need to be targeted and this may require different samples and/or testing requirements.

Similarly, the ISAv survey provides no information about the occurrence of bacterial kidney disease or other salmon pathogens unless they are also specifically included in the survey design.

It is also important to recognize that although it is possible to target multiple diseases with a single targeted survey, the survey design for different diseases and purposes may not be compatible, so inclusion of multiple diseases is not always feasible. In particular, surveys to demonstrate freedom from a disease rarely provide good data for estimating prevalence and vice versa. In situations where there are multiple diseases of interest but with a different purpose to the surveillance it is best to design separate surveys best to achieve the different purposes. In some situations it may be relatively simple to extend a survey, for example, where it is simply a matter of doing another test on the same sample. However, if different samples are required this will increase the complexity and cost of the surveillance, so should only be done if the secondary disease is of sufficient importance.

General surveillance

General surveillance is surveillance not focused on any particular disease, but rather capable of detecting any disease or pathogen.

General surveillance is ongoing work, which maintains continuous observation over the endemic disease profile of a susceptible population, so that unexpected changes can be detected and acted upon as rapidly as possible. In addition, laboratory diagnostic data may be used to define a threshold level of undiagnosed syndromes that would trigger in-depth investigations to try to characterize them. For example, if gill disease in fish exceeded a given prevalence, this could trigger a diagnostic investigation to determine whether or not this is indicative of a new disease. Such surveillance of disease syndromes (common clinical signs) could also be collected from field officers or harvesters/farmers.

The passive disease investigation systems described earlier represent a form of general surveillance. In this case, affected animals may be subjected to a wide variety of investigative tools and tests to arrive at a diagnosis, so that any of a wide range of diseases (including previously undiagnosed diseases) may be detected through this system.

An important feature of general surveillance is that it is able to detect new or emerging diseases in addition to detection of diseases that are already known to be endemic in the population. This is a clear difference from targeted surveillance, which is only able to detect the specific disease or agent being targeted. This arises from the different tests used for disease detection in targeted versus general surveillance.

1. For targeted surveillance specific tests for the disease of concern are used, usually to provide a simple yes/no categorization. For example:
   - i. polymerase chain reaction (PCR) tests for agent DNA;
   - ii. ELISA serological tests for antibodies to the agent; or
   - iii. culture of the agent on artificial or cell-culture media.
2. For general surveillance, primary tests are of a more general nature and usually able to detect multiple different diseases, which may then be confirmed by specific follow-up tests. For example:
   - i. clinical examination;
   - ii. post-mortem examination; or
   - iii. histopathology.

As general surveillance describes the current disease profile, it can also be used to help inform and develop targeted surveillance projects.

Both general and targeted surveillance are necessary components of a local or national animal disease surveillance programme. A wholly targeted programme is not feasible, because it would be too expensive to carry out on more than a select few diseases. General surveillance is useful for both detection of new and exotic diseases and for monitoring the situation with known endemic diseases. General surveillance can also increase awareness of disease, and can also help establish links between farmers and those providing clinical and preventive health care. Where these elements are weak, or not yet established (e.g. in newly developing livestock sectors), there is a stronger case for targeted surveillance. Since resources for targeted surveillance are always limited, risk assessments should be used to design effective targeted surveillance programmes. If the effort is spread thinly across all farms then the frequency and/or intensity of surveillance will be insufficient for a prolonged period of time. Effort should focus on populations at greatest risk of exposure to the targeted pathogen/disease.

Different types of surveillance are often better suited for different purposes, as summarized in Table 12.1. For example, general surveillance is the main method by which new and exotic diseases are detected, while targeted surveillance is more useful for detecting cases of disease or demonstrating freedom from a specific disease of concern. Both general and targeted surveillance activities can provide useful information to help describe endemic disease occurrence.

One exception to the categorization in Table 12.1 is that in some cases, targeted programmes can be used for detection of known diseases that are thought to

Table 12.1. Relationship between surveillance objectives and surveillance types.

	Surveillance type	
Surveillance objective	General	Targeted
1. Detect exotic/emerging diseases	✓	
2. Detecting cases of specific diseases		✓
3. Describe endemic diseases	✓	✓
4. Demonstrate freedom		✓

be exotic to the population. For example, in the case of BSE in Canada or the USA, targeted surveillance programmes were in place to demonstrate freedom in accordance with standards described in the OIE *Code* at the time (Objective 4). However, in both countries, BSE was detected (Objective 1), because the disease was already present in the respective populations. This is an example of the dichotomy of disease detection and freedom – targeted surveillance set up to demonstrate freedom from a specific disease may detect the disease if it is present and conversely targeted surveillance to detect a specific disease of concern can provide useful data for demonstrating freedom from the disease (assuming it is not detected).

12.4.3 Data source versus disease focus

It is important to remember that the above definitions for active, passive, general and targeted surveillance are simply ways of trying to classify surveillance activities. It is also important to realize that these categories are not mutually exclusive and that most activities can be categorized by both data source and disease focus, as shown in Table 12.2. In addition, some activities do not fit neatly into a single category and may have some characteristics of more than one category.

12.4.4 Population coverage

Another important characteristic of a surveillance system is its population coverage, or the degree to which all elements of the population are included in the system.

The population coverage of a surveillance system is the proportion of the population of interest that is included in the surveillance system.

Comprehensive (or complete) coverage occurs where the entire population is included in the surveillance, indicating a census approach. Conversely, incomplete coverage implies that a sampling approach has been used, so that not all members of the population are included in the surveillance.

For example, a farmer-reporting system can be assumed to have comprehensive coverage if it can be assumed that every animal in the population may be observed by a farmer during a given time period and that if observed the farmer might notify abnormalities detected.

An active survey of the population will have complete coverage if every member of the population is surveyed (such as a survey of all aquaculture farms in a region,

Table 12.2. Examples of surveillance activity classification.

	Origin of information	
Disease focus	Active	Passive
Targeted	Structured serological survey to estimate prevalence of bovine brucellosis	Use of dairy factory bulk milk cell counts to assess progress in mastitis control programmes
General	Survey of veterinary practitioners about disease diagnoses	Field veterinary investigation of farmer-reported disease events

where the farm is the unit of interest). More commonly, a population survey relies on a sample from the population, so that only some animals are selected, and therefore has incomplete coverage.

It is also important to note that while a surveillance system might be considered to have complete coverage, such as the farmer-reporting system mentioned above, not all animals in the population will have equal likelihood of being detected. The sensitivity (probability of a positive report if disease occurs) of the surveillance may vary considerably among individuals.

In extensive production systems, animals may be observed only occasionally and often from a distance, so that the likelihood of detecting disease is much lower than for more intensive systems, where animals are observed closely on a daily basis.

Even if a farmer observes something abnormal, not all farmers are equally likely to notify or have it investigated.

Surveillance systems with high population coverage are usually better than low-coverage systems for early detection of incursions of exotic or emerging diseases. This is because we cannot always predict where exotic or new diseases will occur, so the higher our coverage of the population the more likely we are to detect it. However, achieving high population coverage usually relies on lower-cost methods, such as farmer reporting or clinical disease investigation, rather than active sampling and testing of animals. This results in lower sensitivity for detection of individual infected animals, but better overall sensitivity and earlier detection because of the inclusion of the whole population in the surveillance system, which is uneconomic and impractical for an active sampling scheme.

12.4.5 Representativeness

Another important characteristic of a surveillance system is its representativeness of the population of interest.

The representativeness of a surveillance system is a measure of how well the surveillance sample resembles the population of interest in regards to some characteristic(s) of interest.

Representativeness can be measured in terms of systematic error (bias) and random error (precision). When a system has complete coverage, it is, by definition, completely representative of the population, because the surveillance sample and the population of interest are the same.

When surveillance has incomplete coverage (i.e. based on sampling of the population), whether or not it is likely to be representative is determined by how it is selected (see Chapter 8, Sampling Populations).

The major distinctions of importance for sampling approaches are:

- Random (or probability-based) sampling methods are the most reliable way to achieve a representative sample.
- Non-random sampling methods, such as convenience, purposive or haphazard sampling usually result in a non-representative (biased) sample.
- An extreme form of non-representative surveillance is when the surveillance is focused on only a portion of the population, such as where risk-based surveillance is used (see below).

Representative surveillance is important if we wish to make inference about the population, such as estimating the prevalence of disease or the confidence of detecting disease if it were present. Representativeness is less important if we do not intend to make any inference from the surveillance results.

For example, if the aim of the surveillance system is purely for early detection of a disease incursion (such as from a neighbouring infected country), representativeness of the surveillance is not essential and we can focus efforts on the areas and animals considered most likely to be infected. However, if we wish to use the resulting data to quantify our confidence that the country or region is free of the disease, representativeness becomes much more important.

12.4.6 Risk-based surveillance

Risk-based surveillance is where surveillance is intentionally biased towards parts of the population that are considered to be at higher risk of disease, or which are more likely to give a positive test result if infected. Risk-based surveillance is usually more efficient than simple representative sampling for detecting diseases or demonstrating freedom from disease.

Risk-based surveillance is a form of stratified surveillance, where the population is stratified according to a known or hypothesized risk factor and sampling within strata is not proportional to stratum size.

If sampling within risk groups (strata) is representative of the risk group (e.g. simple random sampling within strata), it may be possible to adjust for the biases to produce an unbiased estimate of the sensitivity of the surveillance system. Conversely, if sampling within strata is not representative (convenience or haphazard), such adjustments are not possible and any estimates are likely to be biased.

For example, if free-range piggeries are considered to have poorer biosecurity than intensively housed piggeries, such piggeries might be considered as being a higher risk for classical swine fever (CSF). Therefore biasing our surveillance towards free-range piggeries provides an opportunity for earlier detection and also, assuming we do not find the disease, greater confidence that the pig industry as a whole is free of CSF, compared to if we did the same amount of surveillance using representative sampling. If we can quantify the difference in disease risk between free-range and housed piggeries it may also be possible to quantify the sensitivity of our risk-based surveillance.

The main benefit of risk-based surveillance compared to conventional representative surveillance systems is increased efficiency and resulting cost-savings. In general, a smaller sample size can be used for risk-based surveillance to provide equivalent system sensitivity to conventional representative surveillance. Alternatively, for a fixed sample size, risk-based surveillance will provide higher system sensitivity than conventional representative surveillance.

Although risk-based surveillance normally relies on preferential sampling of high-risk subpopulations, it is also feasible to target risk groups with a lower probability of infection than the general population. In this case sample sizes will be higher than for conventional representative sampling. However, if the cost per unit is low, the benefits of low cost, convenience and high coverage may outweigh the disadvantage of increased sample size.

For our CSF example, sick animals are usually not sent to abattoirs in developed countries and so animals at abattoirs are likely to be at lower risk of disease than animals in the general population. However, some animals may be subclinically affected or become sick in lairage and can be detected at either ante-mortem inspection or at routine meat inspection of the slaughtered pigs. Therefore, although the risk of disease in slaughter pigs might be very low, the very large numbers of pigs being processed through routine inspection means that the meat inspection could have a reasonably high system sensitivity for the detection of CSF, if it were present.

Because risk-based surveillance relies on knowledge of the risk factors for the disease of interest, if nothing is known about likely risk factors or data on potential risk factors are not available, risk-based surveillance is not possible.

In practice, three types of factors can be used for identification of high-risk groups for risk-based surveillance, as follows:

- causal factors for the disease, such as farms with poor biosecurity or animals with signs of disease;
- factors that are caused by the disease, for example, animals with diarrhoea are more likely to have Johne's disease than those that do not; and
- non-causal factors that may be associated with disease, for example, smaller farms may be less interested and experienced and may therefore have poorer biosecurity than larger farms and also may be easier to identify.

12.4.7 Surveillance system sensitivity

One of the primary measures of the performance of a surveillance system for disease detection or demonstrating freedom is its sensitivity, the probability of detecting disease if it is present at a level equal to or exceeding a specified threshold.

System sensitivity is the probability that infection will be detected in the population of interest by the surveillance system, given that it is infected at a prevalence equal to or greater than the design prevalence(s).

System sensitivity is equivalent to the level of confidence of detecting the disease if it were present in the population at the specified level. By convention, the target system sensitivity for a surveillance system is usually 95%, although this can be varied depending on circumstances and on how important it is to have a high level of confidence.

For example, a representative surveillance system for bovine brucellosis in dairy herds using a bulk milk tank antibody test might have a system sensitivity of 95% for a prevalence of 2%. This means that we are 95% confident that we would detect one or more positive herds in our sample if 2% or more of herds in the population were infected.

If the aim of our surveillance is to maximize system sensitivity (within financial and resource constraints), for example, to satisfy trading partners, there are three main ways to achieve this:

1. Sample more animals – the more animals (or other units) we sample the greater our chance of detecting disease if it is present and hence the greater our system sensitivity. However, as system sensitivity gets closer to 100%, each additional animal provides a smaller increment than the last one, so at some stage additional sampling is not cost-effective.

2. Increasing the unit sensitivity of the system (the probability for each animal sampled that it will be detected (give a positive result) if it is infected). This can be achieved by using a more sensitive test (which might be more expensive) or for a farmer-reporting system by public awareness to increase the likelihood of a farmer reporting if he notices anything unusual in his animals.
3. Use risk-based surveillance to preferentially sample high-risk subpopulations. This provides a higher system sensitivity for the same level of sampling, or equivalent system sensitivity for a lower level of sampling.

12.5 Mechanisms of Surveillance

Scudamore (2002) has described seven different mechanisms of surveillance.

1. Outbreak investigations.
2. Voluntary notification.
3. Compulsory notification.
4. Sentinel surveillance using primary and secondary data sources.
5. Sentinel surveillance using tertiary data sources.
6. Structured surveys.
7. Census.

A brief description of each of the different mechanisms along with advantages and disadvantages is provided in Table 12.3.

12.6 Collecting Surveillance Data

In the previous section we described seven mechanisms for surveillance. These mechanisms describe the broad process of surveillance and the means by which data are collected. In this section we discuss the various types of data that are collected for surveillance purposes.

Common data collected in a surveillance system include:

- disease diagnoses;
- disease indicators;
- syndromes or signs;
- indirect indicators of disease;
- risk factors for disease; and
- ancillary data.

12.6.1 Diagnoses

Diagnoses usually refer specifically to clinical disease in an animal or animals. At the individual animal level, a diagnosis tells us what disease an animal has. For the farmer this helps with decisions about whether to treat or not, what treatment to use and what preventive measures might be required for the rest of his herd or flock. For surveillance, a diagnosis can be used to classify some animals (or farms) as having a particular disease, or not. When aggregated over time and across a region or country,

Table 12.3. Mechanisms of surveillance (adapted from Scudamore, 2002).

Mechanism	Description	Advantages	Disadvantages	Comments	Relative cost
Outbreak investigation	Personnel with appropriate expertise and resources required to investigate outbreaks of unusual disease syndromes	'Syndrome surveillance' provides a route for novel conditions to be identified	Depends on clear, agreed definitions of a 'case' and an 'outbreak' for the particular syndrome of interest and agreed 'intervention levels' Depends on good relationship between industry and investigators and, therefore, misses those sectors without this relationship	Variety of observation points may trigger investigations	Can be high if intervention levels not appropriate
Voluntary notification	Observation of disease is reported to responsible government agency either directly or through routinely reviewed publications or other sources e.g. Unusual clinical syndrome	Provides a route for new and unusual syndromes to be identified Can be effective if farmers, fishermen and others are motivated to report Useful for recording unusual events of limited consequence	Will miss cases due to under-reporting (poor sensitivity) Hard to define or measure the denominator, so trends cannot be evaluated. Indirectly reported disease events only captured by government surveillance programme if information-gathering structure exists	Reports are received when the observed disease is recognized and the observer is aware of the route by which the report can be submitted Can be improved by increasing awareness (e.g. by specific campaigns) and by offering financial incentives, but both increase cost	Low
Compulsory notification	Legal obligation for observer to report specific disease events suspected to be of concern to responsible government agency Such events have a legal definition	Good for syndromes that are easily recognized, particularly if awareness is raised Requirement to notify is uniform across the country	Under-reporting is likely, unless training in awareness of clinical presentation and route of reporting is maintained among the appropriate people	Reports are received when the observed event is recognized or suspected of being 'notifiable' and as being subject to statute, and the observer is aware of the route by which a report should be submitted	Low when prevalence is low

Continued

Table 12.3. Continued.

Mechanism	Description	Advantages	Disadvantages	Comments	Relative cost
	e.g. Notifiable diseases in different countries	Notification facilitates the swift implementation of investigation and control measures Clinical notification enables action to be taken in respect of diseases that are not rapidly or routinely confirmed in a laboratory Location details are supplied with notification, which may assist calculation of infection rates, and comparison of infections over time and geographic area	The level of under-reporting of a particular disease is often biased; there are many reasons why a report may not be made, and these can be different for different areas or types of stakeholder interest Reduced sensitivity for syndromes that resemble endemic disease syndromes Events with non-specific signs may be missed (poor specificity) Adverse impact on stakeholder as a consequence of reporting may act as a disincentive and can increase under-reporting (e.g. where disease prevents export) Where it is not possible to estimate population size, incidence rate and prevalence cannot be calculated	Can be improved with incentives such as compensation	
Sentinel systems – primary and secondary information sources	Key observers are recruited to provide routine returns listing the type, number and other specified details of specified events which are observed. Events of interest are defined and may differ in different periods of time	Can be trained for the purpose, giving good specificity Specialized and trained sentinels can provide sensitive and moderately specific estimates of level of defined events in the population of interest	Not useful for rare events, as sentinels usually cover a small proportion of the population under surveillance (because of costs) Can be difficult to recruit sentinels that are representative of the population of interest, so results may be biased	Observers are recruited appropriate to the event(s) to be surveyed for Specificity can be improved by linking field observers with diagnostic laboratories	Moderate to high

	Sentinels can be primary sources such as industry stakeholders, or secondary, such as animal health personnel	Flexible. Once network recruited and established, syndromes of interest and data to be collected can be varied in response to changing needs Can provide data on common conditions that are not notifiable and for which laboratory diagnosis is not routine An estimate of the population size under surveillance many be available so population based rates can be calculated If sentinel sites are representative, estimates can be generalized to a wider population Additional information that enables interpretation to trends can be collected Can monitor the reason for, and outcome of particular laboratory tests or other health event, so improved interpretation of other surveillance data		To be effective, contact must be maintained and regular feedback provided, so as to retain the commitment of the observers

Continued

Table 12.3. Continued.

Mechanism	Description	Advantages	Disadvantages	Comments	Relative cost
Sentinel systems – tertiary data sources	Contributed data (e.g. from diagnostic laboratories) includes number of diagnoses made for particular diseases with a variable amount of supporting information such as species affected, date of diagnosis, geographic location, specimen type, etc. These can be collated to provide national statistics, which can indicate long-term trends and the effects of interventions	Efficient surveillance method for indicators that cannot be confirmed by primary or secondary data sources (e.g. diseases with non-specific clinical signs) Can be universal, involving all sources, with a broad range of indicators reported, so it is sensitive enough to detect rare but important changes at an early stage (e.g. emergence of new diseases) Can provide information on the relative morbidity due to particular indicators (e.g. causes of poor reproduction) and so guide the setting of priorities Highly specific, where accredited and quality controlled data sources are used, so links between cases reported from different areas can be recognized	Under-reporting is likely (as dependent on primary and secondary data sources for material), so it is impossible to calculate the total number of cases of disease May not be universal. Distribution of contributing laboratories may not be comprehensive, leading to geographical 'blind spots' Cases which are easily diagnosed at primary and secondary level will not contribute to the data, as no need to refer cases or diagnostic material The frequency of diagnosis is biased by the rate at which cases or specimens are referred; if the same factors affect all groups (e.g. economic hardship), relative morbidities will still be valid. However, certain population or disease subgroups may be affected to a greater or lesser degree (e.g. availability of a new vaccine) There is no tertiary diagnostic support for some diseases in some countries		Variable, but usually moderate to high

		Provides a mechanism for identifying cases, which can contribute to further study of priority diseases where more information is required Data on some indicators are not routinely available by any other means			
Structured surveys	A selected sample of the population of interest is surveyed for a particular disease(s) and other possible factors of interest	The population of interest and the information needed can be defined Provided a population list (sampling frame) exists, the data must be collected from a representative sample of the population so prevalence or incidence can be measured The survey can be repeated over time to evaluate trends A range of surveys can be carried out, which are targeted at different populations to define the overall level and distribution of disease Cost can be controlled by restricting the precision of the estimate	Targeted, so can only give population estimates for diseases and factors that are specified in the study design Cannot usually respond to new information, or diseases that are new or unexpected Differences in diagnostic methods or changes over time can limit the comparability of surveys that set out to measure the same thing Can have problems with non-participation Baseline datasets may be incomplete or unavailable Can be very expensive if sample sizes are large and access to remote subpopulations difficult	Small sample-size surveys can give useful results, provided the disease or syndrome of interest is not rare Cost depends on disease characteristics and precision required	Variable, but usually moderate to high
Census	Measurement of an indicator in all members of a defined population (e.g. testing of all shrimp broodstock for WSD)	All members of the defined population contribute information, so true prevalence or incidence can be measured	Requires a mechanism for identifying all members of the population to be counted Expensive		High

the cumulative occurrence of a particular diagnosis can provide useful information about the likely distribution and occurrence of the disease.

Depending on the nature of the system and how the data are collected, the diagnosis may be the result of a clinical investigation and field diagnosis, or it may be the result of a variety of tests in the field and/or laboratory before a final diagnosis is made and recorded. Regardless of how it is achieved, it is the final diagnosis that is the important piece of information in this context.

For example, a government veterinary service might require all of its veterinary or animal health officers to report monthly (or more frequently) on the diagnoses made during the period.

Obviously the accuracy and value of the information derived from reports of clinical disease will vary greatly, depending on the nature of the disease, its severity, the ability of farmers to diagnose and treat without veterinary assistance and the availability of veterinary services to investigate the disease.

12.6.2 Disease indicators

Often, we are not interested solely in clinical disease, but in some characteristic of the animal that is related to disease.

For instance, if we are doing a serological survey to demonstrate freedom from brucellosis, we are seeking to classify animals as seropositive or seronegative. Seropositive animals are unlikely to be clinically diseased at the time of detection – we are simply using the serological status to indicate if the animal has been exposed to the bacteria (or possibly a vaccine) at some time in the past.

Similarly, surveillance to evaluate the progress of a foot-and-mouth disease vaccination programme, by estimating the proportion of animals that have protective antibodies, is not based on a diagnosis of disease, but on the antibody status of the animals.

Both the diagnosis of disease and the classification of animals according to some characteristic (e.g. antibody status), are usually achieved with the use of some type of test. Some tests are laboratory-based, such as:

- an ELISA to measure antibody levels;
- virus isolation; and
- PCR to detect a pathogenic agent.

Whereas other tests can be performed in the field, including:

- clinical diagnosis by a veterinarian can be thought of as a type of test for disease; and
- meat inspection in an abattoir can also be considered as a test.

When a laboratory test is used, the item that is collected for surveillance is normally not the information but a specimen from the animal (blood, milk, a tissue sample, etc.). This specimen has a test applied, to produce a test result. It is this test result that is then recorded, which may or may not be indicative of a disease diagnosis.

12.6.3 Syndromes and signs

In the case of clinical disease, the most commonly collected information is the diagnosis.

In order to make a diagnosis, the animal should be examined by a veterinarian and, if required, specimens submitted for laboratory testing.

This is not always possible, so some surveillance systems are designed to collect un-interpreted data, rather than the diagnosis that would result from its interpretation.

To make a diagnosis, a veterinarian will observe the *signs* shown by a sick animal (such as lameness, coughing, increased heart rate, etc.), and interpret them to decide on the disease causing the problem. This diagnosis will usually be correct, but sometimes might be wrong.

Many of these signs are simple to observe by people without veterinary training and can be reported as the presence of particular signs, rather than a diagnosis.

This is important for a number of reasons including:

- While non-veterinarians are unlikely to make a correct diagnosis, those that work with livestock are often very good at identifying clinical signs – abnormalities in their animals.
- In some cases there are legal restrictions on who can make a diagnosis (usually only qualified veterinarians).
- Village animal health workers are usually not veterinarians but are trained to recognize disease signs.

Also, even with thorough field and laboratory investigation a final diagnosis is not always possible. A surveillance system may therefore collect data on the signs of disease observed.

Changes in the patterns of signs observed in a population may indicate changes in the diseases that cause those signs. For instance, even if the diagnosis is not known, a sudden increase in the number of cases of disease showing signs of coughing probably indicates the introduction and spread of a respiratory disease. This information can be used to initiate a detailed disease investigation to determine what the cause of the coughing is.

To make interpretation and reporting of this type of surveillance simpler, cases are often classified into syndromes according to the key sign or group of signs.

A syndrome is a defined collection of clinical signs, usually relating to particular body systems or characteristics of diseases of concern.

In the above example, the syndrome may be respiratory disease and include any case of disease that shows coughing, difficulty breathing and so on.

Examples of syndromes may include:

- respiratory disease;
- acute febrile illness;
- diarrhoea;
- skin lesions;
- sudden death; and
- lameness.

Both reporting of signs and reporting of syndromes are referred to as syndromic surveillance. Syndromic surveillance is usually designed to help with the detection of changes in disease patterns or the early detection of new diseases. When a change is detected, it is followed up by more detailed investigations in order to determine what is causing the change.

Surveillance may collect data on the signs associated with a case of disease, or the general syndrome that describes that case of disease. The use of syndromes in data collection and reporting is more common than collecting signs. This is because with syndromes there is one data item per case (e.g. respiratory disease), whereas when reporting signs a single case may have many different signs associated with it (e.g. coughing, difficulty breathing, standing with neck extended, increased heart rate), making reporting, collation and analysis of the data more complicated.

12.6.4 Negative reporting

Negative reporting is where the primary data recorded by the surveillance system is the fact that an animal or group of animals were examined and did not have the disease of concern.

A negative reporting system can be based on either laboratory or field data. In a laboratory-based system, all tests undertaken for a specific disease of concern are recorded and reported and if the results are all negative this provides additional evidence that the disease is not present. In some cases, this may also be supported by additional data (e.g. disease syndrome) that the animals were tested because they showed clinical signs suggestive of the disease, further value-adding to the data.

For example, the OIE surveillance requirement to demonstrate a country's negligible risk for bovine spongiform encephalopathy (BSE) requires laboratory examination of brain tissue from a specified number of animals exhibiting neurological or other specified signs. This does not provide any information on what neurological diseases are present, but does provide evidence that BSE is not present, assuming all samples are negative for BSE.

A field-based negative reporting system is a little more complicated, but essentially works on the same principles. Field-based or clinical negative reporting can be used mainly for diseases with typical, easily recognized clinical signs (e.g. foot-and-mouth disease) and preferably diseases that spread rapidly in a susceptible population. In contrast to the laboratory-based system, the presence of clinical signs is not a necessary component to trigger a negative field report. Instead, a system can be established whereby whenever a veterinarian (or other trained animal health officer) visits a farm or village and examines animals (for some unrelated reason), part of their examination includes a brief observation for any obvious signs of the disease (or diseases) of concern. Because these diseases usually have obvious clinical signs, often in multiple animals, they should be easy to detect, if present. Therefore, if signs are not observed during the visit it is unlikely that the herd is infected. These negative findings are reported through established reporting channels and can be collated periodically to provide information on disease status of the country or region.

Documentation of such a clinical negative reporting system can provide valuable reassurance to trading partners about the continued freedom from disease of a particular zone, compartment or country.

12.6.5 Indirect indicators

Most surveillance systems collect data on the disease or health status of animals directly. However, some take a more indirect approach, by monitoring other attributes that may be related to the occurrence of disease in the population.

For example, information provided by drug companies, distributors and feed supply stores on the sales of particular types of veterinary drugs and/or medicated feeds can be used for indirect surveillance for the occurrence of disease in the population.

Like syndromic surveillance, changes in the patterns of drug sales and medicated feed sales are likely to be good indicators that there is a change in the pattern of disease. However, this does not say what the disease is. Any observed changes must therefore be followed up by a detailed investigation to assess if there is really an increase in disease and if so, what is causing the disease.

Surveillance for indirect indicators of disease is often grouped together with syndromic surveillance as a technique to assist with the early detection of disease. Therefore the ideal indicators are those that change early in the disease process. For example, the most common direct surveillance system used to detect disease is based on a farmer reporting to a veterinarian when they have a disease problem. However, before the farmer calls the vet, they may try to treat the problem themselves.

If a new widespread problem affects a population, it may be possible to detect the problem earlier through the use of drug sales than by waiting for veterinary reports, which may only come some time later.

In human disease surveillance, thermometer sales and business sick-leave records have been found to be good early indicators of disease patterns in the population.

Indirect indicator surveillance is normally active surveillance, where the veterinary authorities establish a relationship with the holders of the data (e.g. drug suppliers) and ask that updates on sales be provided at regular (e.g. daily or weekly) intervals for analysis.

Another increasingly common form of indirect surveillance is through monitoring Internet traffic on or about a particular disease, particularly for human diseases but also to a lesser extent for animal diseases. There is now a number of online agencies that monitor disease-related topics on the Internet, such as searches relating to influenza symptoms or diagnoses. These are then mapped in close to real-time and can be analysed to detect clusters in space and time. Alternatively, some government agencies use similar electronic monitoring of Internet searches, and other content, looking for keywords relating to diseases of interest (e.g. highly pathogenic avian influenza), to try to establish systems for early detections of outbreaks.

12.6.6 Risk factors

Most surveillance seeks to collect information about disease or a disease-related state, including indirect surveillance which measures indicators of disease that occur early after the onset of disease. Another approach to surveillance is not to measure disease at all, but to measure the risk factors that may be involved in causing the disease. This type of surveillance seeks to provide alerts before an outbreak of disease so preventative measures can be put in place.

For example, vector surveillance for *Culicoides* spp., the biting midge that is the vector for bluetongue, can provide early warning of likely outbreaks of bluetongue virus infection. Insect trapping sites provide surveillance information on the presence or absence of the disease vector and can be useful for monitoring changes in distribution of the disease over time.

Another example is the monitoring of risk factors for development of algal blooms. Under certain conditions, algal blooms can develop, which may produce toxins that can either kill aquatic animals or contaminate aquatic products making them unsafe for humans to eat. Surveillance systems can be established to monitor sunlight and water temperature to assess the risk of the development of the blooms. Alternatively, the surveillance could directly measure the amount of algae present, and whether they are toxic or not.

External risk factors or factors not having a direct biological effect on the occurrence of disease in animals can also be considered for enhancing surveillance activity.

For example, in some regions movement of animals from one area to another during religious festivities has resulted in the increase or resurgence of foot-and-mouth disease outbreaks and other important transboundary animal diseases.

Alternatively, data on prices and livestock movements can be used to predict times of increased risk and the location of potential new disease outbreaks.

12.7 Approaches to Surveillance

Approaches to surveillance are many and varied, depending on the disease of concern, the nature of the population of interest, the aims of the surveillance and the resources available. This section aims to provide a brief outline of some of the more common approaches.

12.7.1 Farmer disease notification

Many countries maintain a list of notifiable diseases that are considered important for a variety of reasons. Farmers are required by law to notify if they suspect the presence of one of these diseases and may be prosecuted and suffer financial penalties for failure to do so. However, despite the potential penalties, many farmers fail to notify, either through ignorance or deliberate lack of cooperation.

Farmer disease notifications can be useful for detecting infected farms for action but depend strongly on farmer cooperation for their success. Therefore they are best suited to diseases that are easily recognized by the farmer, that have a significant production impact and that might be difficult for the farmer to control in isolation.

For example, footrot in sheep is a severe, debilitating disease of sheep that spreads easily through trade in asymptomatic carriers or by straying of sheep between properties. It is therefore quite difficult for individual farmers to prevent its introduction, particularly in regions of high prevalence. However, the disease has been successfully controlled in New South Wales, Australia through a programme of notification and cooperative group action to control the disease, with support and advice from government agencies.

Farmer disease notification is a targeted, active surveillance system with comprehensive coverage of the population.

12.7.2 Veterinary diagnostic system

Farmers (or other animal owners) are the primary source of information on sick or diseased animals. However, it is not always easy to access this information and farmers vary substantially in their ability and willingness to provide surveillance data. It is also often difficult to obtain information from farmers in a timely manner. One way of achieving this is through on-farm diagnostic investigations of disease events.

Such investigations may be provided free of charge or subsidized (subject to meeting eligibility criteria) by government veterinary services, or may occur through the farmer's decision to have a disease event investigated by a private veterinarian. In either case, the investigation is often supported by free or subsidized laboratory testing, usually for exclusion of specific diseases of concern. Data collected in this way can then be channelled through either the veterinary diagnostic laboratory or from the field service to a central database for collation and analysis.

For example, a government interested in maintaining surveillance for anthrax in livestock could provide a free (or subsidized) investigation service for animals that die suddenly, including free laboratory screening for anthrax. Depending on financial constraints and other surveillance priorities (or the need to ensure throughput of samples) additional testing to establish a diagnosis could also be subsidized.

The resulting data from such a system will be a mix of disease exclusions (negative test results for specific diseases) and of positive diagnoses. Depending on how the system operates it may be based on either field or laboratory reports or both.

A decision by farmers to seek veterinary assistance depends on a range of factors, including:

- farmer awareness of the service;
- cost to the farmer;
- farmer attitudes to the government services;
- legal requirement to notify authorities when a specified disease is suspected or confirmed and penalties for not complying with this requirement;
- concerns about potential adverse effects that may arise if a specific disease were to be confirmed (such as quarantine and trade restrictions); and
- availability and proximity of the service to the farmer.

Farmer participation can be improved by ensuring a readily available and reliable service at low cost to the farmer, and by promoting awareness of the system and minimizing adverse impacts on farmers.

While a veterinary diagnostic system can provide useful information, analysis and interpretation must be undertaken with considerable care due to the inherent biases in the system related to whether or not the farmer will recognize a problem and whether they seek veterinary assistance or not.

The major advantages of the veterinary diagnostic system are that:

- It has complete coverage of the population so that, at least potentially, any animal in the country could be sampled, although with varying likelihood.
- It is capable of detecting any disease, including exotic or emerging diseases, not just the ones we know about.
- It can be relatively inexpensive and the cost can be varied by manipulating the level of subsidized or free service provided.

A veterinary diagnostic investigation system is primarily a general, passive surveillance system with comprehensive coverage of the population. However, veterinary diagnostic systems can include targeted components, for example where free testing is offered for specific diseases of interest (that might not otherwise be tested for).

12.7.3 Abattoir surveillance system

Another approach to surveillance for some conditions is through abattoir examination and inspection. In many countries, all animals being slaughtered for human consumption undergo compulsory inspection to ensure they are safe for eating. Usually this involves an ante-mortem inspection to ensure they are apparently fit and healthy before slaughter, followed by visual and manual inspection of tissues and organs on the slaughter floor, looking for signs of disease or other conditions that might render the carcass unsuitable for human consumption.

Abattoir inspection relies primarily on visual and manual inspection of animal pre- and post-slaughter and is therefore only likely to detect clinical disease or (usually chronic) diseases that produce obvious gross lesions that can be detected in the carcass.

Because abattoir inspection is already in place in many abattoirs, it can provide a very useful source of surveillance data. The main advantages of abattoir surveillance include:

- It is inexpensive – the system is already in place for meat inspection purposes and adding data collection is an incremental cost only.
- There is a high throughput of animals and consequently a relatively high coverage of the population is possible.
- It is usually possible to collect additional tissue or blood samples for follow-up testing if necessary.
- It may be possible to provide feedback to farmers about conditions found in their animals that are affecting production and/or product quality (e.g. liver fluke, cysticercosis, hydatidosis, etc.).
- Abattoir surveillance can sometimes be extended to target specific diseases of animal health interest that may not otherwise be routinely covered by meat inspection, either through specific examination for gross lesions or by sampling blood or tissues for laboratory testing (e.g. tuberculosis, brucellosis).

Using abattoirs as a source of surveillance data also has significant disadvantages, including:

- The source population is strongly biased to healthy animals and usually also to either young or old animals.
- Routine data collection is limited to diseases with obvious gross lesions in slaughtered animals.
- Data collection on additional diseases (or specific sample collection) may be logistically difficult in the environment of a busy abattoir.
- The nature and quality of the data collected can be quite variable.
- For some conditions, data are limited to the presence of a lesion and diagnosis of the cause may not be possible without further testing or investigation (e.g. lymph node granuloma), while for others a specific diagnosis is possible (e.g. hydatidosis).
- Data collection and collation depends on the data management systems in individual abattoirs and may not be in consistent formats or in many cases may be paper-based records requiring substantial effort for data entry.

Abattoir surveillance is often a form of passive, general surveillance but can also be utilized as the basis for active, targeted programmes for specific diseases.

Because the infrastructure is already in place and animals can be sampled at little additional cost, compared to field sampling of an equivalent number of animals, such targeted programmes can be extremely cost-effective. Targeted abattoir programmes can also be very useful for case-detection for on-farm follow-up. However, the downside is that the study population (animals being slaughtered) is not representative of the general population and therefore any estimates of disease prevalence or confidence of freedom should be treated with caution.

Abattoir surveillance can provide useful data on the occurrence of chronic diseases such as liver fluke, hydatidosis, caseous lymphadenitis, cysticercosis, etc. The results can be used to monitor the effectiveness of voluntary control programmes for these diseases or can be fed back to producers to make them aware of the potential losses they are experiencing and to encourage them to implement on-farm control measures.

A common example of a targeted abattoir surveillance programme is the examination of lymph nodes of cattle at slaughter for evidence of tuberculosis (TB) granulomas. This can provide an important source of surveillance data for bovine TB, initially for case-detection for on-farm testing and follow-up as part of a broader control or eradication programme and subsequently to provide supporting evidence for freedom of the local cattle population from TB.

Abattoir sampling is also an important mechanism for monitoring meat and other products for the presence of residues of potentially dangerous chemicals. Many countries implement routine sampling protocols, whereby a set number of samples is collected each month, selected randomly from abattoir throughput. These samples are then tested for residues of specified chemicals (such as organochlorine or organophosphate pesticides, heavy metals, etc.). This serves as a monitoring process for the levels of these chemicals and also for detection of farms producing residue-affected animals for further investigation and action. In addition to random sampling, some farms with a known history of residues may also be identified for regular testing whenever they send animals for slaughter, until authorities are confident that the residues have been eliminated.

12.7.4 Veterinary negative reporting system

Veterinarians and lay animal health officers regularly visit farms or villages and examine animals for a variety of reasons. In most cases, these visits are undocumented, except for in the veterinary practice records or the diaries of government veterinary and animal health staff. However, if this data can be captured and utilized it can be a powerful source of information to support a case for freedom from some diseases.

A veterinary negative reporting scheme provides a mechanism for capturing these data, usually for a specified disease or small group of diseases. At its simplest, veterinarians and animal health staff complete a brief report (preferably into a centralized database) of any farm visits, including location or farm identifier, the date of the visit and confirmation that the disease or diseases of interest were not present in animals at the time of the visit. Over time, the potentially large number of records of farm visits where disease was not detected provide strong evidence that the disease is not present.

Obviously, for maximum effectiveness, it is important that the disease or diseases of interest present with obvious and consistent clinical signs. Diseases with subtle or variable signs are less likely to be noticed and a negative report would therefore carry less weight. For the same reason highly infectious diseases that affect multiple animals in a short period are better suited to this form of surveillance than diseases that are sporadic and likely to go unnoticed.

Main advantages of a veterinary negative reporting system include:

- It is a relatively low cost leveraged value because veterinarians and other animal health staff are visiting farms and seeing animals anyway, so the only cost is the additional cost associated with reporting.
- It provides good coverage of the population, at least in areas where veterinarians and animal health staff are operating.
- It provides documented evidence that the disease is not present.

Disadvantages of a veterinary negative reporting system include:

- Reporting provides an additional impost on busy veterinarians resulting in poor and inconsistent compliance.
- It is only suitable for a limited range of diseases that are easily recognized at a casual examination.
- It may be subject to problems with implementation where busy veterinarians complete a negative report (because they are asked and perhaps paid to) without really looking at the animals or asking about disease history from the farmer.
- It is only suitable for known exotic diseases – not suited to monitoring of existing endemic diseases.

A veterinary negative reporting scheme is a form of passive targeted surveillance – it is passive because it relies on veterinarians and others visiting farms and seeing animals for reasons other than the collection of surveillance data and targeted because it usually targets specific diseases of interest.

An example of a negative reporting surveillance programme would be for a country undergoing eradication of foot-and-mouth disease and where there might already be some regions that are FMD-free zones. In these areas, veterinarians and official animal health staff would be asked to report the absence of FMD from animals on any farms they visit. This data would provide twofold benefits: first that a system was in place for early detection of breakdowns and second to reassure livestock industries and trading partners that the zone was truly free of FMD.

12.7.5 Sentinel herds or flocks

To be a sentinel is to keep watch, usually to warn of impending danger. Sentinel herds or flocks are a simple means of setting up an early-warning scheme for a disease incursion or the extension of the distribution of a disease. A sentinel herd is usually a small number of immunologically naive animals that are maintained together and sampled on a regular basis to test for seroconversion or examined for clinical signs of target diseases. Often, these animals are part of a commercial herd and are maintained as part of that herd throughout the monitoring process, so that there is no additional cost in maintaining the animals.

The animals are usually selected at a young age and screened to ensure they have not already been exposed to the disease. They are then visited on a regular basis, which may be as frequent as weekly or as infrequent as quarterly (or less), depending on the disease, time of year and importance of early detection. At each visit, the animals are checked for clinical signs of disease and samples taken to check for antibodies and evidence of seroconversion.

Sentinel herds are therefore useful to provide early warning of disease incursion or expansion and also provide some evidence for freedom from disease. They can also help define the distribution of disease, but are less useful for estimating disease prevalence.

Sentinels can also be used following an eradication programme to determine whether the measures employed were effective. Naive animals are introduced to the farm or herd and monitored for a period of several weeks to determine whether they develop clinical disease or seroconvert, indicating eradication was ineffective. If, at the end of the sentinel period, they remain unaffected and seronegative, eradication is assumed to have been successful and the farm can be fully restocked and quarantine measures relaxed.

Advantages of sentinel herd surveillance include:

- Provision of strong evidence for occurrence (or freedom) for the particular disease in the sentinel group.
- High specificity for the disease(s) of interest.
- Useful for defining geographic spread of disease where spread is predictable and on a front, such as vector-borne diseases.
- Provision of evidence of temporal and spatial dynamics of disease.

Disadvantage of sentinel herd surveillance include:

- The cost of maintaining animal groups and sampling including identification, initial eligibility testing, travel, sampling and laboratory testing.
- Difficulties in maintaining manageable groups of sentinel animals at different locations, including isolated areas and commercial livestock enterprises.
- The sentinel herd concept may only be useful for selected diseases and not useful for others; the approach also has relatively poor population coverage (possibly only one location in a region with perhaps several hundred farms), so works best for diseases likely to impact multiple farms in an area simultaneously.

Sentinel herds are an example of active, targeted surveillance – active because they are primarily planned and implemented specifically for the purpose of collecting surveillance data and targeted because they usually target specific diseases.

A common use of sentinel herds is for monitoring the distribution and early warning of outbreaks of arboviruses such as bluetongue or ephemeral fever. Sentinel cattle herds are established across the known range of the vectors and extending into presumed vector-free areas. These herds are then sampled on a periodic basis to determine when exposure occurs and to monitor any changes in vector (and hence disease) distribution.

Sentinel flocks (using chickens) are also used to monitor for arboviruses affecting humans, such as Ross River fever and Murray Valley encephalitis in Australia. The vectors of these viruses feed happily on chickens as well as on humans, so that detection of seroconversion in sentinel chickens provides an early warning for potential human outbreaks.

12.7.6 Sentinel veterinary practices

Sentinel veterinary practice networks are another form of sentinel disease surveillance. Such networks are increasingly common in developed countries and provide a means of monitoring endemic diseases and for detection of new or emerging diseases.

To set up a sentinel practice network, veterinarians (or veterinary practices) are recruited and usually paid to report on livestock health-related activities. This can be as simple as reporting disease investigations and diagnoses that meet certain criteria on a regular basis. Alternatively, it is possible to also recruit practice clients and undertake regular monitoring on these farms, in much the same way as for sentinel herds, except with more comprehensive data collection, including for example production-related data.

Sentinel practice networks have a lot in common with the veterinary diagnostic system but have a more pro-active involvement of the veterinary practitioner. In a veterinary diagnostic system, the practitioner is simply a conduit between the farmer and the laboratory and is primarily concerned about diagnosis and treatment. In a sentinel practice situation this role is changed and the practitioner takes on an additional role as a primary provider of data. This means that a sentinel practice approach is more useful for obtaining data on diseases or production parameters that do not rely on a laboratory diagnosis. It also means that the sentinel practitioner can be expected to provide more information about the case (history, clinical signs, etc.) than might normally be the case for a diagnostic laboratory submission.

Advantages of sentinel practice surveillance include:

- Relatively low cost since payment to practitioners may be based on marginal time required for additional reporting, rather than for the full cost of an investigation.
- Application to a broad range of target diseases or syndromes including new, emerging, exotic and endemic diseases as well as production measures.
- Application for diseases that do not require laboratory testing for diagnosis.

Disadvantages of sentinel practice surveillance include:

- The imposition of extra work and reporting on busy practitioners.
- Difficult in keeping participants motivated.
- Problems at the receiving end associated with workload in collating results and reporting back to participating practices to provide feedback and maintain interest and commitment.

Sentinel practice networks are a form of targeted surveillance with both active and passive aspects. They are passive because they rely on farmers calling on veterinary services to assist with diagnosis and treatment of disease problems, but active in that they are actively seeking additional data from the practitioner over and above what would normally be expected. They are generally targeted at a range of specific diseases and/or syndromes, but because of the enhanced relationship through the network can be useful for early detection of trends or occurrence of new syndromes, thus providing an enhancement to general surveillance.

An example of a sentinel veterinary practice network is the UK's National Animal Disease Information System, encompassing 60 veterinary practices and six veterinary colleges (http://www.nadis.org.uk).

12.7.7 Surveys

Planned surveys can be undertaken of farmers and their animals to determine if disease is or has been present and to collect other related information. This is usually a time-consuming and expensive process and the quality of the resulting data depends on the nature of the disease and the timing and scale of the survey. Usually, the better the quality of the survey data required, the more expensive it will be to collect. Surveys involving sampling and testing of animals generally provide better quality data than questionnaire surveys of farmer knowledge and opinion, but are more expensive and are limited by the capability of available tests.

For example, a serological survey will provide information on seroprevalence of a disease, but may not distinguish between vaccination response and previous infection or tell anything about timing of exposure. On the other hand, surveys of farmer recollection and opinion without sampling of animals are usually cheaper, but are subject to recall bias and are only suitable for diseases or syndromes that are easily recognized and likely to be remembered by the farmer.

Surveys can be undertaken for a variety of purposes, including estimating disease prevalence, demonstrating disease freedom, or evaluating risk factors for disease. Surveys may also be representative or risk-based, where herds or animals that are considered at highest risk are preferentially sampled.

Advantages of structured disease surveys include:

- ability to design and implement the sampling strategy specifically to meet the aims of the survey;
- ability to deliver (unbiased) estimates of disease prevalence or system sensitivity;
- application for diseases that can be readily identified by laboratory testing of blood or faecal samples, making it suitable to determining previous exposure to disease; and
- ability to be easily repeated at appropriate intervals to establish temporal disease trends or maintain confidence of freedom.

Disadvantages of structured disease surveys include:

- demands in resource inputs because of design requirements to achieve representative sampling;
- problems with poor response rates if farmers are not willing to cooperate;
- difficulties in ensuring a truly representative sample in many cases, particularly if information on the population of interest is lacking; and
- requirement for more sophisticated analytical techniques to estimate system sensitivity for risk-based methods (or in some cases, estimation may not be possible at all).

An example of a planned survey would be to plan a survey for estimating prevalence of brucellosis-infected dairy herds, based on bulk-milk testing for *Brucella* antibodies.

Structured surveys are a form of active, targeted surveillance.

12.7.8 Syndromic surveillance systems

Syndromic surveillance is surveillance based on a disease syndrome, rather than a specific diagnosis. A syndrome is simply a specified collection of clinical signs, usually relating to one or more body systems. It is usually possible to relate each syndrome to one or more disease of interest.

Syndromic surveillance data can be collected in much the same way as specific disease data, through veterinary diagnostic investigations, sentinel practice networks or planned surveys. The main difference is that with syndromic surveillance it is usually changes in the temporal and spatial pattern of reports that is of interest, rather than specific event reports.

For example, a syndromic surveillance system could be set up through the veterinary diagnostic system, whereby individual laboratory submissions are classified according to one or more syndromes. One syndrome is likely to be respiratory signs. A single case of respiratory signs in poultry is unlikely to trigger any interest or investigation. However, multiple cases in a short time period from a small geographic area could be sufficient to trigger further investigation in case it was avian influenza or Newcastle disease.

Because syndromic surveillance is based on disease syndromes, rather than diagnoses, it is also a useful tool for detection of new or emerging diseases. For example, if a cluster of neurological disease cases occurs in time and space and is negative to testing for common neurological conditions, this could trigger further investigation to see if it is a new condition or an incursion of a disease not previously seen in the area.

Advantages of syndromic surveillance include:

- relatively low cost because of use of existing data collection channels;
- capacity to detect new diseases or incursions of exotic diseases;
- ability to collect and analyse data and report in near real-time; and
- flexibility to manage syndromes that may be narrow or very broad in definition and that can include indirect measures of disease or production indices as target measures.

Disadvantages of syndromic surveillance include:

- Dependence of data quality on the original data collection method.
- Limitations in syndrome definitions may mean that syndromes can sometimes be vague and non-specific.
- Early detection of changes in temporal and spatial patterns can be difficult unless there are large quantities of data being entered.
- Small numbers of cases of diseases of concern can be obscured by background noise associated with common diseases that share the same syndrome.
- It can take some time to establish background seasonal and spatial patterns of disease.

An example of syndromic surveillance is where every disease-related laboratory submission is classified according to one or more syndromes. The data are then analysed on a daily basis using special pattern-detection algorithms, looking for changes in temporal and spatial patterns. In the previous example, if neurological diseases are relatively uncommon, a cluster of new disease might be identified quite quickly. However, for a new or emerging disease with diarrhoea as a primary presenting sign, it might take some time to identify the new syndrome if diarrhoea is a relatively common syndrome in the population.

Syndromic surveillance is a form of passive general surveillance, because it utilizes existing data collection pathways and is not usually targeted at specific diseases.

12.8 Deciding on an Appropriate Surveillance Strategy

Deciding on the most appropriate strategy for surveillance is a complex process and depends on a range of factors. Key considerations are the objectives of the surveillance, the budget or financial constraints and the availability of existing data sources that you might be able to use.

In most cases, the surveillance is required to help make decisions about animal health management. The importance and timing of these decisions often determine the priority that must be placed on the surveillance and therefore often the budget. If it is important and an answer is needed promptly more funding will often be available.

There are no strict rules for deciding an appropriate surveillance strategy. The following points are offered as guidance for those who may be tasked with developing a surveillance strategy.

1. Are there any data already available that might be available and useful? If it exists, it is often better to try and obtain existing data and evaluate it for suitability. Even if it is not suitable for the immediate purpose it will at least guide you as to what you might expect to find and may help in planning or your surveillance.
2. Is the surveillance disease-focused or more general? If the surveillance is for a particular disease or diseases you will need some form of targeted surveillance, such as through a sentinel practice network or a targeted survey. If it is not focused on a specific disease but needs to be able to detect a range of diseases, including emerging or exotic diseases, a general surveillance scheme is required, such as the veterinary diagnostic system.
3. Are precise estimates of prevalence or system sensitivity required? If precise estimates of disease occurrence (or absence) are required an active survey is the only reasonable alternative in most cases.
4. Does the disease exhibit typical clinical signs or lesions? If affected animals have typical gross lesions easily detected at slaughter, an abattoir-based surveillance system may be suitable. Conversely, if the disease presents as a typical combination of clinical signs, syndromic surveillance or negative veterinary reporting may be appropriate.
5. Is the data required as a one-off or on a regular basis? A one-off structured survey is usually easier to justify than an ongoing programme of repeated surveys. If surveillance is expected to be ongoing, another alternative may be more appropriate.
6. Is it feasible to use abattoir sampling for the disease? If quantitative estimates are not required, for example for case-detection rather than prevalence estimation, abattoir sampling may be cheaper and more convenient than on-farm sampling.
7. Are resources limiting? If resources are limiting some form of passive surveillance, such as a veterinary diagnostic system or sentinel veterinary practices, may be easier to manage than a more resource intensive approach.

12.9 Basic Requirements for a National Surveillance Programme

The basis of all good surveillance programmes is observant and skilled people with appropriate support resources who understand what is normal, are alert to changes and can describe the abnormalities they see.

Investigations of suspected disease occurrences which eventually result in meaningful surveillance information require:

- appropriately trained and motivated personnel;
- standardized field and laboratory methods supported by quality control; and
- access to manuals and training opportunities.

The precise design and structure of a surveillance programme depends on its purpose. However, all surveillance programmes have some basic common features, including:

- clearly stated objectives;
- a list of diseases of concern;
- the capability and capacity to undertake investigations to the required level of diagnostic certainty;
- specifications for methods of collection of the information required; and
- a system to collect, record and collate data, as well as report findings.

12.9.1 A clear purpose and objectives

The following section provides information on approaches to achieve each of the four general objectives of surveillance early in this chapter.

Detect new and exotic infectious diseases in animals

All countries should have a system in place that gives early warning of new and exotic animal diseases, as a minimum requirement. Such surveillance is based on comprehensive general surveillance activities that provide the reference baseline for endemic pathogens within any given area. If this system is working well, new or exotic disease can be detected by field investigation, although confirmation will almost always require laboratory follow-up and/or confirmation by a reference laboratory.

Once a new or exotic pathogen is detected, targeted surveillance will be required to define its distribution and the magnitude of the problem, track its spread, assess feasible control options and, where appropriate, demonstrate successful eradication.

Detect cases of selected diseases and pathogens

In some instances, activities associated with the control or eradication programme will provide all the necessary information to detect cases of the disease of concern. For example, where all farms in an area participate in the control programme, they will participate in periodic testing to provide information both for control and surveillance purposes. However, where some farms in an area are not part of the control programme, additional surveillance activities may be needed to detect cases. Alternatively, an active programme of surveillance through abattoir inspection or at other processing plants can be used for detecting cases of diseases of public health concern.

Describe the distribution and occurrence of diseases relevant to disease control and domestic and international movement of animals and products

Defining the general geographic distribution of specific diseases can often be determined from the general surveillance activities, provided they are sufficiently comprehensive and include sufficient sample sizes from all geographical areas where susceptible host populations occur. However, general surveillance cannot provide precise evidence for the geographical distribution of the disease agent, nor the infection/disease levels present. This information can only be gathered using *targeted surveys* and specific diagnostic techniques.

Demonstrate freedom from pathogens and diseases relevant to domestic and international movement of animals and products

The existence of comprehensive general surveillance activities, which have the ability to diagnose the pathogen(s) of interest, provides the initial evidence of freedom from diseases of national/international concern. Any historical records available can be used to reinforce the hypothesis of freedom being tested by the current surveillance programme. Historic records can also be used to develop preliminary surveillance programmes, although results may necessitate modification of the programme where conditions (environmental or human) have changed host susceptibility. For significant (high-risk) diseases, active, targeted surveillance methods may be required to formally quantify system sensitivity and confidence of freedom for a particular pathogen. Methods of analysis for risk-based surveillance and for incorporation of historical data are now also available (Martin *et al.*, 2007).

12.9.2 List of diseases

Each country has its own specific diseases of concern. A minimum list would be those notifiable to the OIE, which are relevant to the particular country's resources or trade interests.

12.9.3 Capability and capacity

A plan for the development of disease surveillance capabilities and capacity at the national and regional levels should be developed.

12.9.4 Information specifications

The information generated from surveillance activities should be aligned to the objectives of the programme and the characteristics of the disease(s) being evaluated.

Basic information

In the case of an emergency report on a disease outbreak or incident, the basic information that needs to be conveyed includes:

- the disease(s) suspected;
- the exact geographical location(s) of the outbreak(s);
- the contact information for affected sites;
- species affected;
- approximate numbers (estimated percentages) of sick and dead animals, where this can be calculated (other units may be used e.g. paddocks, farms);
- brief description of history, clinical signs and lesions observed;
- date(s) when the disease was first noticed at the initial outbreak site and any subsequent sites;
- details of any recent movements of susceptible animals to or from the affected site;
- any other key epidemiological information, such as disease in surrounding wild populations, environmental factors (abnormal rain, drought, etc.), possible vectors (birds, human activities, etc.); and
- initial disease control actions taken.

Important exotic and other emergency animal diseases should be notifiable under legislation within the country.

In the case of endemic diseases, it may simply be a case of reporting the presence or absence of a particular disease in a particular area or, in more sophisticated systems, an attempt may be made to estimate the prevalence of the particular disease.

12.9.5 Data management and reporting

To provide access to surveillance findings, some form of information repository or national/regional registry is required, from which various communications can be produced as required.

Various animal health information systems may be required. A national system is required to collect, store and use the data required to establish and maintain zones or for national and international reporting obligations. This is principally presence/absence data for mandatory reportable diseases within a country. Data required for risk analysis may be stored at a regional or local animal support facility (veterinary, governmental, or research), and may be independent of, or linked to, data repositories for surveillance. Generally, corporate or individual client information is retained by the direct animal health service provider (extension officer, local veterinarian or government animal health services). Such information is kept separate from the national database, but kept accessible in case of the need to respond to a disease emergency (no point in having mandatory reporting if you cannot access the location contact details).

Animal health information systems may range from information gathered by stock-owners, passed by word of mouth, stored in the memory, analysed mentally, and further reported by word of mouth, to national networks that use computerized data management and analysis systems to link a broad network of government agencies and diagnostic laboratory resources.

National disease reporting

Special emergency disease reporting mechanisms for potentially serious disease outbreaks or incidents are an essential component of surveillance designed to provide an early warning system. These reporting mechanisms (usually part of a more comprehensive contingency plan) should allow critical epidemiological information to be transmitted quickly and accurately to the local and national authorities responsible for animal disease control (preferably, the same day of detection). This means that field and laboratory staff involved in surveillance need to have the necessary contact information (with a list of alternatives) so emergency disease reports can be acted upon with minimal delay.

A national disease reporting system should be based on the day-to-day disease investigation activities by field officers and diagnostic laboratories. Such a reporting system, by necessity, requires feedback loops. An example of information flow in such a system is shown in Fig. 12.3. At the first stage of investigation, sufficient data are collected to assist the industry stakeholder with their problem. Only a small proportion of the field information is required by the next administrative level, and likewise 'up the line', however, an audit trail should be maintained of all records generated at each stage of reporting. Thus, although the national system may contain only a very brief summary of each investigation, the full information can be accessed if required.

International disease reporting

Most countries report disease occurrence in some way. There are various international levels of formal reporting, the most important for animal diseases being through the World Organisation for Animal Health (OIE). The OIE has the responsibility for developing international standards for animal disease control for diseases deemed of international trade importance and has obligatory disease reporting requirements for member countries that need to be addressed within any national animal disease control programme.

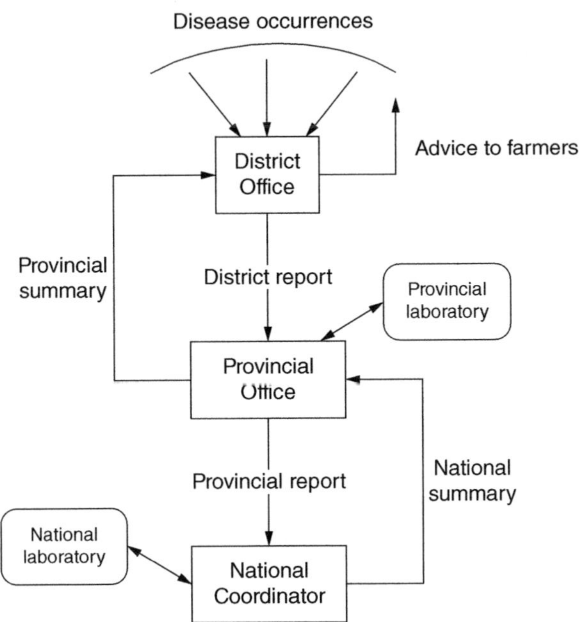

Fig. 12.3. Example of information flows in a national disease reporting system.

In brief, countries should notify OIE within 24 h of any of the following events:

- the first occurrence or re-occurrence of a disease notifiable to the OIE, if the country or zone of a country was previously considered to be free of that particular disease;
- important new findings, which are of epidemiological significance to other countries;
- a provisional diagnosis of a disease if this represents important new information of epidemiological significance to other countries; or
- if there are new disease findings of exceptional significance to other countries.

Thereafter, monthly reports are sent to OIE to update information on the evolution of the disease incident, until the disease has been eradicated or the situation has stabilized.

Annual reports from member countries are sent to OIE listing absence or presence data, as well as any information on changes in status of diseases notifiable to the OIE, or findings of epidemiological importance to other countries for diseases that are not listed.

In addition, there are requirements to report any significant changes in the status of infected zones of relevance to other countries.

12.10 Managing Surveillance Data

To be useful and usable, surveillance data need to be in a consistent format and readily accessible for analysis. Ideally, standard reports and analyses should be pre-set and able to be run on demand. Another essential feature of managing surveillance data is ensuring that quality is maintained and that they are error-free. Unfortunately, the better the data management system for ensuring data quality and ease of reporting the more expensive it is likely to be. However, investment in the additional cost for a reliable and robust system usually pays off in the long term through savings in time spent grappling with a substandard system to clean data and produce reports.

12.10.1 Spreadsheets

Spreadsheets are an inexpensive and flexible option for data management. They have the advantage of flexibility in data entry and structure, and have inbuilt analytical and graphics tools. However, spreadsheets provide only minimal control over data entry, so that data quality is often an issue requiring constant attention. In addition, using spreadsheets runs the risk of having multiple spreadsheets for a project, often maintained by different people and circulating spreadsheets for checking and analysis by other people creates problems of version control – which version is the correct one (or are any of them). In addition, while graphics are often excellent and easy to use, spreadsheets are not suited to more sophisticated analyses, so separate analytical software may be required depending on the reporting requirements for the programme. As a result, any savings from using an inexpensive and flexible spreadsheet are lost in the additional time and effort required for data checking and analysis. Spreadsheets may be useful for small projects with only relatively small amount of well-defined data but should be avoided for larger and more complex datasets.

12.10.2 Desktop database

A better alternative to using spreadsheets is to use a dedicated desktop database. This has the significant advantage that data entry can be much more strictly controlled, resulting in fewer data-entry errors and overall improved data quality. It is also usually relatively inexpensive, although there may be some additional set-up costs compared to using spreadsheets. In the long run the extra cost of getting the database set up properly more than pays for itself in improved efficiency and data quality. Most modern desktop databases have powerful query tools and can produce complex reports, although this is a fairly specialized activity. In many cases use of separate dedicated reporting tools is preferable, particularly if complex reports and graphics are required. Because of the centralized nature of a desktop database this usually means that data entry is centralized as well, which is good for data-entry quality and consistency but may place a significant load on a small number of people. Remote data entry is possible but also gets more complicated and can lead to transcription errors.

12.10.3 Online database

Over the last decade or two the power and capability of online databases has increased dramatically, as has accessibility to the Internet at reasonable cost and speed. This now makes a centralized online database a very attractive option, particularly if access by field staff or remote users is important. While there is a significant set-up cost, data quality can be strictly controlled and reporting can be automated to produce complex reports, graphs and maps on demand. The other significant advantage of an online database is that remote data entry is possible, so that those collecting the data can be responsible for data entry and quality, further reducing transcription and data-entry errors. The downside of online data management is that there is a significant development cost and lead time and it is important to fully understand the data structures and reporting requirements from the beginning.

References

Cameron, A.R. (1999) *Survey Toolbox – A Practical Manual and Software Package for Active Surveillance of Livestock Diseases in Developing Countries*. Australian Centre for International Agricultural Research, Canberra, Australia.

Martin, P.A.J., Cameron, A.R. and Greiner, M. (2007) Demonstrating freedom from disease using multiple complex data sources: 1: a new methodology based on scenario trees. *Preventive Veterinary Medicine* 79(2–4), 71–97.

OIE (2011) *Terrestrial Animal Health Code.* World Organisation for Animal Health (OIE), Paris, France.

Scudamore, J.M. (2002) *Partnership, Priorities and Professionalism – A Proposed Strategy for Enhancing Veterinary Surveillance in the UK.* Veterinary Surveillance Division, Department for Environment Food and Rural Affairs, London.

13 Regional Animal Health Programmes

13.1 Introduction

Many animal diseases are endemic in a population and are either not sufficiently serious to warrant control, or are amenable to well recognized treatment, control or preventive measures implemented at the farm or individual level. However, where diseases are less easily controlled at the individual or farm level, or where there are overflow effects to other producers which they cannot manage on their own, coordinated action at a regional, provincial or national level may be required to provide effective control or eradication. In extreme cases, some diseases are sufficiently costly to justify attempts to eradicate them from the population. For example:

- Milk fever and grass tetany are affected by seasonal and management factors and are generally managed at farm and individual animal levels.
- Clostridial diseases of sheep and cattle are widespread and generally controlled by on-farm vaccination programmes.
- Internal and external parasites in sheep and cattle are generally managed at the farm level, but can be very costly on an industry basis (many millions of dollars per year) and on-farm control may be supported by regional programmes providing technical advice and support.
- Some diseases, such as ovine brucellosis or caprine arthritis-encephalitis virus, affect only some herds or flocks, and can be managed at a regional or industry level through voluntary quality assurance (QA)-type programmes.
- Control of Johne's disease in many countries is moving towards voluntary, industry-based programmes.
- Zoonotic disease such as anthrax, rabies, bovine spongiform encephalopathy and highly pathogenic avian influenza are subject to strict regulatory programmes in many countries.
- Brucellosis and TB in cattle have been eradicated from Australia and are subject to national eradication programmes in some countries.
- Exotic disease outbreaks in some countries are usually subject to emergency eradication programmes (e.g. foot-and-mouth disease) in countries where the disease does not usually occur.
- Global freedom from rinderpest was declared in 2011, following a lengthy eradication programme.

The occurrence of most animal diseases is affected by a wide range of factors associated with the host (e.g. breed, species, age), the agent (e.g. strain virulence, methods of transmission, etc.) and the environment (e.g. housing, nutrition, management). In developing a regional control or eradication programme it is important that these factors are understood and manipulated to achieve the desired goal.

For any regional animal health programme to be successful it is essential that the disease is amenable to control and that the programme:

- is appropriate to the circumstances of the particular disease of concern;
- is properly justified and supported;
- has a clear vision, objectives and targets;
- is properly designed and planned; and
- utilizes appropriate tools and methods, which are correctly applied.

The aim of this chapter is to provide an understanding of the key epidemiological concepts involved in the development and implementation of effective national or regional animal health programmes.

13.2 Why Have a Regional Programme?

Regional disease control or eradication programmes have been an important facet of livestock production since at least the 18th century. Early programmes were directed at eradication of outbreaks of severe diseases such as rinderpest and foot-and-mouth disease from Europe and the UK in the 18th and 19th centuries. Also in the 19th century, Australia eradicated sheep scab from its national flock, while in the mid- to late 20th century contagious bovine pleuro-pneumonia brucellosis and tuberculosis were also eradicated from the Australian cattle population. More recently, in 2011 international freedom from rinderpest was proclaimed after a protracted eradication campaign. This is only the second time global eradication of a disease has been achieved (following the eradication of smallpox in the mid-20th century) and the first time for an animal disease.

Up until the mid-20th century, the main reason for attempting animal disease control or eradication programmes was because of the severe economic impact of epidemic diseases on affected farmers and industries. As the dependence of national economies on livestock industries has declined, particularly in developed countries, and awareness of public health increased, the rationale for development of regional animal health programmes has broadened.

Regional or national programmes may be implemented for a variety of reasons, including to:

- control or eradicate diseases with severe productivity and economic (including trade) consequences (e.g. foot-and-mouth disease);
- protect or maintain trade in animals and animal products (e.g. enzootic bovine leucosis in dairy cattle);
- protect human health from zoonotic infections (e.g. bovine spongiform encephalopathy, bovine tuberculosis, anthrax);
- maintain product quality (e.g. chemical residues);
- protect unaffected producers or regions from disease that may be endemic in other regions (e.g. footrot, ovine brucellosis, Johne's disease, cattle tick);
- reduce indirect effects of disease on unaffected producers who are not in a position to take action themselves to effectively prevent or control the impacts of the problem on their enterprise (e.g. chemical residues, Johne's disease); and
- reduce the impact of disease on affected herds and flocks (e.g. mastitis, internal parasites in sheep).

Table 13.1. Characteristics of conditions suited to farm-level or regional control (adapted from Hanson and Hanson, 1983).

Farm-level control	Regional control
Spread can be stopped by a physical barrier such as a fence	Physical barriers of limited effectiveness in preventing spread
Rate of transmission is slow enough to allow intervention before the entire herd is infected	Transmission is too fast for intervention before the entire (or majority of) herd is infected
Carriers are readily detectable on-farm	Apparently healthy carriers can only be detected by laboratory tests
No public health, food safety or product quality implications	Condition is a public health, food safety or product quality risk
Low or no mortality rate	High morbidity and high mortality rates
Highly effective vaccine or treatment is available	Vaccine or treatment is only poorly to moderately effective

An important aspect of diseases requiring regional or group action to control or eradicate is that they are often diseases where producers can take individual action if they wish, but where the risk of re-infection or break-down of control because of external factors is sufficiently high to discourage individual action.

For example, many sheep producers in the Australian state of New South Wales were reluctant to attempt eradication of footrot in sheep until a regional programme started and provided some reassurance that they were not likely to get re-infected.

Table 13.1 lists the characteristics of conditions that determine whether a disease is more suited to individual farm or regional control.

13.3 Types of Programmes

Regional animal health programmes can vary substantially in their design, the tools used and the way they are implemented, depending on the rationale and objectives of the individual programme. Programmes can be broadly classified according to their objectives as either eradication or control programmes.

13.3.1 Eradication programmes

Eradication programmes are generally directed at the elimination of a disease agent from a region. This is usually achieved by the implementation of measures directed at reducing prevalence on infected farms and interrupting spread from infected to uninfected farms.

Eradication programmes are usually based on a strong regulatory framework, with significant government input to the management and implementation of the programme. Funding for eradication programmes may be largely from governments, or shared by governments and affected industries, depending on the nature of the disease and the capacity and willingness of governments (and industry) to contribute.

In cases of endemic diseases, eradication may be preceded by a period of control to reduce the prevalence of disease to a level where eradication becomes feasible and economical.

13.3.2 Control programmes

In this context, control implies any programme directed at reducing the level of morbidity, mortality or production losses due to a disease, regardless of how this is achieved.

Control can be achieved by:

- treating diseased animals;
- preventing infection occurring; or
- reducing the impact of disease in infected animals.

Control programmes tend to be ongoing while the disease or the reasons for its control persist. In contrast, eradication programmes tend to be time-limited.

Disease control programmes are directed at reducing the prevalence or impact of a disease, whereas eradication programmes are directed at elimination of clinical disease or the causal agent from a region within an acceptable time frame.

In contrast to eradication programmes, control programmes can be based on a number of different approaches, depending on the nature of the disease of concern and the objectives for the programme.

13.3.3 Regulatory programmes

Some control programmes may be supported by government regulation to allow enforcement of compliance. Regulations may relate to movement controls, animal treatments, destruction of animals and compensation. Regulatory programmes are more common for diseases that have a public good component, such as zoonotic diseases. Over time, if a control programme is successful it can be extended and adapted into an eradication programme. Examples of diseases where regulatory control programmes are used include anthrax, rabies and bovine spongiform encephalopathy.

13.3.4 Voluntary (industry-based) programmes

As governments in developed countries move away from regulation of the livestock industries, there has also been a move towards voluntary or industry-based control programmes. These programmes rely on farmers complying voluntarily with recommended practices to reduce disease risk to themselves and other producers, rather than using regulations to enforce compliance. Voluntary programmes depend heavily on an effective communication and education programme to change the behaviour and attitudes of farmers and their advisors and to get farmers to adopt the recommended practices.

Voluntary programmes may have some regulatory support (e.g. legislative support for the use of vendor declarations or movement controls), but are being used increasingly as an alternative to regulatory programmes, particularly where most of the benefits of the programme flow to producers rather than consumers or the general public. Examples of voluntary programmes include the early stages of enzootic bovine leucosis eradication in dairy cattle in Australia and Johne's disease control programmes in many countries.

13.3.5 Assurance-based programmes

Assurance-based programmes rely on on-farm implementation of a quality assurance approach to management and production on some farms to provide a source of quality-assured stock for other producers. Quality assurance programmes require participating farmers to implement a range of recommended practices to achieve a quality outcome and are supported by an audit process to ensure compliance and demonstrate programme integrity. Stock from qualifying farms may be assured as low-risk for a particular disease or for chemical residues, depending on the programme(s) in which they participate and the level they have achieved.

Although assurance-based programmes may not significantly reduce the regional prevalence or impact of the disease or condition of concern, they can reduce further spread by providing sources of low-risk stock for producers who wish to avoid introducing unwanted diseases to their farm. They can also be used as part of a broader regulatory or voluntary control programme. Examples of assurance-based programmes include the various Johne's disease Market Assurance Programs in Australia and similar programmes in other countries, as well as industry-based product quality programmes.

13.4 Prerequisites for a Successful Programme

Before embarking on a potentially difficult, costly and often controversial disease control or eradication programme, it is essential to evaluate the proposed programme in terms of its technical feasibility and likelihood of success.

The critical elements required for a successful disease control or eradication programme are summarized below (from Yekutiel, 1981 and Thrushfield, 1995). Although it may be possible to successfully control or eradicate a disease without meeting all of the criteria listed, the likelihood of failure increases as more criteria remain unfulfilled.

1. Adequate knowledge about the cause of the disease and its epidemiology. Knowledge of the cause (at least in epidemiological terms) and the epidemiology of a disease is essential for the development of effective strategies for the prevention of transmission and spread of the disease and for the application of screening tests to detect cases.
2. Adequate veterinary infrastructure and resources, including administrative and operational personnel. Adequate infrastructure and veterinary staff are essential for the effective implementation of a programme. Inadequate staffing of the programme is likely to result in failures in the application of the selected control measures and significant delays in meeting programme objectives.

Important components of the infrastructure required for a successful programme include:

- field veterinary staff;
- lay staff to assist with field activities;
- administrative staff to manage the programme and maintain databases and reporting capability;
- regulatory staff to implement and enforce legislative support measures;
- diagnostic facilities and staff; and
- research facilities and staff.

3. Accurate, reliable and economical diagnostic tests. Reliable and economical tests that have been adequately characterized for sensitivity and specificity are essential for the identification of infected animals and herds or flocks for appropriate follow-up action. Reliable tests are also required for herd/flock classification and identification of low-risk replacement stock. A good understanding of test sensitivity and specificity and factors that may affect these characteristics is also required for the development of appropriate testing and surveillance strategies.
4. Epidemiological features that facilitate case detection and effective surveillance. Diseases that are mainly subclinical or for which diagnostic tests have a poor sensitivity are likely to be difficult and expensive to detect, making the reliable identification of cases and implementation of control measures difficult. Diseases that can be detected through screening of routinely available samples or by simple testing at the herd/flock level (e.g. abattoir screening, bulk milk samples) are more suited to an effective programme than diseases that require on-farm testing of large numbers of individual animals for the identification of infected individuals and/or herds/flocks.
5. Control measures that are simple to apply, relatively inexpensive and highly effective at preventing transmission of infection. Any control or eradication programme depends on the implementation of one or more control measures to interrupt transmission and reduce prevalence. While it is possible to control and even eradicate diseases with imperfect tools (e.g. brucellosis, TB), the more effective the measures are, the more likely a programme is to succeed. The less that is known about disease transmission and on-farm control measures, or the harder it is to control on-farm, the more difficult it will be to control the disease on a regional or national level. Measures must also be effective at preventing spread between farms, as well as at reducing or preventing transmission on infected farms.
6. A reliable source of sufficient numbers and quality of disease-free replacement stock for those destroyed or culled during the campaign. Any programme requiring slaughter or compulsory culling of infected stock is heavily dependent on a source of disease-free replacements. If disease prevalence is high, this becomes more difficult. Also, if available tests have a poor sensitivity it may be difficult to reliably identify low-risk animals or populations as a source of replacements.
7. Support for the programme amongst producers and the general public, and cooperation by producers with the requirements of the programme. If there is not a high level of commitment to the programme among producers it is likely to be affected by criticism, unrest and even active resistance, hampering implementation and potentially undermining the effectiveness of the programme. This is even more important for voluntary programmes, where farmer education, support and compliance are critical for programme success.
8. A specific and valid reason for eradication or control, and the programme should be justified by an independent cost–benefit analysis. Without a clear and well-argued rationale for eradication or control, any programme is likely to lack the support of producers, industry leaders and governments. The most common reasons for eradication or control have been discussed previously, but include public health effects or the cost of the disease to the industry or community. If eradication is proposed, there also must be a valid reason for recommending eradication rather than control.

For a programme to be supported, a social cost–benefit analysis will generally be required, demonstrating that the programme is economically justifiable and that the expected returns (in terms of savings in cost of disease or productivity losses) exceed the cost of the programme over the longer term.

9. Supporting legislation to enable the programme to proceed, including provision for compensation. Appropriate legislation is required to implement movement controls, compulsory slaughter, compensation and other measures included in regulatory-type programmes. However, even in voluntary programmes, some level of legislative backing may be required to provide a legal basis for area declarations and movement restrictions and for enforcement of programme requirements.
10. The ecological consequences of the programme must be assessed and addressed. There is increasing public concern over environmental and ecological issues, such that they must now be an important consideration in any animal health programme. If the proposed programme is likely to have adverse environmental or ecological effects it is unlikely to be supported by governments or the general public. However, programmes that have a positive impact on the environment (e.g. by reducing the feral animal population) are likely to be well-supported.
11. Adequate funding committed to the programme. Without adequate funding, any animal health programme is doomed to failure. In the current economic climate, governments are reluctant to commit large amounts of public money unless there is a positive return on their investment and an obvious public benefit from the programme. Where the livestock industries are the major beneficiaries of disease control, they are also expected to be the major funders in some countries. A requirement for industry contribution also raises the issue of how to collect money from producers at a state or regional level, usually through some form of levy at sale or slaughter.

13.5 Disease Control Tools

There are a number of disease control tools that can be used, either alone or in combination, as part of control or eradication programmes. These tools are generally used to manipulate the agent/host/environment interaction to reduce the opportunity for spread of infection or exposure to a chemical agent.

For infectious diseases, maintenance of infection in a population depends on:

- the presence of infectious individuals and herds;
- the presence of susceptible individuals and herds; and
- contact between infectious and susceptible individuals and herds.

Disease will persist in the population while these conditions remain. Disease control tools are used in four main ways.

1. To detect the disease agent.
2. To reduce the number of infected hosts.
3. To increase the resistance to infection of susceptible hosts.
4. To reduce contact between infectious and susceptible hosts.

13.5.1 Detecting the disease agent

Surveillance

Because of the substantial cost involved, surveillance programmes used for disease control often encompass several diseases at the one time. Surveillance is discussed briefly here in the context of disease control and eradication. More extensive general information about surveillance is provided in separate sections.

Important questions that are often asked directly or indirectly as part of control programmes, and which can be answered by well-structured surveillance, are:

- Is the frequency of the disease remaining constant, increasing or decreasing?
- What is the relative frequency of one disease compared with another?
- Are there differences in the geographical pattern of the condition?
- Does the disease have any impact on productivity and/or profitability?
- Is the disease absent from a particular herd, region, or nation?
- Is a control or eradication programme cost-effective?

The potential sources of data for surveillance programmes include clinical evaluations, laboratory reports, slaughter inspection data, screening tests, owner reports and on-farm screening programmes.

Surveillance programmes may be developed at a number of different levels, depending on the level of need for the information. Some examples are listed below:

1. Individual farms – these usually include monitoring of economically significant production parameters, such as mortality rates, somatic cell counts in milk as an indicator of mastitis, growth rate, milk production, mortality rates, etc. Monitoring of temporal patterns of these variables is important for early detection of potential disease problems or failure of on-farm control programmes.
2. Region or state – this may involve testing to:

- establish regional freedom from particular diseases, which may give individuals collective financial/production advantages over competitors;
- identify infected herds/flocks for control action;
- identify infected animals for specific control actions; or
- determine prevalence and distribution of disease.

3. National – national surveillance programmes can be very costly. To help defray costs these programmes may predominantly be based on passive surveillance (investigation initiated by the owner) or involve testing of only a sample of the national herd. Passive surveillance schemes are in place in many countries for the early detection of foreign and/or emerging diseases. Such schemes depend on recognition and reporting by livestock owners or veterinarians of suspicious disease signs.

Surveillance to identify infected animals or infected herds/flocks is an essential component of any control or eradication programme at a regional, state or national level. For such programmes, surveillance could be targeted at individual animals on-farm (e.g. test-and-slaughter programmes for brucellosis or bovine tuberculosis eradication), or could use aggregate samples, such as bulk milk or pooled faeces, or could use off-farm sampling such as through milk factories or abattoirs (e.g. milk-ring testing to identify brucellosis-infected herds). Farmer notification of suspected cases also forms an important component of surveillance for case detection. For surveillance to be effective, an economically justifiable test with known sensitivity and specificity should be used (see Chapter 7 on Application of Diagnostic Tests). Once an infected animal or farm has been identified, further action is likely using one or more of the other tools discussed below.

Tracing

Tracing of livestock movements is an important tool particularly for the detection of infected herds or flocks. For disease control purposes, tracing usually involves the identification of potentially infected farms through the tracing of movements of infected or exposed animals. Further testing is usually undertaken on the identified farms to establish their true infection status. If a farm's infection status cannot be determined immediately, quarantine measures may be imposed until the situation is resolved.

Tracing can involve any of the following activities:

- identification of the property of origin of animals identified as infected or suspect through testing at abattoirs or sale-yards (abattoir/sale-yard trace-back);
- identification of the property of origin of animals suspected as a potential source of infection on an infected farm (trace-back);
- identification of farms that have received possibly exposed animals from an infected farm (trace-forward);
- identification of farms with animals potentially exposed during movement of infected animals, such as at sale-yards or during transport;
- identification of neighbouring farms or other farms potentially exposed to an infected farm by local movement of animals or infectious material; and
- identification of vehicles used to transport potentially infected animals or vehicles, people or other fomites that have had possible contact with infected animals or environments.

Tracing activities are made much easier and more reliable by the consistent use of unique animal identification and identification of sale animals to the farm of origin. Without reliable animal identification, effective tracing and hence adequate disease control becomes very difficult and the development of national animal identification systems, including transaction databases, has greatly facilitated tracing capabilities in many countries.

In the absence of a comprehensive database of animal movements, tracing relies on interviews with the owners of infected or exposed animals to identify potential animal or other movements that might have spread infection. Investigations may also include discussion and examination of records from livestock agents, stock selling centres, milk processors and abattoirs.

Effective tracing can also consume large volumes of resources for both the identification of movements to/from infected farms, and also the subsequent identification and investigation of the source or destination properties. However, examination of tracing records can often help understand the epidemiology and distribution of a disease during an outbreak. An excellent real-world example of the use of tracing in understanding disease spread is provided by the equine influenza virus outbreak in Australia in 2007. A special issue of the *Australian Veterinary Journal* was published in 2011 containing a large number of scientific papers and abstracts all relating to aspects of the outbreak and its subsequent control (Jackson, 2011).

Moloney *et al.* (2011) provide a visual summary of horse movements supporting the hypothesis that movement of infected horses from four key locations prior to the implementation of movement controls explained almost all of the geographic spread of the disease. In each of these four situations the infected case horses themselves only directly infected relatively small numbers of other horses but these in turn then contributed to further spread of the infection.

13.5.2 Reducing the number of infected hosts

Slaughter

Slaughter of individual infected animals, in-contact animals or entire herds may be an option, depending on the nature of the disease and the programme involved. Slaughter of infected animals and herds has an immediate effect of reducing the number of infected animals in the population, thereby reducing opportunities for further spread of the disease. However, this comes at a significant cost in terms of surveillance to detect the infected animals and the costs of compensation and disposal if the animals are not salvaged through normal slaughtering.

Depending on the type and scale of the programme, slaughtering of stock can be undertaken in a number of ways.

1. Immediate destruction of infected and in-contact animals (e.g. foot-and-mouth eradication programmes, bovine spongiform encephalopathy). In such emergency situations, slaughter may also be accompanied by destruction of carcasses, disinfection of premises and a period of quarantine before restocking, to reduce the risk of agent survival and transmission to other animals.
2. Compulsory slaughter of infected animals only may be required for infectious diseases where eradication is the objective. Test-and-slaughter programmes have frequently been used in the past for regional eradication of infectious diseases such as bovine brucellosis and bovine tuberculosis.
3. Herd depopulation may be used in extreme situations or for problem herds where eradication using other methods has failed (e.g. foot-and-mouth disease, bovine spongiform encephalopathy in the UK; problem herds for bovine tuberculosis and brucellosis late in the Australian brucellosis and tuberculosis eradication programmes).
4. Slaughter or early culling of individual animals may also be used in non-emergency situations as part of a voluntary or regulatory control programme for some diseases (e.g. footrot or ovine brucellosis in sheep, chronic mastitis in dairy cows).

Animal treatments

Where available, treatments (either therapeutic or preventive) can be used to treat infected or exposed animals and reduce prevalence. For example, antibiotic preparations can be used to treat mastitis cases and teat disinfection preparations can be used to prevent new infections occurring.

13.5.3 Increasing resistance of susceptible hosts

Vaccination

Vaccination is an important tool for the control and eradication of many diseases, and can be used in two main ways.

1. Routine on-farm disease control. Vaccines are available for many economically important diseases of livestock and are commonly used as part of routine on-farm disease

control for diseases such as clostridial diseases, leptospirosis, vibriosis, Marek's disease and many others.
2. Prevalence reduction. Vaccines can be very effectively used to reduce the prevalence of disease (both on-farm and at a regional level) as part of a regional control or eradication programme, by increasing the level of herd immunity. This can be used solely for control purposes, or as a prelude to eradication, with eradication attempts only proceeding subject to reducing prevalence of infection to an acceptable target level. For example, a key aspect of the brucellosis eradication programme in Australia was the use of Strain 19 vaccine to reduce prevalence in high-prevalence regions before eradication commenced.

Progress of a disease in a population is affected by herd-immunity effects. From a population perspective, herd immunity is the immunologically derived resistance of a group of individuals to attack by disease based on the resistance of a large proportion, but not all, of the group. Herd immunity may arise from innate immunity (although this may not always have an immunological basis), natural infection or vaccination.

Herd immunity will slow the rate of transmission of a disease within a population, with the magnitude of the effect depending on the level of herd immunity. If herd immunity is high, infection may fail to establish or can be eliminated from the population. It is not necessary for all individuals in a group to be immune to eliminate infection. The level of herd immunity (proportion of immune animals in the population) must simply be sustained at a level that exceeds a critical threshold value at which the contact rate between infectious and susceptible individuals is insufficient to sustain the epidemic. This means that if a minimum critical proportion of animals can be kept immune to infection, a disease can be eliminated from the population. For many infectious diseases, effective vaccination rates of 70–80% provide sufficient herd immunity to prevent an epidemic being sustained.

Genetic manipulation

Many diseases have some level of genetic resistance or susceptibility. For these diseases it may be possible to breed for resistance to infection (e.g. internal parasites in sheep). However, any such breeding programme is likely to be long term, and must consider competing priorities for selection on production traits.

13.5.4 Reducing contact between infectious and susceptible hosts

Quarantine

Quarantine is the physical isolation of infected or potentially infected animals to prevent further spread of infection. Quarantine can be applied to farms that are known or suspected to be infected to prevent spread of infection to other farms. It can also be applied within farms to prevent spread between infected and uninfected groups of animals, or to isolate introduced animals until the farmer can be confident that they are disease free. Occasionally groups of farms may also be quarantined, particularly if they are potentially exposed to a highly infectious disease.

Movement controls

In a similar way to quarantine of infected farms, regional or inter-property movement controls can be used to reduce the risk of spread of infection from areas of high prevalence to areas of lower prevalence. These movement controls can be supported by official disease 'zones' and regulatory requirements for movements between zones, or by a less-regulated approach and voluntary implementation of recommended movement controls to minimize disease spread by farmers.

If a regulatory programme is implemented it is appropriate not only to have regulatory support for movement controls (including quarantine), but also the willingness and resources to enforce the regulations. Under such programmes it may be necessary to have regulatory staff available to maintain movement check points, check movement documentation, carry out sale-yard inspections and enforce other regulations, as appropriate. However, regulation does not necessarily mean that the programme will be complied with. In fact, a voluntary programme with effective education and ownership of the programme by farmers may be more effective than an unpopular regulatory approach.

In a less-regulated or voluntary programme, it is still important to know the level of farmer compliance with recommended control measures. Therefore, even in completely voluntary programmes it is essential to monitor or audit compliance rates against targets on a regular basis.

If farmer compliance is poor, the programme is unlikely to succeed and progress and future options should be urgently reviewed.

Vector control

For vector-borne diseases, control measures may be more easily directed at the vector than at the actual disease agent. For example, effective control of tick fever in cattle in many parts of Australia is achieved mainly by controlling its cattle-tick vector. Similarly, effective long-term control of liver fluke in sheep and cattle can be achieved by either eliminating the snail vector or restricting access of stock to the snail's habitat area. Vector control also should include consideration of mechanical vectors such as syringes/needles, which can be important vectors for some diseases such as enzootic bovine leucosis or caprine arthritis-encephalitis virus.

Management changes

For some diseases, grazing management strategies can be used to reduce exposure of susceptible animals to contamination. For example, many internal parasite control programmes are based on grazing susceptible young animals on pastures that have previously been grazed by low-risk older animals. Similar strategies have been tried for control of Johne's disease, although low-risk animals may be difficult to identify, and may be a different group to animals that are low-risk for parasites.

Many diseases are also affected by factors under the control of the farm manager, such as housing, nutrition, stocking rates, feeding practices, etc. For these diseases, effective control can often be achieved by changing management practices or housing to reduce the transmission or impact of the disease. For example, inadequate ventilation is an important contributor to respiratory disease in pigs, so that severe respiratory disease problems can often be overcome by improving shed ventilation. Similarly, bovine Johne's disease transmission relies on ingestion of contaminated faecal material by susceptible calves, so that the incidence of Johne's disease in dairy cattle can be reduced by changing management to minimize the exposure of young calves to adult faecal contamination.

Biosecurity

While quarantine is an important measure for preventing the spread of disease, quarantine measures are often focused particularly on infected or at-risk herds and flocks. With the increased emphasis on industries, and farmers individually, taking responsibility for managing their own disease risks, the use of biosecurity measures is an important disease control measure.

In practice, biosecurity comprises two quite separate components, bio-exclusion, aimed at keeping diseases out and biocontainment, aimed at preventing onward transmission from infected herds or flocks.

Bio-exclusion is the implementation of measures to prevent the introduction of unwanted pathogens into a livestock (or other) population.

Biocontainment is the implementation of measures to prevent the onward transmission of unwanted pathogens from a (potentially) infected livestock (or other) population.

In contrast to quarantine measures, bio-exclusion measures are focused on disease-free farms, and are made up of a range of measures designed to keep disease out. These can include isolation of introduced stock, only sourcing introductions from farms with a specified level of testing or assurance, disinfection of equipment and clothes/boots coming on to the farm, management of boundary fences and contact with neighbouring stock, vaccination, testing of introductions and any other measures designed to keep disease out or for early detection and response to disease introduction.

Conversely, biocontainment measures are aimed at control of disease on infected farms to reduce prevalence and other measures to reduce the likelihood of onward transmission. Although quarantine is one important biocontainment measure, biocontainment is broader than just quarantine and includes a range of other measures, including many of the same activities as for bio-exclusion. Specific additional measures include vaccination, culling or treatment of affected animals, selling animals for slaughter only, testing animals prior to sale, disinfection of people and equipment leaving the farm, maintenance of boundary fences, etc.

Disinfection

For highly infectious diseases such as foot-and-mouth disease, disinfection of premises and potential fomites (including veterinary equipment) is an essential component of any control or eradication programme. Disinfection can also be an important part of on-farm biosecurity programmes to keep farms free of disease.

13.6 Supporting Activities

13.6.1 Communication, education and training

Support of producers and the general public for the programme and compliance of producers with programme requirements are essential requirements for a programme's success. Without an effective communication and education programme, high levels of producer support and particularly of producer compliance are unlikely to be achieved. Programme messages must be simple and consistent, and in many cases a substantial effort will be required to change the attitudes of farmers and their advisors to disease control and also their actions in managing disease risk. Education and training are also critical elements, to inform and educate producers and advisers about technical aspects of the disease and the programme.

This is increasingly important with the shift from regulatory to voluntary programmes, so that farmers are being asked to voluntarily change their practices to reduce disease risk, possibly at a significant short-term cost to themselves.

13.6.2 Risk assessment

Traditional disease control programmes have relied on regulatory management of quarantine and movement controls to limit the spread of disease, with the underlying assumption that the measures imposed would be effective. Movement controls were generally based on a perceived no-risk approach to prevent spread of infection.

With the move towards more voluntary programmes and the recognition that there is no such thing as a no-risk policy, risk assessment has become an important aspect of any control or eradication programme. A risk assessment approach makes a thorough understanding of the epidemiology of the disease much more important, so that the true risk associated with various options can be properly evaluated and communicated.

It is also important to note that in risk analysis terminology, risk includes elements of both likelihood of occurrence of an event and the expected consequences, should it occur. This is in contrast to the epidemiological definition of risk, which relates to likelihood of occurrence only.

The increasing move to a risk-based approach and voluntary control programmes has occurred because we are dealing with increasingly complex and challenging disease issues requiring more sophisticated and complex responses. This has also coincided with an environment of decreasing government expenditure on disease control, placing increased reliance on the livestock industries to fund and manage programmes with fewer government inputs.

In this changing environment, control of livestock movements has become an essential part of risk management, both at the farm and regional levels. As such, any movement controls should be objective, scientifically based and subject to a risk assessment. Key elements of this approach include the following:

- What are the potential scenarios for the spread of the disease?
- What is the likelihood of disease spread under each scenario?
- What is the potential impact of disease spread under each scenario?

- What is the acceptable level of risk (probability of spread and impact if it occurs) under various circumstances (the acceptable risk for a transaction within a high-prevalence area is likely to be substantially different from that for a low-prevalence area)?
- What tools are available to manage the risk?
- What combination of tools and measures is required to reduce the risk to an acceptable level for each circumstance?
- Development of a transparent and simple process for managing livestock movements.
- Involvement of all stakeholders in the process and communication of results and recommendations to producers.

For such a process to be effective it is essential that producers are involved in programme development and that there is widespread communication with the farming community. For such a programme to be successful, it is important that producers take ownership of the programme and accept responsibility for managing the risk of infection on their farm, rather than relying on regulations to protect them.

13.6.3 Economic analysis

Just as a cost–benefit analysis is essential in determining whether or not a programme is worthwhile in the first place, it is also essential that any programme is subject to ongoing economic analyses. Such analyses should be directed at determining if the achievement of the programme objectives is still economic, as well as determining which are the most economical and cost-effective of a range of potential control options.

13.6.4 Animal identification

Identification of individual animals to their property of origin (and even their property of birth) is an essential component of an effective surveillance programme for the detection of infected herds and flocks.

For example, abattoir inspection of adult sheep is an important part of surveillance for ovine Johne's disease in Australia. Australia's flock identification system allows rapid tracing of the origin of sheep that are inspected and found to be either positive or negative, so that an inspection history can be built up for each flock and region over time, providing better levels of assurance for low-risk flocks and areas and allowing estimation and monitoring of flock-prevalence on an area basis.

Many countries now have mandatory cattle identification and passport systems in place to support traceability of animals and product in the wake of the bovine spongiform encephalopathy outbreak.

Identification of animals to the property of origin is important both at the abattoir and for sales between properties, to support rapid tracing of animal movements in cases of emergency disease outbreaks, such as for foot-and-mouth disease or bovine spongiform encephalopathy or for chemical residue incidents.

Permanent individual identification of animals on farms is also an important and useful tool in any programme that depends on animal testing or examination. Unique animal identification allows animals requiring further action (such as culling or treatment) to be easily identified for such action as may be required.

13.7 Designing an Appropriate Animal Health Programme

The challenge for designing an animal health programme is to bring together the most cost-effective mix of tools to achieve the desired goal.

Key issues in planning and designing an appropriate regional animal health programme include:

- What is the current situation (how common is the disease, what inputs and tools are available, etc.)?
- What is the desired situation?
- Is a regional programme the right approach?
- Is a regional programme feasible and likely to be successful?
- Is the proposed programme likely to be a voluntary or regulatory type of programme?
- What control tools are available for use in the programme that are likely to be effective for the disease of concern?
- What level of resourcing is available for implementing the programme?
- Is the proposed programme feasible and likely to be successful?
- Who are the main beneficiaries of the programme?
- How will the programme be funded?
- How will the programme be managed?

In most cases, any programme will be made up of a one or more of the various tools discussed above, with the specific choice of tools depending on the available resources and the range of measures that are likely to be effective in the circumstances. Once the appropriate tools have been identified, and the ways in which they will be applied have been determined, detailed business and operational plans for the programme should be developed.

The programme plan describes the overall management and operations of the programme and should:

- define the overarching goals or aims of the programme;
- identify specific objectives against which progress can be measured and reported;
- provide a detailed description of how the programme will be managed;
- define roles and responsibilities for participating organizations and key personnel;
- include a detailed budget and funding sources for the programme;
- identify supporting legislation and regulatory powers required or available to support the programme;
- identify the resources required for implementation and where these resources will come from;
- define timelines, targets and monitoring processes to evaluate progress of the programme; and

- provide decision points and criteria for key decisions as to whether to continue, modify or abandon the programme.

In some cases a programme plan may be split into a business plan, covering broad goals, management, responsibilities and funding and a separate operational plan (often reviewed annually), which provides the specific details of targets, resourcing and day-to-day operational activities of the programme.

13.8 Monitoring Programme Performance

The success of animal health programmes is highly variable, depending mainly on the factors outlined previously. However, if programme performance is not monitored and regularly reviewed, stakeholders will not know whether it is succeeding or not. Therefore, ongoing monitoring of programme performance and review of achievements against targets and objectives is essential for any animal health programme.

It is also important that performance is monitored against both financial and animal health objectives. A programme can be operating very efficiently on a financial basis and remain well within budget, but fail to achieve any of its animal health objectives, and vice versa, either of which represents significant failure of the programme.

As part of the planning process, milestones should be set, at which progress can be reviewed against targets. Failure to meet targets at a review point should trigger a response to identify why targets are not being met and to implement measures to correct any deficiencies. In some cases the programme business or operational plans and budgets may need review and refinement, or in severe cases a major overhaul of the programme may be required.

References

Hanson, R.P. and Hanson, M.G. (1983) *Animal Disease Control*. Iowa State University Press, Ames, Iowa.

Jackson, A.E. (ed.) (2011) Equine influenza in Australia in 2007. *Australian Veterinary Journal* 89 (Suppl. 1), 173 pp.

Moloney, B., Sergeant, E.S.G., Taragel, C. and Buckley, P. (2011) Significant features of the epidemiology of equine influenza in New South Wales, Australia, 2007. *Australian Veterinary Journal* 89, 56–63.

Thrushfield, M. (1995) *Veterinary Epidemiology*. Blackwell Science, Oxford, UK.

Yekutiel, P. (1981) Lessons from the big eradication campaigns. *World Health Forum* 2, 465–490.

14 Introduction to Risk Analysis

14.1 Introduction

Risk is defined as the combination of the likelihood of occurrence and the likely severity of the consequences of an adverse event.

Risk analysis is the process of identifying what might happen, how likely it is to happen and how bad it would be (consequences) if it did happen.

Risk analysis usually includes thinking of things that might lower the risk to an acceptable level (risk management) and letting others know about these things (risk communication).

We all use risk analysis at an informal and personal level all of the time. When someone considers an action such as crossing a busy road they will usually consider the risks and may choose to cross where they are or move to a safer place such as a pedestrian crossing and wait until the walk signal is displayed.

14.1.1 Risk analysis in livestock health and biosecurity

Import risk analysis

Much of the development of risk analysis in animal health has been in the area of import risk analysis (IRA). IRA methods are trade-based, focus on differences between importing and exporting countries as a way of identifying possible hazards, and concentrate on sanitary methods as options for risk management.

The OIE describes four components of risk analysis as shown in Fig. 14.1 (Murray *et al.*, 2004).

Note that IRA is simply a specific application of a more generic risk analysis process that can be applied to any situation where decisions are made that require management of uncertainty.

Risk analysis for reasons other than trade

The risk analysis process or selected parts of it can be used in other areas of biosecurity or animal health programmes.

Preparedness planning for animal disease outbreaks

Preparedness planning for animal disease outbreaks involves two fundamental components: early warning, and early and effective reaction.

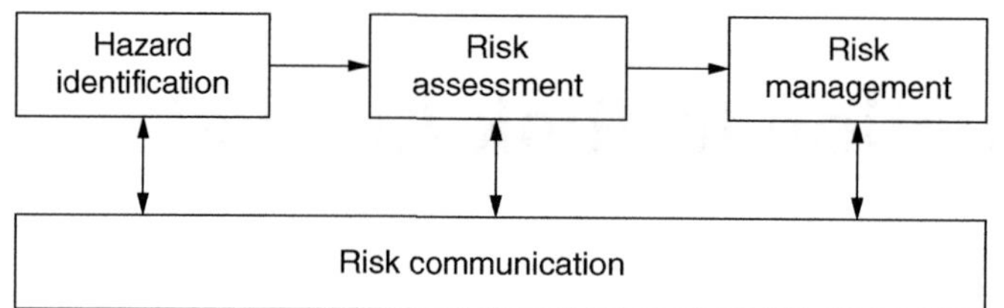

Fig. 14.1. The four components of import risk analysis.

The risk analysis components of hazard identification and risk assessment can be used to identify the major risks to a particular country or area. Risk management planning can then be conducted to develop strategies about how to detect outbreaks quickly and to respond to an outbreak if it occurs.

Benefits of these activities include better understanding of the pathways and likelihoods of disease entry, and gaps in resources and capacity for both surveillance and response at hotspots or points of elevated risk.

In consequence, advice can be provided to decision makers concerning:

- which emergency diseases have the greatest need for preparation of contingency plans;
- where and how border controls and quarantine procedures need to be strengthened;
- where and how disease surveillance activities need to be strengthened; and
- the need for:
  - training courses (veterinary and animal health technicians); and
  - farmer awareness and publicity campaigns.

14.2 Framework for Risk Analysis

A risk analysis framework is the set of components that are used to conduct risk analyses in a consistent and objective manner. One definition of risk analysis framework indicates that it is the guidance on the systematic application of legislation, policies, procedures and practices to risk analysis. A good general review of risk analysis in animal health has been produced by Cribb *et al.* (2011).

A number of risk analysis frameworks exist. The general processes are very similar, indicating there is a common, inherent structure in risk analysis and management. However, differences do exist in terminology, which means that it is important to use simple terms in a consistent manner and to define the terms used.

14.2.1 OIE import risk analysis framework

We will pay most attention to the OIE IRA framework, because:

- it deals with animals and animal products;
- it has been widely used and evaluated IRA; and
- it can be adapted to non-IRA situations.

Import risk analysis is covered in both the Aquatic and Terrestrial Animal Health Codes (OIE, 2012a,b).

Although using the IRA framework, we will spend most of our time applying it to non-IRA situations, to deliver recommendations on:

- The likelihood of an organism or disease:
  - entering;
  - establishing; and
  - spreading in a country.
- The likely impact on:
  - animal health;
  - plant health;
  - human health;
  - the environment; and
  - the economy.
- The options for managing identified risks.

These types of questions are very important for all countries in managing livestock diseases, even when there is no importation of animals or animal products.

Expanded details of the OIE IRA framework (for terrestrial animals) are shown in Fig. 14.2.

14.2.2 Guiding principles of risk analysis

The following principles have been adapted from those used by Biosecurity New Zealand (Biosecurity New Zealand, 2006) to define the nature and performance of their risk analysis programme:

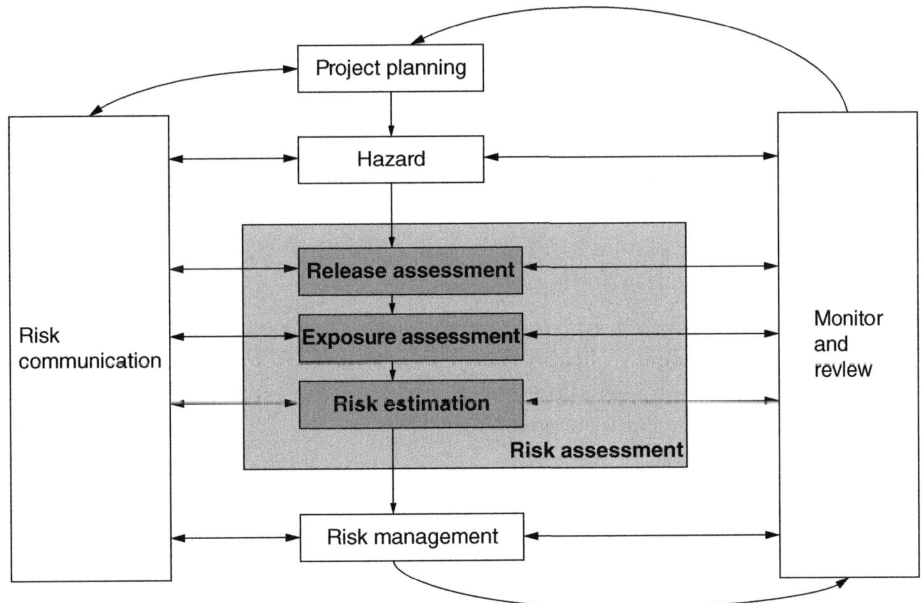

Fig. 14.2. Diagrammatic outline of the OIE import risk analysis framework (adapted from Murray *et al.*, 2004).

- Effective: that each risk analysis accurately measures the risks to the extent necessary and identifies mitigation options that achieve a level of protection appropriate for the relevant country.
- Transparent: that the reasoning, assumptions and evidence behind the risk analysis, and areas of uncertainty and their possible consequences to the findings, are clearly documented and made available to stakeholders.
- Comprehensive: that the full range of values, including economic, environmental, social and cultural, is considered when assessing risks and determining mitigation options.
- Risk management: that zero risk is not obtainable and as such risk is managed through deciding in each instance what should be considered an acceptable level of risk.
- Precautionary: that the risk analyst will incorporate a level of precaution in the import risk analyses to account for uncertainty; for instance when making a professional judgement on whether available information is sufficient, when making assumptions, and when selecting risk management options. Where there is insufficient information, provisional measures may be recommended recognizing the obligation to seek additional information.
- Science-based: the risk analysis should be based on the best available information that is in accord with current scientific thinking. The risk analysis process and the determination of the appropriate risk management techniques should not be compromised by pressures of trade or protection.
- Compliant: that the risk analysis process and methodology meet the needs of and comply with a specific country's domestic legislation and international obligations.
- Consistency: the risk analysis should be based on a well-described methodology so that all risk analyses performed according to the methodology will achieve an expected and predictable standard with minimal variation in methodology. Note that a risk analysis methodology incorporating the characteristics listed above will contribute to consistency in the resulting risk analyses.

14.3 Planning for Risk Analysis

A risk analysis should be planned and managed in the same way that it is necessary to plan for any major project, including:

- The amount of time required for project planning is proportional to the size and complexity of the project.
- A reasonable estimate is to allow at least 10% of the estimated project time for planning and management purposes.

14.3.1 Project management

Project management involves setting the boundaries and rules for the particular project.

Project planning involves developing clear descriptions of the roles, responsibilities and activities for people involved in the project and that will result in the project producing the required outcomes on time, within budget and to the agreed standards.

Responsibilities of the project manager

The project manager has the following responsibilities:

- completing the project plan, including identification of major project risks;
- identifying project team members to ensure all required skills are present/available;
- establishing a risk communication strategy;
- ensuring adequate technical oversight of project team members as they complete the project;
- commissioning internal and external review by suitable experts of the draft risk analysis report;
- managing a repeated process of response from project team members to external review and additional review as required until the project is deemed to have been completed and all issues adequately dealt with;
- obtaining approval from the project sponsor(s); and
- publishing the final version of the risk analysis.

14.3.2 Scope

Defining the scope of the project is an important part of planning.

Focus

A risk analysis can focus on any or all of the following:

- Organism or disease:
  - the appropriate scientific name should be used when reference is made to an organism or disease agent.
- Goods or commodity:
  - may be of plant or animal origin;
  - may be inanimate objects; or
  - of interest in a risk analysis if it has potential to cause an adverse impact to animal and human health or the environment.
- A pathway:
  - pathways include all biological pathways for the entry or spread of a particular organism or disease.
- Method or mode of movement:
  - packaging;
  - containers; or
  - any vessel (ship, plane, truck, etc.) that may be associated with movement of a good or commodity.

Application

The extent of the analysis's application should be defined. For example, an import risk analysis can apply to imports from one country, multiple countries or one or more regions.

Objective

The objective of the risk analysis problem must be defined. This is one of the most important outcomes of the scoping process and involves defining the risk(s) in which you are interested.

For example, consider the importation of a group of cattle. You may be interested in the risk of those particular cattle introducing any infectious pathogen to livestock in your country. Alternatively, you may be interested in the risk per year of introduction of foot-and-mouth disease virus into your country from importation of cattle.

These are two quite different questions and will clearly have a major impact on the scope and how you go about doing the risk analysis.

14.3.3 Method

The method to be used in the risk analysis must be determined. The possible approaches are:

- qualitative;
- quantitative; or
- semi-quantitative.

Qualitative risk analysis

Qualitative risk analysis is:

- suitable for the majority of risk analyses;
- the most common type of assessment done to support routine decision making;
- may be extended or reworked into quantitative analyses where:
  - sufficient data are available; and
  - the need exists.

Some experts feel that all risk analysis problems should be developed initially as qualitative risk analyses.

Further, rigorous quantification of risk as is required for quantitative assessment may not be possible, and it is not necessary to quantify risks for an effective risk-management process to be developed.

Finally, the major outcome of interest for a risk analysis is often not any precise estimate of risk but rather a deeper understanding and insight into the factors that contribute to risk, the pathways through which they may operate, and complexities and uncertainties associated with relationships between various factors.

It is these insights that often benefit the decision makers and policy makers who may be grappling with questions surrounding trade or livestock biosecurity.

Quantitative risk analysis

Quantitative risk analysis may be used to:

- gain further insights into a particular problem;
- identify particular steps; and
- compare sanitary measures.

All aspects of the risk model must be able to be expressed numerically. This is usually done by using point estimates that are drawn from a distribution. This is repeated many times, and the distribution of the results are recorded.

The result of a quantitative risk analysis is expressed as a number, which can present challenges for interpretation and communication. Numbers generated from a quantitative risk analysis are not necessarily more objective, and the results not necessarily more precise, than findings from a qualitative risk assessment.

It is important that stakeholders understand what has been done, so you must maintain and report comprehensive documentation of:

- information;
- data;
- uncertainties;
- methods; and
- results.

Note that the complexity of many problems and the lack of rigorous and valid scientific data for all component parts of a risk analysis generally mean that all models (both qualitative and quantitative) contain varying levels of uncertainty and subjective assessment.

Semi-quantitative analysis

In semi-quantitative analysis, qualitative scales are given values. For example, numbers (or ranges of number) such as 1, 2, 3, 4 may be assigned to negligible, low, moderate and high likelihoods or consequences.

The objective is to produce a more expanded ranking scale than is usually achieved in qualitative analysis, rather than suggesting realistic values for risk such as is attempted in quantitative analysis.

Since the value allocated to each description may not bear an accurate relationship to the actual magnitude of consequences or likelihood, the numbers should only be combined using a formula that recognizes the limitations of the kinds of scales used.

Care must be taken with the use of semi-quantitative analysis because the numbers chosen may not properly reflect relativities and this can lead to inconsistent, anomalous or inappropriate outcomes. In addition, the analysis may not differentiate properly between risks, particularly when either consequences or likelihood are extreme.

14.3.4 Risk evaluation criteria

Risk evaluation criteria are terms of reference and are used to evaluate the significance or importance of risks. They can be used to determine whether a specified level of risk is tolerable.

The simplest risk evaluation criteria divide risks that need treatment from those that do not. This gives attractively simple results but does not reflect uncertainties in estimating risks or in defining the boundary between those that require treatment and those that do not.

It is important to recognize that political and economic judgements may be used in addition to risk analysis results in determining criteria and priorities for treatments.

Terms such as tolerable or acceptable risk are used to identify thresholds of risk that individuals may be prepared to 'tolerate' in return for specified benefits.

On occasion, risk evaluation criteria may be based on consequence alone. This is likely to be restricted to hazards that are expected to be rare but that may be associated with very severe consequences. As a result, a decision may be made to implement some form of risk treatment or risk avoidance, even though the likelihood of the event is extremely low, simply because of the desire to avoid the consequences.

A common approach is to divide risks into three bands (adapted from Standards Australia/Standards New Zealand, 2004):

1. An upper band where adverse risks are intolerable whatever benefits the activity may bring, and risk reduction measures are essential whatever their cost.
2. A middle band (or grey area) where costs and benefits are taken into account and opportunities balanced against potential adverse consequences.
3. A lower band where adverse risks are negligible or so small that no risk treatment measures are needed.

For risks with significant potential health, safety or environmental consequences, this is expressed as the 'as low as reasonably practicable' (ALARP) concept, illustrated in Fig. 14.3. ALARP is a level of risk that is broadly tolerable to stakeholders and that where further risk reduction is deemed to be either more expensive than is warranted given the benefits or is not practical to implement.

The ALARP concept is also applicable for other risks, and balances the ideas of practicality (Can something be done?) with the costs and benefits of action or inaction (Is it worth doing something in the circumstances?).

These two aspects need to be balanced carefully if the risks being treated are related to an expressed or implied duty of care.

The width of the cone indicates the size of risk, and the cone is divided into bands as discussed above:

- When risk is close to the intolerable level, the expectation is that risk will be reduced unless the cost of reducing the risk is grossly disproportionate to the benefits gained.
- Where risks are close to the negligible level, action may only be taken to reduce risk where benefits exceed the costs of reduction (Fig. 14.4).

Risk evaluation criteria must be consistent with the findings of the context/scope setting component of the process. They may be based on threshold measures of risk, consequence and likelihood.

Appropriate level of protection

The Agreement on the Application of Sanitary and Phytosanitary Measures (commonly referred to as the SPS Agreement) of the World Trade Organization (WTO) refers to the term 'Appropriate Level of Protection' or ALOP. The ALOP is the level of protection deemed appropriate by a member country when conducting import risk analysis. This is similar to the ALARP term used in generic risk management applications.

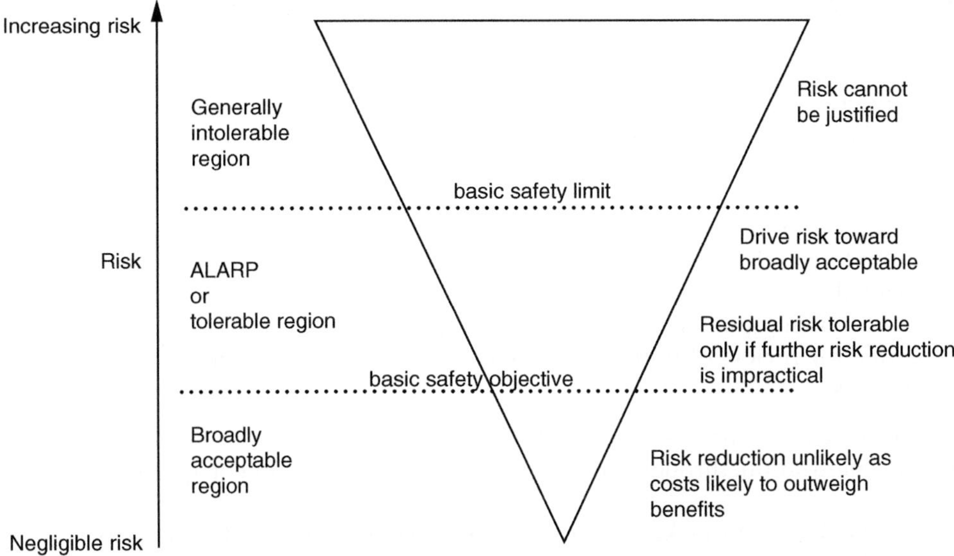

Fig. 14.3. Illustration of the 'as low as reasonably practicable' (ALARP) concept (adapted from Risk Management Guidelines Companion to AS/NZS 4360:2004).

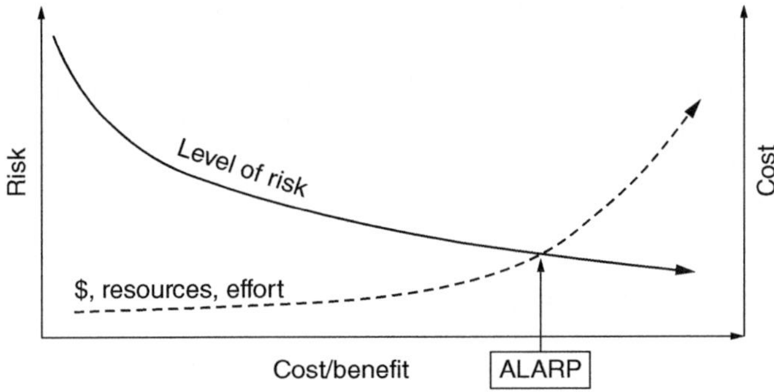

Fig. 14.4. Costs/benefits of risk mitigation: illustration of the point where risk and resources achieve optimal balance concept (adapted from Talbot, 2011).

However, in determining their ALOP, the SPS Agreement obliges members to be transparent and consistent. By this, members cannot use different levels of protection for different products with the same risk, or insist on different measures for the same product from different exporting countries with similar risks. Through consistency and transparency, many of the arbitrary or disguised restrictions on trade are overcome.

This is not to say that a member country must determine a single ALOP that applies to all imports. Members may choose to apply a higher ALOP to risks to human health than for animal or plant health. A further principle is that having determined the ALOP, a member is required to select the quarantine measure that is least restrictive to international trade, while still ensuring the required level of health protection. This is a key provision under the SPS Agreement.

14.3.5 Expert review

Review of the draft report by experts (commonly called peer review) is very important to ensure the analysis is scientifically credible and based on the most current information available. In many countries this is a formal process with internal review by someone within the biosecurity area, followed by external review, often involving international experts.

Reports from reviewers are then provided to the project team member and every issue raised by each reviewer must be responded to, and both the issue and response documented.

The following points have been suggested by Biosecurity New Zealand (2006) as suitable for review of import risk analyses and serve as a guide for any form of risk analysis.

1. Is the logic of the process clear to the reader? Can the reader follow the steps from hazard identification, through the risk assessment to formulation of appropriate measures?
2. Does the document make a clear distinction between facts and assumptions?
3. Does the report include reference to scientific literature? Have any important publications been overlooked? Are the citations accurate? Do they accurately reflect the findings of the underlying papers?
4. For quantitative risk analyses:
   i. Does the report clearly outline the scenario being modelled and the modelling approach used?
   ii. Is the modelling approach and model structure plausible, logical and appropriate?
   iii. Are the assumptions, parameter values and any data used in the model(s) appropriate?
   iv. Are you aware of any data or information that have been overlooked but which might be appropriate in the quantitative assessment?

14.3.6 Communication strategy

All risk analyses should have a communication strategy that describes how the project will be reported to stakeholders and decision makers.

Risk communication involves movement of information in two directions: to inform stakeholders of the activities and findings, and to seek information and feedback from others.

Communication material will need to be developed for stakeholders with differing interests, needs and understanding, so that all stakeholders receive appropriate information and the opportunity to provide feedback.

It is important to develop clear lines of communication to allow feedback and opinion from all stakeholders and ensure that all stakeholder views are taken seriously and are seen to be addressed.

The processes, findings and reports from risk analysis projects must be presented in a way so that stakeholders can understand the process and the reasons for the conclusions reached (often described as transparent).

The analysis must be well documented and supported with references to the scientific literature and other sources of information, including relevant agreements or standards and any expert opinion or other relevant material.

The analysis must provide a reasoned and logical discussion that supports the conclusions and recommendations.

Not all stakeholders will agree with the findings of a risk analysis report. An effective, open and clear communication strategy that is implemented right from the initiation of a risk analysis project should ensure that all stakeholders recognize that their concerns have been addressed and everyone can understand the reasoning behind the conclusions of the final report, whether they agree with the final report or not.

14.3.7 Monitoring and review

A risk analysis is based on information, data and assumptions concerning all of the factors that may contribute to risk. Most of these factors are dynamic, meaning that they can change at any time.

New advances in scientific knowledge may change our understanding of a hazard or raise alternative methods for detection and treatment.

Changes in transport and human behaviour may mean that more of a product or live animals are moved from one location to another, altering risk pathways.

It is important to recognize that while a risk analysis should be based on current information, the nature of the world means that the analysis will rapidly become out of date once it is published.

Therefore, there is a need to review and update the risk analysis as necessary. Information supporting the risk analysis should be periodically reviewed to ensure that any new information that becomes available does not invalidate the decision(s) taken. For example, if beef imports were accepted from a particular country based on disease-free status for various diseases and then a foot-and-mouth disease outbreak occurred in the exporting country, the process would need to be reviewed and the trade decision revisited.

Once risk treatments are imposed as a result of a risk analysis, there is also a need to monitor the treatments to ensure they are effective. For importation of animals or animal products, this is typically done by inspection of the product on arrival.

14.3.8 Keep it simple!

Careful planning including clear definition of scope of the project and risk criteria are essential to effective risk analysis and allow the project team to ensure that the report is as simple as possible.

Each organism or disease should be discussed only to the extent necessary to enable the reader to gain an appreciation of likelihood of entry, establishment or spread of hazard(s) and of their associated potential consequences.

If, for example, it is concluded that the likelihood of a hazard entering the country is negligible, there is no need to undertake an exposure, establishment and consequence assessment and explore risk management options. It is not necessary to offer detailed description of clinical syndromes, pathology, treatments, etc., unless these have a direct bearing on the likelihood of detecting infested commodities or organisms, or managing disease or organism risks.

14.4 Hazard Identification

14.4.1 What is a hazard?

A hazard in the context of livestock health is something that is potentially harmful to humans, animals, plants or the environment.

Hazards are likely to be organisms or disease-causing agents, but could include pests such as introduced species (ants, bees, spiders, screwworm, mites), poisons or toxins, or vectors that may be capable of carrying other disease-causing organisms.

14.4.2 Listing hazards

When compiling a list of potential hazards it is suggested that the initial list be as comprehensive as possible. Each identified organism can then be assessed against criteria to determine if it is a potential hazard.

The following criteria for listing hazards have been adapted from Biosecurity New Zealand (2006).

1. Is the organism or disease absent from the importing country and present in the exporting country?

- This can be a complex issue to answer with confidence.
- Information should be verified where possible and will depend in part on the ability of a particular country's animal health services to detect and diagnose a disease or to determine with suitable confidence that the country is free from a particular disease.

2. Is the organism or disease associated with the commodity or movement pathway in some way?

- If the organism is not associated with the product or the particular movement pathway under consideration then it is not considered as a hazard:
  - Recombinant vaccine products are unlikely to be contaminated with bacteria because of their method of production.
  - Gastrointestinal parasites are unlikely to be associated with processed, frozen semen being considered for importation.

3. Organisms or diseases that are present in both the importing and exporting countries may still be classified as a hazard if they meet one or more of the following criteria:

- The organisms may act as vectors for other pathogens or parasites which themselves are not present in the importing country.
- The organisms may be different in some way to those isolates already present in the importing country such as by:
  - genetic differences;
  - different strains or subtypes;
  - differences in pathogenicity;
  - difference in host association; or
  - differences in severity of disease.

4. The organisms or diseases may be already present in the importing country but the import under consideration may increase the existing hazard in some meaningful way:

- An organism may be present but confined to one small area and if imports were brought into the country there could be risk of increasing the distribution of the hazard.

5. The organism may be present in the importing country but subject to control and eradication measures, or be listed as an unwanted or notifiable organism.
6. The organism may be present in the importing country but there may be insufficient information currently available about the organism(s), so that a conservative approach might be to rule that it is a potential hazard.

14.4.3 Sources of information

For import risk analysis, development of the hazard list involves investigation of diseases present in the exporting country and consideration of any hazards associated with movement of product from the exporting country to the importing country.

The process of making the list involves reviewing national and international databases on disease occurrence such as the World Organisation for Animal Health (OIE). This provides information on current disease status and disease notifications for member countries and specific information about diseases of importance. The OIE's World Animal Health Information Database (WAHID) allows the user to select an exporting and importing country, then reports the OIE-listed diseases present in the exporting but not the importing country.

Preparation for hazard assessment often involves collecting a large amount of information about the animal health capacity (veterinary services and laboratory support, surveillance systems, infrastructure, etc.) in the country of origin, as well as information on diseases of interest that may be present in the country of origin.

In addition, searches should be conducted of the mainstream published scientific literature for information on previous risk analyses and relevant scientific publications.

It may also be useful to seek out expert opinion from suitably qualified and experienced individuals on topics related to the particular issues being investigated.

14.5 Risk Assessment

14.5.1 Introduction

The risk question developed during the scoping and planning phase of the process should define the unwanted consequences that are being considered in the risk analysis.

Hazard identification provides a list of things that are capable of causing harm.

The next component of risk analysis is risk assessment, which involves outlining the pathways or sequence of events that would need to take place in order for the unwanted consequence to occur. The pathways may be broken into components associated with assessment of release, exposure and consequence.

An understanding of the epidemiology of the disease(s) or hazards of interest is necessary to outline the pathways. In some cases, it is also necessary to understand common behavioural practices. For example, preparation of foodstuffs and feeding of food scraps to pigs may be important events in a pathway for risk of entry of foot-and-mouth disease into a country.

A starting list of chronologically ordered events that are likely to be included in a pathway for IRA for an infectious disease includes:

- animals in the exporting country (or animal products) infected with the agent;
- the agent survives commodity handling, treatment, or in-transit time;
- the commodity and associated agent is exposed to susceptible animals or man;
- the agent is transmissible via one or mode mode(s) of transmission;
- exposure to the agent induces infection (entry and development or multiplication of the agent);
- infection induces disease(s);
- disease spreads; and
- disease is detected.

There has been considerable debate over whether risk-reducing measures should be included in these initial pathways or whether they are part of risk management.

Biosecurity New Zealand (2006) suggests that the initial pathways should ignore any hazard management measures such as vaccination, testing, treatment and quarantine (either in the country of origin or the importing country) as these may change over time. They recommend, instead, that all such measures should be incorporated into the risk management options. The term unrestricted has been used to describe the risk before selecting or applying any risk reduction options such as diagnostic testing, quarantine and further processing.

However, others recommend that any measures that are normally implemented by the importing country should be included as part of the pathways described in risk assessment. This is simply part of the process of describing the risk pathway as it is in its usual and current form.

14.5.2 Components of risk assessment

A risk assessment consists of four inter-related steps.

1. Likelihood of entry (called a release assessment by OIE).
2. Likelihood of exposure and establishment.
3. Assessment of consequences.
4. Risk estimation.

14.5.3 Assessing likelihood

Whatever type of analysis is used (qualitative, quantitative, or semi-quantitative), some form of measurement of likelihood is necessary for the release and exposure assessments.

The main types of measurement scales for expressing likelihood are nominal and ordinal.

- Nominal scales use words to describe levels of likelihood.
- Ordinal scales use numbers to represent categories (e.g. 1 = low, 2 = moderate, 3 = high); the numbers only indicate order and do not represent a numerical measure of risk (see Table 14.1 for example).

Table 14.1. Ordinal scaling and adjectives used to qualify an estimated probability (of release, exposure, or occurrence) and the severity of the consequences (Dufour *et al.*, 2011).

Ordinal scaling	Adjectives used	Abbreviation
0	Null	N
1	Nearly null	NN
2	Minute	M
3	Extremely low	EL
4	Very low	VL
5	Low	L
6	Not very high	NVH
7	Quite high	QH
8	High	H
9	Very high	VH

Numerical scales use numbers to measure likelihood, which means that the component must be able to be measured or estimated using real numbers.

Attempts have been made to quantify descriptive terms used to express likelihood. This is difficult, as words tend to mean different things to different people, and it can be hard to obtain agreement about terminology.

There is no agreed international standard for qualitative assessment of likelihood; nevertheless, recent work published in the OIE's journal can be used as a guide (Table 14.1). Note particularly that the same scale or scheme is used to describe different items (likelihoods, which are probabilities, and the severity of consequences, which are not).

14.5.4 Combining likelihoods

Risk pathways usually involve multiple steps, each of which will have an associated likelihood. In order to come up with an assessment of likelihood for the entire pathway, the individual likelihoods need to be combined. The approach used for combining likelihoods depends on the risk analysis method used:

- **Qualitative** – an overall assessment can be made after consideration of the pathway as a whole, or after considering both release and exposure components together.
- **Quantitative** – the individual likelihoods are multiplied together; each likelihood must be estimated as being conditionally dependent on the preceding steps in the pathway (What is the probability of step X occurring, given that all preceding events have already occurred?).
- **Semi-quantitative** – when likelihood categories are assigned to probability ranges, the midpoint of the ranges can be multiplied together to combine categories. The result is assigned to a category according to the range in which it fell.

Dufour *et al.* (2011) present a matrix for combining likelihoods for the probabilities of release and exposure for use in qualitative risk analyses (Fig. 14.5). This approach uses a ten-point ordinal scaling system with associated text definitions to assess probability of release, probability of exposure and the combination of the two (release and exposure), called the probability of occurrence.

		Probability of release									
		N 0	NN 1	M 2	EL 3	VL 4	L 5	NVH 6	QH 7	H 8	VH 9
Probability of exposure	N 0	0	0	0	0	0	0	0	0	0	0
	NN 1	0	1	1	1	1	1	1	1	1	1
	M 2	0	1	1	1	1	2	2	2	2	2
	EL 3	0	1	1	1	2	2	2	3	3	3
	VL 4	0	1	1	2	2	3	3	3	4	4
	L 5	0	1	2	2	3	3	4	4	5	5
	NVH 6	0	1	2	2	3	4	5	5	6	6
	QH 7	0	1	2	3	3	4	5	6	7	7
	H 8	0	1	2	3	4	5	6	7	8	8
	VH 9	0	1	2	3	4	5	6	7	8	9

Fig. 14.5. Combining a probability of release with a probability of exposure to produce an estimate of occurrence of the event. See Table 14.1 for explanation of abbreviations.

14.5.5 Release assessment

Release assessments (also called entry assessments by some groups) describe the pathways of movement of a potential hazard from its country of origin into the importing country and the likelihood of this occurring.

The release assessment process typically involves identification and detailed description of each of the pathways by which a hazard may move from the exporting country into the importing country.

Pathways are often described diagrammatically using scenario trees. The likelihood of progression of a potential hazard can then be estimated at each step along the pathway, leading to an overall likelihood of entry of each potential hazard along each potential pathway.

As with the hazard identification, the release assessment for each hazard should be clearly presented.

The risk analysis may be concluded at this point if the likelihood of the potential hazard being able to enter into the importing country is deemed to be negligible.

Factors for consideration

Biosecurity New Zealand (2006) provide a list of factors that could be considered during a release assessment.

1. Biological factors including:

- Susceptibility of a commodity or pathway to infection or contamination by the potential hazard.
- Means of transmission of the potential hazard:
    - Horizontal transmission:
        - direct (contact, airborne spread, ingestion, coitus); and
        - indirect (mechanical and biological vectors, intermediate hosts).
    - Vertical transmission (from an infected female to a fetus or egg).

- Infectivity, virulence, stability or reproductive strategy of the potential hazard.
- Outcome of infection or contamination (sterile immunity, incubatory or convalescent carriers, latent infection).
- In the case of diseases, routes of infection (oral, respiratory, percutaneous, etc.) and predilection sites of the potential hazard.

2. Country of origin factors, including:

- Incidence and prevalence of hazard in the country of origin (annually or seasonally).
- Evaluation of the exporting country's pest and disease management systems, including surveillance.
- Seasonal timing.
- Existence of hazard-free areas and areas of low hazard prevalence in the exporting country.

3. Commodity/pathway factors, including:

- Ease of contamination.
- Effect of relevant processes (e.g. refrigeration) and production methods in the country of origin, country of destination, or in transport or storage.
- Volume and frequency of movement of commodity to be imported along the pathway.
- Speed and conditions of transport and duration of the life cycle of the hazard in relation to time in transport and storage.
- Vulnerability of the life-stages during transport of storage.

Use of scenario trees in release assessments

Scenario trees are a useful tool for risk analysis because:

- They help us understand the steps that are required for an event to happen.
- They help us describe alternative pathways for an event to happen.
- They allow us to estimate the likelihood of each individual event.
- The give us a mechanism for making an overall assessment of likelihood, based on the likelihood of each individual step.
- They are useful to help communicate the possible risk pathways to others.

An example is provided in Fig. 14.6.

Rules for the branches of scenario trees:

- The branches are mutually exclusive (there is no overlap).
- The branches are comprehensive – there can be more than two, but all contingencies must be covered.
- The sum of the likelihoods (if used) must equal one.

14.5.6 Exposure assessment

Exposure assessments (sometimes referred to as exposure and establishment assessments) describe the biological pathway(s) necessary for exposure of animals or humans in the importing country to the hazards identified and processed in the release (entry) assessment step and the likelihood of these exposures occurring.

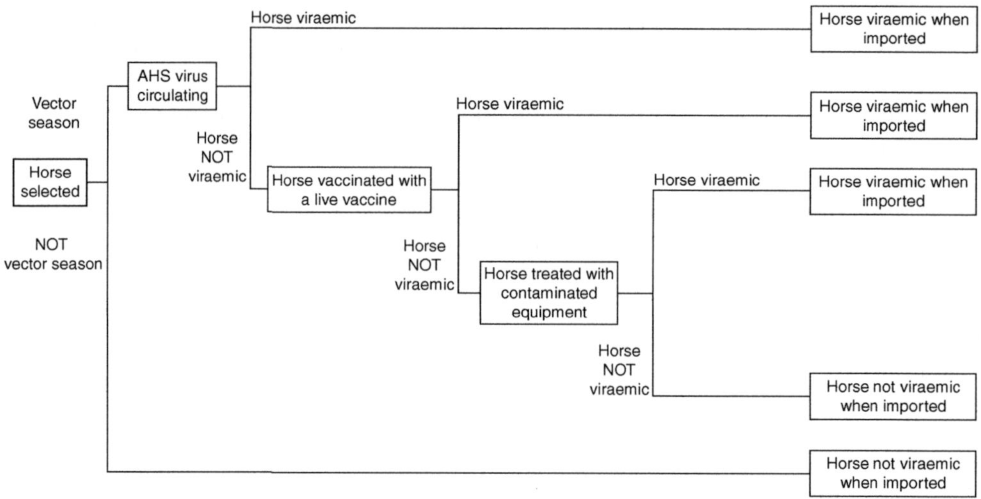

Fig. 14.6. Scenario tree example – a release assessment outlining the biological pathways necessary for a horse to become infected and harbour African horse sickness (AHS) virus when imported into New Zealand (Biosecurity New Zealand, 2006).

Remember that exposure is not always the same as infection. Exposure is necessary before infection can occur, but exposure may not necessarily result in infection. Factors affecting whether exposure results in infection may include the level of exposure (dose), pathogenicity of the hazard and degree of susceptibility of the host. Other causal factors may also influence the outcome of exposure for an individual animal.

Factors for consideration

Biosecurity New Zealand (2006) provide a list of factors that could be considered during an exposure assessment.

1. Biological factors including:

- Means of transmission of the potential hazard:
  - Horizontal transmission:
    - direct (contact, airborne spread, ingestion, coitus); and
    - indirect (mechanical and biological vectors, intermediate hosts).
  - Vertical transmission.
- In the case of diseases, route of infection (oral, respiratory, percutaneous, etc.) and outcome of infection (sterile immunity, incubatory or convalescent carriers, latent infection).
- Infectivity, virulence, stability or reproductive strategy of the potential hazard and potential for the hazard to survive and reproduce in the new environment.
- Adaptability and stability of the potential hazard.
- Demographics of the potential hazard.
- Minimum population needed for establishment – if possible, the threshold population that is required for establishment should be estimated.
- Susceptibility of the environment likely to be exposed to the potential hazard, to adverse impacts such as infection/infestation, predation, competition or hybridization.

2. Risk analysis area factors including:
- Presence of potential hosts including intermediate or alternate hosts, vectors or habitats and how abundant or widely distributed they may be.
- Geographical and environmental characteristics including rainfall, soil and temperature.
- Presence of potential competitors or predators that could reduce the likelihood of establishment.

3. Commodity/pathway factors including:
- Intended use of the commodity (e.g. for planting, processing or consumption).
- Unintended use of the commodity (e.g. offal fed to dogs or pigs).
- Quantity of the commodity to be imported on a pathway or pathways.
- Proximity of entry, transit and destination points to suitable hosts or habitats.
- Likelihoods of repeated introductions maintaining a permanent non-breeding population of the potential hazard.
- Waste disposal practices – risks from by-products and waste.
- Time of year at which import or entry takes place.

Use of scenario trees in exposure assessments

As for the release assessment, scenario tree pathway diagrams can be used to illustrate the biological pathways necessary for the exposure or establishment of the hazard.

Some hazards may have more than one pathway for exposure or establishment; in such cases, a scenario tree must be developed for each pathway.

An example of a scenario tree diagram for the exposure assessment for the infection of susceptible animals in New Zealand with African horse sickness virus following the entry of a viraemic imported horse is shown in Fig. 14.7.

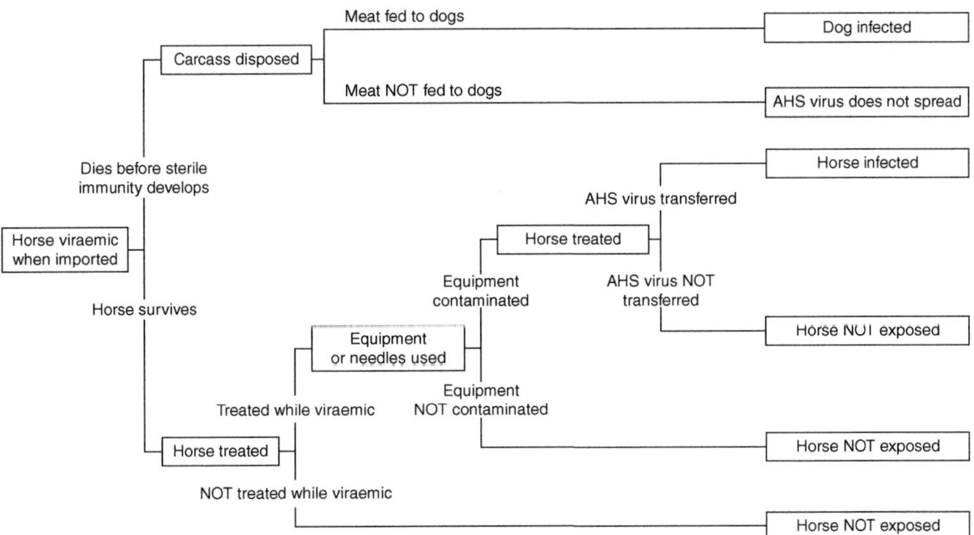

Fig. 14.7. Scenario tree example – an exposure assessment outlining the biological pathways necessary for susceptible animals to become infected with African horse sickness (AHS) virus in New Zealand (Biosecurity New Zealand, 2006).

14.5.7 Consequence assessment

A consequence assessment describes the consequences of a given exposure to a hazard and the likelihood of them occurring.

For livestock diseases the first consequence of interest is successful infection of at least one animal. In many cases it will include an assessment of the likelihood of spread of the potential hazard within the country. This can be used to estimate how rapidly a hazard's potential economic, societal and/or environmental impacts may be expressed. It also has significance if the potential hazard is liable to enter and establish in an area of low potential consequence and then spread to an area of high potential consequence.

Detailed analysis of the estimated consequences is not necessary if there is sufficient evidence (or it is widely agreed) that the introduction of the hazard will have unacceptable consequences.

However, it will be necessary to do a more detailed analysis if the level of consequence is unknown or uncertain, or when the effect of a risk management option must be assessed.

The extent to which the consequences must be considered will be directed by the scope of the project (determined earlier), which will be influenced by relevant legislation (e.g. Biosecurity Act, or similar). It may be necessary to consider animal, human and environmental health, as well as aesthetic, cultural, social and possibly economic conditions that are affected by these factors.

The OIE (2012b) provides examples of consequences that may be assessed.

1. Direct consequences, including:
   i. Animal infection, disease and production losses.
   ii. Public health consequences.
2. Indirect consequences including:
   i. Surveillance and control costs.
   ii. Compensation costs.
   iii. Potential trade losses.
   iv. Adverse consequences to the environment.

Note that a consequence assessment may be repeated at difference levels in the population (e.g. farm/village, district, regional, national).

Use of scenario trees in consequence assessments

Once again, scenario trees can be used to assist understanding of consequences, particularly as it is important to assess not just what the different potential consequences may be and how severe they are, but also to assess how likely they might be (Fig. 14.8).

Measuring consequences

In a qualitative risk analysis, descriptive terms may be used to evaluate consequences. These terms may be similar (or identical) to those used to measure likelihood, but it should be remembered that these are distinctly different matters.

As noted above, Dufour *et al.* (2011) used the same terms to describe consequences as they did to qualify probabilities (of release, exposure or occurrence) (Table 14.1). The methods used by Dufour *et al.* (2011) to evaluate consequences will not be suitable

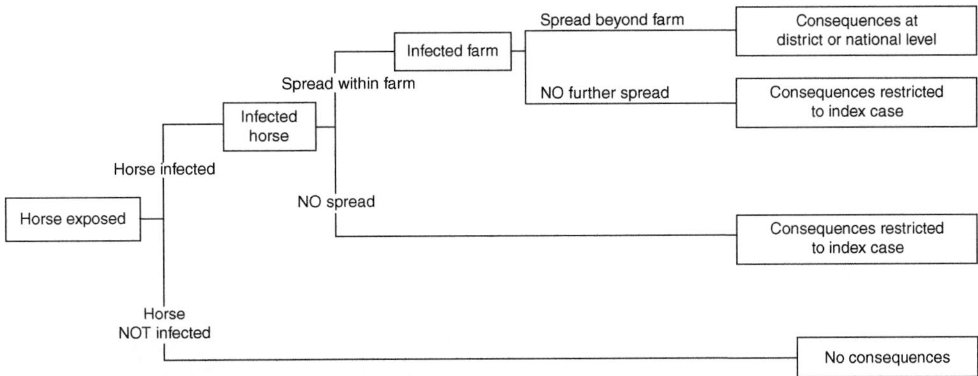

Fig. 14.8. Scenario tree example – a consequence assessment using the African horse sickness example in New Zealand (Biosecurity New Zealand, 2006).

for all situations, but they provide a simple, achievable model that can be adapted or extended to suit other situations. Note that in this example, the relative likelihood of the difference scenarios is captured only in the 'likelihood of disease spread' aspect.

14.5.8 Risk estimation

Combining measures of likelihood and consequence

Combining the estimated probability of an adverse event occurring with the consequences of such an occurrence provides an estimate of risk, which can be used for decision making.

Typically, estimates of likelihood are combined with consequences using a matrix approach. For consistency, it makes sense to use the same general framework for risk estimation as for other components of risk analysis. We will refer to the approach described by Dufour *et al.* (2011), using probability of occurrence (likelihood) from Fig. 14.5 and combining it with consequence to produce a risk estimate (Fig. 14.9).

We repeat that likelihood and consequences are different types of information, and combining them to fill in the matrix is not a matter of mathematical calculation but rather a matter of judgement that depends on one's attitude to risk and the science-based information that is available to make that judgement.

As an example, the following points reinforce the subjective nature of risk estimation.

A more risk-tolerant person would move all the category boundaries in a risk matrix such as Fig. 14.5 towards the bottom right reflecting tolerance of higher risk. A more risk-averse person would move them towards the top left. A person who gives relatively more weight to the severity of the consequences would make the diagonal boundaries between risk categories slope less steeply.

Variability and uncertainty

When analysing risk, it is important to understand and represent uncertainty and variability.

Consequence		Probability of occurrence									
		N	NN	M	EL	VL	L	NVH	QH	H	VH
		0	1	2	3	4	5	6	7	8	9
0	N	N	N	N	N	N	N	N	N	N	N
1–3	NN	N	NN	NN	NN	NN	NN	NN	NN	NN	NN
	M	N	NN	NN	NN	NN	NN	NN	NN	NN	M
	EL	N	NN	NN	NN	NN	NN	NN	NN	M	EL
4–6	VL	N	NN	NN	NN	M	M	EL	EL	VL	VL
	L	N	NN	M	M	EL	EL	VL	VL	L	L
	NVH	N	M	EL	EL	VL	VL	L	L	NVH	NVH
7–9	QH	N	L	L	L	NVH	NVH	NVH	QH	QH	QH
	H	N	NVH	NVH	NVH	QH	QH	QH	H	H	H
	VH	N	QH	QH	QH	H	H	H	VH	VH	VH

Fig. 14.9. Combining a likelihood (probability of occurrence) and consequence to produce a risk estimate. See Table 14.1 for explanation of abbreviations.

Variability refers to the spread of values that a variable can take due to chance or random error. Collecting more data does not reduce variability in a quantitative model, but allows it to be represented with more precision.

Uncertainty indicates the spread of values that a variable can take because we lack knowledge about the possible values. Collecting more data or information about a variable can reduce uncertainty.

In the model used by Dufour *et al.* (2011) for expressing probabilities of release and of exposure, and to assess the severity of consequences, intervals were used to express uncertainty in the estimated probabilities or consequences. For example, the probability of importing a disease into a country might be considered to lie between two and three (2–3) on an ordinal scale that ran from zero to nine.

After the completion of the draft risk estimation, it is useful to review the uncertainties and assumptions identified during the hazard identification and risk assessment stages. This assists in determining which inputs are critical to the outcomes of the risk analysis and may identify particular information gaps that might need to be further investigated to reduce the level of uncertainty prior to making a final decision about risk management.

Repeating risk estimation

If the result of an unrestricted risk estimation (that is, without application of any sanitary measures) is above the level deemed to be acceptable, then the effect of risk management measures must be assessed (and risk estimation repeated) to determine whether the risk can be reduced to a level that is acceptable.

14.6 Risk Management

Risk management describes the process of deciding measures to reduce or avoid the risks associated with the particular hazard(s) being considered. The guiding principle of risk management is to reduce risk to below an acceptable level. It is not appropriate to argue for zero risk. Figure 14.10 provides an outline of the risk management process.

The need for risk management to be implemented will be based on the risk assessment findings.

However, it is important to recognize that risk management decisions will consider a wide variety of scientific and non-scientific input information including social, political, economic and environmental information in addition to risk assessment. Any final decisions may be strongly influenced by political and social inputs.

Risk management is typically carried out by regulatory authorities with legislative mandates.

Risk management is generally regarded as being best managed in a process that is independent from risk assessment. The reasons for this are mainly because risk assessment can be considered to be a technical and science-based process whereas risk management incorporates a wider range of non-technical inputs and in particular value judgements related to public perceptions of risk. Separating the two components ensures that risk assessment can be clearly identified as a science-based and separate process, and not influenced by the value judgements that may influence risk management.

14.6.1 Objectives for managing risk

Risk management objectives should be clearly defined in terms of the desired level of risk reduction and protection and should be very specific.

As an example, two risk management objectives for African horse sickness (AHS) are provided here:

- An objective of ensuring that infected animals are not imported is not sufficiently specific to guide risk analysis.
- A more specific objective may be to effectively manage the risks of AHS; measures should ensure that horses are neither incubating the disease nor viraemic when imported.

14.6.2 Options for managing risk

Specific information on risk management options for most of the major livestock diseases of importance to trade are listed in the OIE's Terrestrial and Aquatic Animal Health Codes.

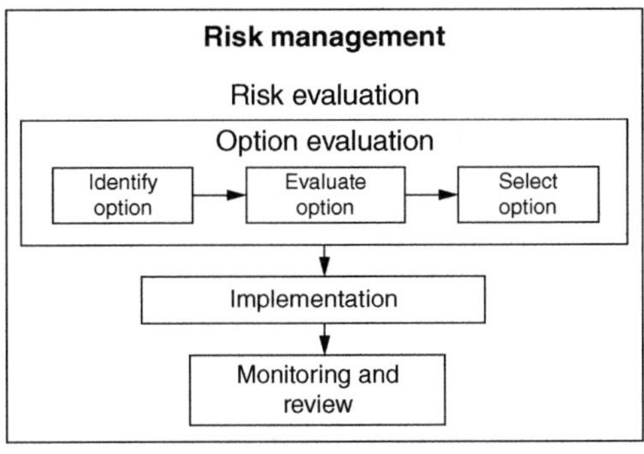

Fig. 14.10. The elements of risk management.

It is important to choose one option or a combination of options that specifically addresses the identified risks associated with entry, exposure and spread in order to reduce risk to an acceptable level.

The principle of equivalence of sanitary measures requires governments to recognize that there may be more than one way of ensuring that a product is safe.

If an exporting country can demonstrate that the safety of its product is equivalent to that required by the importing country, despite not being produced according to the standards normally required by the importing country, then the entry of that product should be permitted. The responsibility is on the exporting country to provide the necessary scientific evidence to show that the product is equally safe.

14.6.3 Selection of risk management options

Murray *et al.* (2004) recommends that selection of risk management options should ensure that:

- The option(s) are based on scientific principles.
- Measures identified by international standard setting bodies (e.g. OIE) are considered:
  - if there is a scientific justification that an international measure does not effectively manage the risks, measures that result in a higher level of protection may be applied; and
  - if there is sufficient justification that measures less stringent than those recommended in international standards can effectively and acceptably manage identified risks, the less stringent measures should be applied.
- The option(s) are applied only to the extent necessary to protect the life or health of humans, plants and animals and the environment.
- Negative trade effects are minimized.
- The option(s) do not result in a disguised restriction on trade.
- The option(s) are not applied arbitrarily.
- The option(s) do not result in discrimination between exporting countries where similar conditions prevail.
- The option(s) are feasible by considering the technical, operational and economic factors affecting their implementation.

If after considered review of available information it is felt that there are no suitable options that can provide confidence of reducing risk to acceptable levels, then the final decision may be to not allow the activity (importation) to proceed.

14.6.4 Implementation of risk management options

Risk management measures may be implemented in the country of origin or in the importing country.

Measures implemented in the country of origin may include:

- requiring demonstration of freedom from a specific hazard (at farm, regional or national levels);
- restricting movement to periods of the year when a disease is not active;

- requiring pre-export quarantine and testing; and
- specifying particular processing or treatment procedures to reduce risk.

Measures implemented in the importing country are often related to post-entry quarantine and testing either before, during or after entry into the country.

Clear and comprehensive records must be maintained of the risk management deliberations and findings and a summary of the measures to be implemented.

There will also be a need for ongoing monitoring and review to ensure that any risk management measures are achieving the results intended, for example, through thorough inspections or audits.

14.7 Risk Communication

The communication strategy that outlines how the project will be reported to stakeholders and decision makers should be developed as part of the planning process. It is a vital part of all risk analyses. This can be seen in Fig. 14.11, which is included here as it provides an excellent summary of the typical (import) risk analysis process.

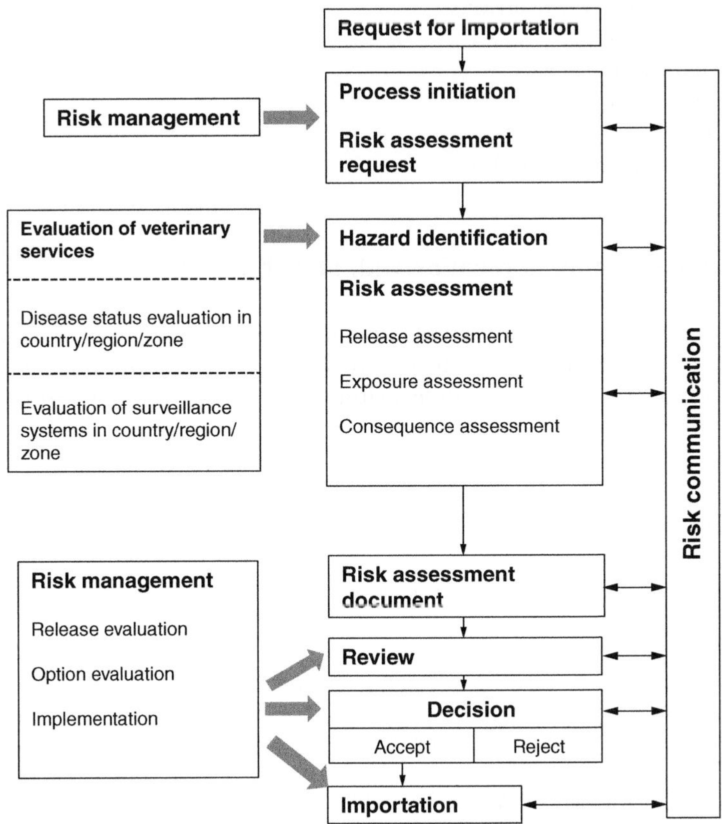

Fig. 14.11. Summary of relationships between hazard identification, risk assessment, risk management and risk communication in the import risk analysis process (adapted from The Expert Panel on Approaches to Animal Health Risk Assessment, 2011).

14.7.1 Stakeholders in risk analysis

A stakeholder is any person or group of people who can affect or are affected by the risk analysis. The process of identifying stakeholders should begin in the planning and scoping stage of the risk analysis.

A list of stakeholders should be maintained and updated as necessary. Stakeholders may include:

- Government veterinary services:
  - risk analysis team or group; and
  - senior staff outside of the group.
- (Other) government agencies responsible for:
  - legislation and compliance;
  - quarantine;
  - trade;
  - social programmes;
  - human health;
  - wildlife; and
  - others.
- Non-government organizations:
  - local (grass-roots);
  - international;
  - industry; and
  - sport.
- Members of the general public.

14.7.2 Methods of communication with stakeholders

Communication to stakeholders can be done in many ways. Each country must determine the most efficient and cost-effective methods for their circumstances. Possible communication methods may include printed materials, meetings and workshops, electronic communications, mass media, Internet-delivered information and others.

References

Biosecurity New Zealand (2006) Risk analysis procedures (version 1). Ministry of Agriculture and Fisheries, Wellington.

Cribb, A., Dohoo, I. R., Donahue, D., Fairbrother, J.M., Frank, D., Hall, D.C., Hurd, H.S., Laycraft, D., Leighton, F.A., Leroux, T., Pfeiffer, D. and Sargeant, J. (2011) *Healthy Animals, Healthy Canada: The expert panel on approaches to animal health risk assessments*. Council of Canadian Academies Ottawa, Canada.

Dufour, B., Plee, L., Moutou, F., Boisseleau, D., Chartier, C., Durand, B., Ganiere, J.P., Guillotin, J., Lancelot, R., Saegerman, C., Thebault, A., Hattenberger, A.M. and Toma, B. (2011) A qualitative risk assessment methodology for scientific expert panels. *Revue Scientifique et Technique Office International des Epizooties* 30, 673–681.

The Expert Panel on Approaches to Animal Health Risk Assessment (2011) *Healthy Animals, Healthy Canada*. The Council of Canadian Academiesm Ottawa, Canada. Available at:

http://www.scienceadvice.ca/uploads/eng/assessments%20and%20publications%20and%20news%20releases/animal%20health/final_ah_web_report_eng.pdf (accessed 1 November 2014).
Murray, N., Macdiarmid, S., Wooldridge, M., Gummow, B., Morley, R.S., Weber, S.E. and Giovannini, A. (2004) *Handbook on Import Risk Analysis for Animals and Animal Products*. OIE (World Organisation for Animal Health), Paris, France.
OIE (2012a) Aquatic Animal Health Code. OIE (World Organisation for Animal Health), Paris, France. Available at http://www.oie.int/international-standard-setting/aquatic-code/access-online (accessed 8 July 2014).
OIE (2012b) Terrestrial Animal Health Code. World Organisation for Animal Health (OIE), Paris, France. Available at http://www.oie.int/international-standard-setting/terrestrial-code/access-online (accessed 8 July 2014).
Standards Australia/Standards New Zealand (2004) *Risk Management Guidelines Companion to AS/NZS 4360:2004*. Standards Australia/Standards New Zealand, Sydney/Wellington.
Talbot, J. (2011) As Low as Reasonably Practical (ALARP). Available at http://31000risk.blogspot.com.au/2011/04/as-low-as-reasonably-practicable-alarp.html (accessed 1 November 2014).

15 Spatial Epidemiology

15.1 Introduction

Proximity can influence the occurrence of both infectious and non-infectious diseases (Pfeiffer *et al.*, 2008). For example, spatial or temporal proximity may increase the probability of contact between infectious and naive individuals resulting in an increased probability of infectious disease transmission. Likewise spatial proximity to an environmental risk factor may increase the local occurrence of a non-communicable disease. Hence consideration of spatial and temporal information during assessment of disease (or infection) is often important to avoid errors (confounded inferences) about risk factors for disease. Fortunately, the development of powerful computers, suitable software and readily accessible spatial data has led to the rapid uptake and development of spatial methods in epidemiology.

Spatial epidemiology is the description and analysis of geographic variations in disease with respect to demographic, environmental, behavioural, socio-economic, genetic and infectious risk factors (Elliott and Wartenberg, 2004). This definition could be expanded to include temporal factors because temporal considerations are often a critical and interlinked part of spatial epidemiology, especially in infectious disease transmission (Cowled *et al.*, 2009a).

Spatial epidemiological analyses can be categorized into several key areas as discussed in a spatial epidemiology text (Pfeiffer *et al.*, 2008):

1. Visualization (e.g. mapping the distribution of disease).
2. Cluster detection (e.g. detecting aggregations of disease events).
3. Visualizing disease risk across an area.
4. Identifying risk factors (cause of disease).
5. Risk assessment and management of disease.

The ability to conduct all these techniques would enhance a veterinarian's ability to investigate animal disease and infection in the field.

Some of the five key areas identified above are technically complex and require skill and experience in spatial epidemiology. It is unrealistic to expect field veterinarians to conduct the full range of spatial epidemiological analyses. However, it is feasible for veterinarians and other field animal health staff to be able to apply simpler spatial methods to field data on animal disease. Visualization is useful for a number of reasons, for example, to understand the extent of endemic disease or outbreaks, to assist directing resources to relevant places, to assist design of surveillance and control programmes, to begin to formulate hypotheses about the cause of disease and to concisely communicate information to others (i.e. with maps).

This chapter will begin with a concise description of a case study of wild pigs and *Salmonella* that will be used to demonstrate concepts throughout. The chapter will then discuss the major steps involved in visualizing disease data and some simple queries. Finally, a summary of more complete spatial epidemiological analyses that could be pursued to analyse the case study will be presented. Interested readers are referred to the EpiTools website (http://epitools.ausvet.com.au), where the wild pig dataset can be downloaded along with detailed notes on how to conduct visualization and queries in Quantum GIS (QGIS). The intent is to assist field veterinarians to learn basic applications in a geographical information system (GIS).

15.2 Case Study: *Salmonella* in Wild Pigs in Australia

Wild pigs (*Sus scrofa*) are an introduced invasive species in Australia. They are found across nearly 40% of the continent (Choquenot *et al.*, 1996) and number in the tens of millions (Hone, 1990). Recently, research occurred to investigate infection transmission in wild pigs in a remote area of north-west Australia, the Kimberley (Cowled *et al.*, 2009b, 2012a,b; Ward *et al.*, 2013). The objective was to investigate risk factors for transmission of infection in wild pigs using *Salmonella* as a model. Part of this dataset will be used here to demonstrate visualization, queries and hypothesis generation for field veterinarians. Specifically, the location of 109 sampled feral pigs along with their *Salmonella* status will be mapped and explored against a number of putative risk factors.

15.3 How to Visualize Animal Health Information

15.3.1 Geographical information systems

A geographical information system (GIS) is computer software that links geographical information (where something is) with descriptive information (what something is) (ESRI, 2012). A GIS is useful to explore geo-referenced animal health information and to easily create useful and informative maps.

To understand GIS software it is important to understand conceptually how a GIS works. GIS software allows many separate tables to be opened and worked on at once. These tables can contain routine data that you would find in any spreadsheet or table in a database (i.e. they do not need to be geo-referenced). However, the tables can also contain geographic information that geographically indexes features of the table to a location. Each table generally represents different features of a landscape. For example, one table may represent rivers in a jurisdiction and another table may represent the location of wild pigs that were sampled for *Salmonella*. These tables are known as layers. If the layers represent features that are located in the same space, the layers can all be visualized on the screen together, thus creating a map. This can be explored interactively with various GIS tools, such as select, pan or zoom tools. Alternatively, the map can be exported as an image.

The layers can also be analysed by the user of a GIS, most commonly with queries selected by clicking with a mouse or through command line interfaces or structured query language scripts. Queries are a very useful feature of GIS and are essentially what distinguishes a GIS from simpler mapping software. Queries can occur within a single layer. An example may be: 'Show the location of all wild pigs that are female'.

Queries can also occur across multiple layers and this generally involves geographic queries. An example may be: 'Show all the sampled wild pigs that are located within 1 km of a river'.

There are many different GIS software packages available, all with relative advantages and disadvantages. Often the starting point for distinguishing different software is through cost. Commercial software can be feature rich and very powerful but may also be expensive. Examples include Mapinfo (PitneyBowes: http://www.mapinfo.com) and ArcGIS (ESRI: http://www.esri.com).

Open-source products are generally free and may be similarly capable to some of the commercial software products. Quantum GIS (QGIS: http://www.qgis.org) is an example of a free product that is powerful and user friendly and is the product used for all analyses described in this chapter. QGIS is compatible with a range of other related open-source software including database software (PostgreSQL: http://www.postgresql.org) installed in conjunction with a spatial database extender for PostgreSQL called PostGIS (http://postgis.net). The open source Geographic Resources Analysis Support System GIS (GRASS GIS: http://grass.osgeo.org) is another free program that can be made compatible with QGIS with a GRASS plugin.

Our preference is to manage geographic data with PostGIS and PostgreSQL. Spatial queries can be conducted with structured query language (SQL), which allows fast, repeatable queries that can be recorded and run repeatedly or in batch files to facilitate analyses. Geographically referenced data can then be exported to QGIS for visualization and additional queries. Running GRASS within QGIS adds additional functionality for some applications but for the purposes of this chapter QGIS is excellent for exploring and visualizing spatial data.

15.3.2 Data (layers)

Conceptual understanding of data layers in a GIS

To create a map within GIS software, data are required. As discussed, it is easiest to conceptualize data as geographically referenced tables that are placed on a map as a layer. Each table may have a row for each geographic object (e.g. a sampled wild pig). The table has a number of columns that allow recording of data for each row. This data can be routine and can be browsed by the GIS user. However, the table will also have a geographic column, which is generally hidden when a table is viewed in GIS software. This is used by the GIS software behind the scenes to locate the object on a map and facilitate geographic queries. This allows the table to become a layer on a map, rather than just an ordinary table of routine data.

There are usually several tables or layers open at one time contributing to a screen display (map). In the wild pig case study there are five data layers. Four of these are shown here and a fifth will be introduced later.

1. Sampled wild pigs (Cowled *et al.*, 2012b). See Table 15.1 for an example of the data included.
2. Major rivers in the sampling area (Geoscience Australia, 2006).
3. The mean maximum greenness of the region (a proxy for plant photosynthesis) (ABARES, 2011).
4. The continent of Australia.

Table 15.1. The first five rows of a wild pig location geographic table/layer. Each row represents a single sampled pig. There are data columns for sex, weight and *Salmonella* status. The layer will be used to contribute to a map showing the location of sampled wild pigs, their status and the relationship to putative risk factors for infection. The geometry column is not visible but exists for use by the GIS.

Sex	Weight	*Salmonella* status
Female	68	0
Male	62	0
Female	62	0
Male	90	0
Male	63.5	0

Types of data layers and sources of data

There are two common types of GIS data, vector and raster data.

Vector data represent objects in the form of points, lines and polygons (shapes). For example, the location of a sampled wild pig is a point, a river is a line and the boundary of Australia is a polygon. The gradual layering of these tables of vector data can be observed in Fig. 15.1a–d. It is important that the data layers be placed in an appropriate order in the map to facilitate visualization. For example, if the pig locations in Fig. 15.1c–d were placed below the Australia polygon they would not be visible (unless the polygon was made transparent). A good rule of thumb is to place the largest polygon at the lower level, then smaller polygons, then lines then points on the top of the display.

There are many types of vector data files, but the two most common files are shape files (.shp) and tab files (.tab). There are several associated parts with each shape or tab file. These are generally found in the same directory and have the same name but a different extension. When moving a vector file, ensure that you take all the associated parts or you will no longer be able to open the file.

Raster data present a matrix of shapes, usually squares or rectangles, organized as rows and columns in a grid. Each individual shape or cell (also called pixels) contains a value so that there is a continuous surface of values across the grid. For example, remote sensing using a satellite in the wild pig study area was used to produce a raster layer of the mean maximum greenness for 2010 (the year of sampling). This can be added to the map of wild pig locations, with the raster layer of mean maximum greenness overlying the continent of Australia layer. Figure 15.2 is the same map as Fig. 15.1d, except that an additional raster layer (mean maximum greenness) has been added over the Australian layer, but beneath the major rivers layer. This obscures the Australia polygon but leaves other layers visible. Colour density or shading is then used to represent greenness with increasing colour density (darkness) indicating increasing mean maximum greenness values. The choice of colour can be manipulated by the user.

Again, there are many types of raster files. The mean maximum greenness file was a GeoTiff file (a geo-referenced .tif file).

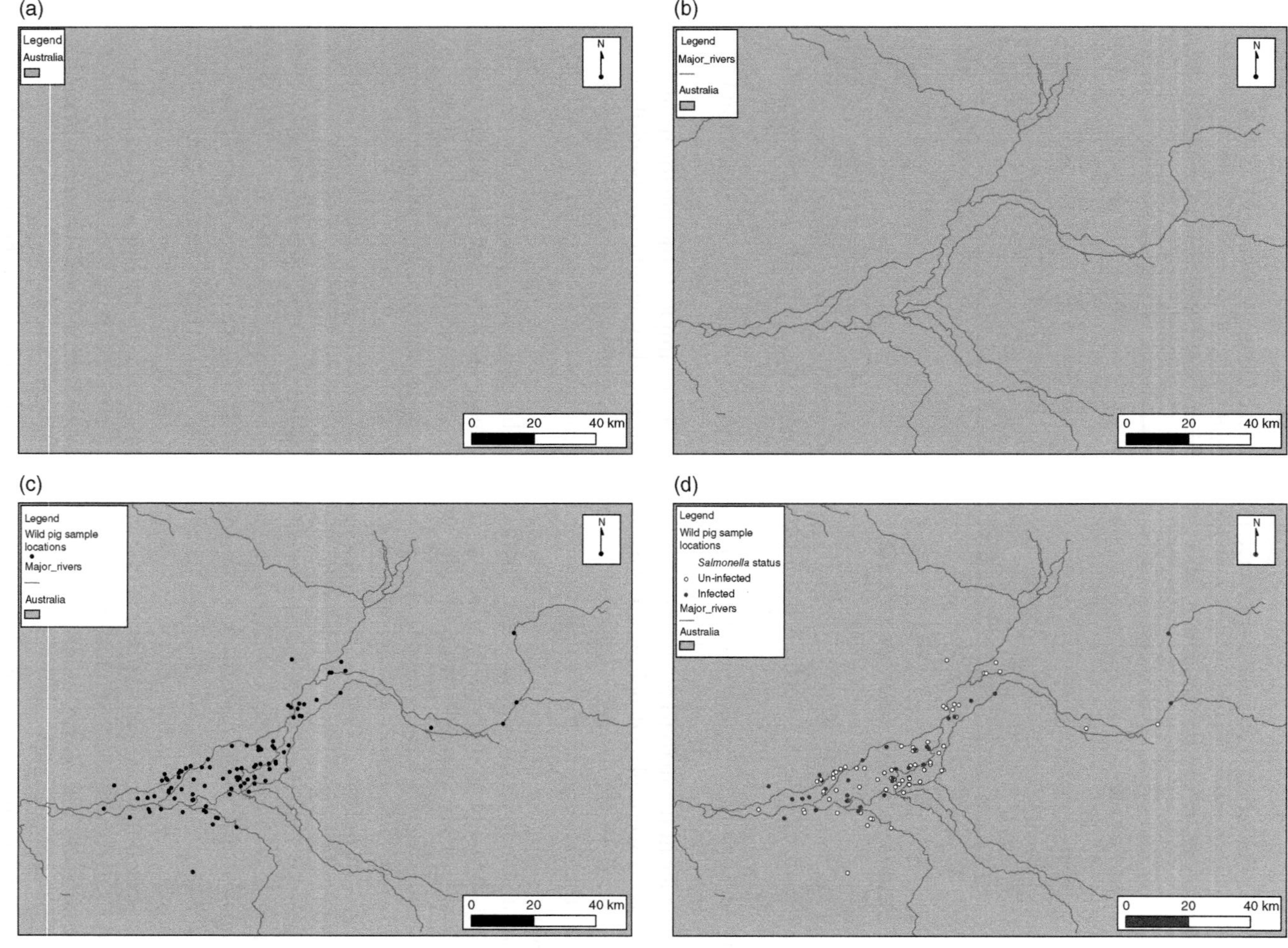

Fig. 15.1. Four maps with increasing degrees of complexity as additional layers are added. (a) A map consisting only of a portion of the Australian continent with no distinguishing features. Note the boundary of Australia is not obvious as it falls outside the study region. All that can be seen is the background of the Australia polygon. (b) Map 1a + layer representing major rivers. The added river layer is line data. (c) Map 1a + Map 1b + layer representing wild pig sampling locations. The added wild pig locations are point data. (d) Map 1a + Map 1b + Map 1c + a colour scheme for wild pig based on *Salmonella* status. The point data are coloured dark or white for infected/uninfected pigs.

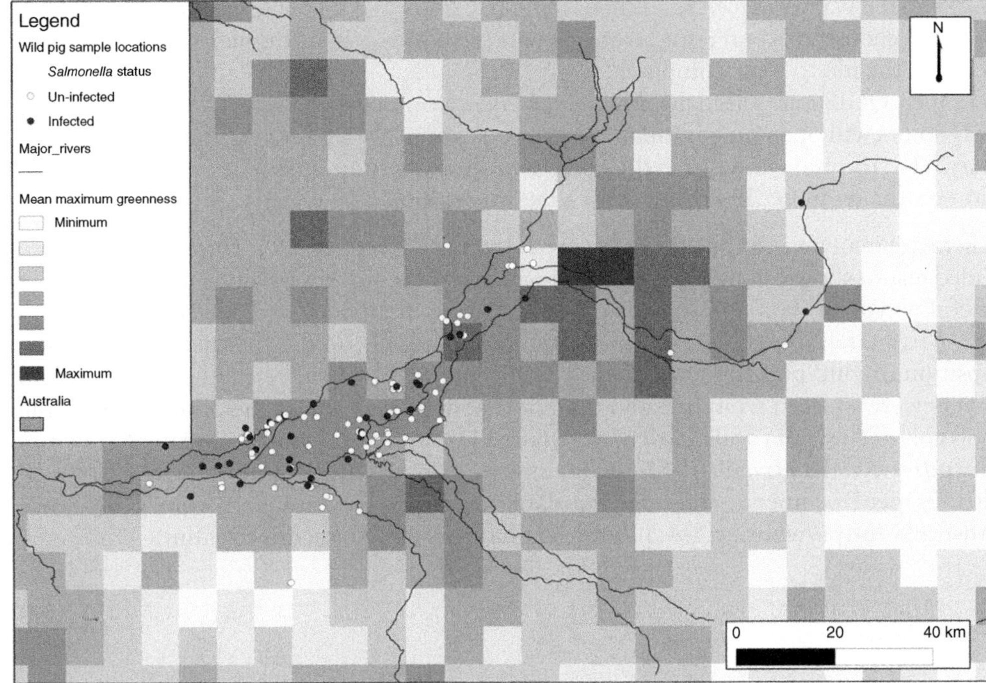

Fig. 15.2. The location and status of sampled pigs against major river systems and the mean maximum greenness.

GIS data types can be produced in very many ways including with remote sensing (e.g. from satellite imagery or aerial photographs), digitization of old maps and with field surveys using global positioning system (GPS) recording.

The GPS in particular is useful for field veterinarians. The GPS interacts with a handheld GPS receiver to allow a user to record positions on the earth's surface. A GPS receiver can be either a purposeful GPS unit or nowadays a mobile device with a relevant app. Using a GPS receiver, we can record the position of sampled animals (such as occurred with the wild pigs sampled in the case study) or other relevant data. These data can then be imported into a GIS, either manually or electronically depending upon permissions and software compatibility.

A detailed example of how to use a mobile app to collect waypoint data is provided below, using GPS Essentials© (Schollmeyer, 2013).

GPS essentials is a free app that works on Android phones. The app can create a location (waypoint) and then export the waypoint in several formats, including Google Earth files (Keyhole Markup Language: .kml files). QGIS can then import .kml files directly.

Start by installing the GPS Essentials app on your Android smartphone. Open the app and proceed through the following steps.

1. Select the Waypoints icon from the start screen.
2. Press the plus button in the waypoint page to create a waypoint and name it something appropriate. You will have to be outdoors with satellite line of sight to do this.

3. Open the Waypoint menu and choose export. Choose the correct format for export (.kml) and then choose to export using an appropriate method (e.g. email the file to your computer).
4. Save the file to your computer.
5. Open QGIS and select the add vector layer icon and browse to the saved file. The waypoints will open on your map. Be cautious about the projection you are using. You may have to resave the file to the correct projection and re-open it, or choose projection on the fly in QGIS settings to see the waypoints.

There are many other apps that may provide similar functionality. This example is provided just to show one approach that can allow you to use your mobile phone to collect useful waypoint data and visualize those data on a map on a separate computer.

Fortunately, much data is also now freely available on the Internet. Although the position of wild pigs in the case study was generated by field research, the other data layers were sourced from free and reputable sources on the Internet. For example, the polygon of Australia and districts was sourced from the Australian Bureau of Statistics (http://www.abs.gov.au/AUSSTATS/abs@.nsf/DetailsPage/1259.0.30.001July%20 2011?OpenDocument) and the line data for rivers was sourced from Geoscience Australia (http://www.ga.gov.au/topographic-mapping/mapconnect.html).

Projections

A map is flat and the earth is an irregular oblate spheroid. It is therefore complex to represent the earth's surface on to a flat map. Projections (or coordinate systems) assist the accurate transmission of the earth's surface on to a flat map. However, the process is never perfect and different types of projections are better depending on what feature of the earth's surface it is most desired to preserve. Two common features that are frequently required to be preserved are the shapes of small areas and the total area of a shape. Area is often the most important for epidemiological studies. There are many different map projections; see Pfeiffer *et al.* (2008) for further discussion.

In our case study we are using GDA94/Australian Albers as the projection. This is a projected coordinate reference system for use in Australia, which focuses on preserving area.

15.3.3 Visualization and interactivity of mapping

An image of data layers forming a map in a GIS display is not static. Instead the map can easily be manipulated, explored, changed and queried. Most GIS software manipulates an image with a number of common tools, including the pan and zoom tools and the layer window. An illustration of these concepts using the zoom tool is provided in Fig. 15.3, which is the same map as Fig. 15.2 except that the zoom tool has focused the view on to a smaller area (or on a subset of the data).

Map images and cartography

Geo-referenced data can be interactively visualized on a GIS display and queried as discussed above. GIS outputs and particularly map images can also be exported as a

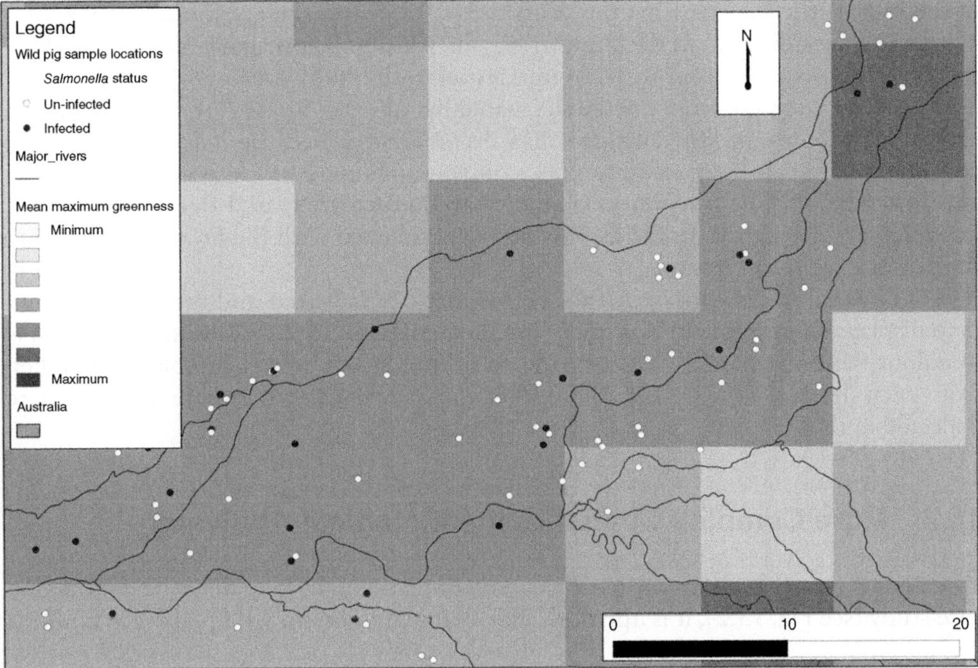

Fig. 15.3. A zoom tool has been applied to Fig. 15.2. The zoom tool allows the image to be focused into a smaller area with fewer pig locations evident. Conversely, the zoom tool could expand the viewing area.

static image file or .pdf file for inclusion in reports and presentations. The export facility in QGIS is termed the print composer. Figures 15.1 to 15.3 were all prepared using the print composer in QGIS.

It is important to include several features on a map to aid in interpretation. These include:

- an indication of the direction of north (indicated by an arrow in the maps within this chapter);
- a scale bar that presents information on how the size of the map relates to the size of the portion of the earth's surface that the map is representing; and
- a legend that indicates what the various symbols or colours on the map represent.

Spatial queries

A key advantage of a GIS is the ability to conduct spatial queries. Individual locations on a display can be queried simply with the information tool. In QGIS more complex queries can be conducted using the open field calculator and by using plugins such as Ftools for vector data and GdalTools for raster data. For example, veterinarians often need to be able to compare the amount of sampling in different areas. One may ask the question in the wild pig case study: How many samples have been taken in each of the four districts comprising the study area? To answer the question, we introduce a fifth GIS layer, districts of the study area, which is a polygon-shape file. See Fig. 15.4 for the locations of the four districts in relation to the study area.

To answer the question one could manually add the number of sampled pigs in each district polygon. However, this has disadvantages because it is slow and time consuming and can be inaccurate (e.g. sample points may be close and overlapping and hence be difficult to count). Therefore an automated spatial query can be conducted as an alternative. In QGIS, this can be conducted with the Ftools plugin using the points in polygon option.

The spatial query generates a shape file that can be saved and then opened on a map display. An example of this query is shown in Table 15.2. An additional option is to colour the districts in a colour theme according to how many samples were taken from each district. In Fig. 15.5, the darker the background, the more samples were collected in that district.

15.4 More Complex Spatial Epidemiological Analyses

Visualizing animal health information can often be useful to help describe data. In the case study (see Fig. 15.2), it is apparent that a large number of wild pigs were sampled

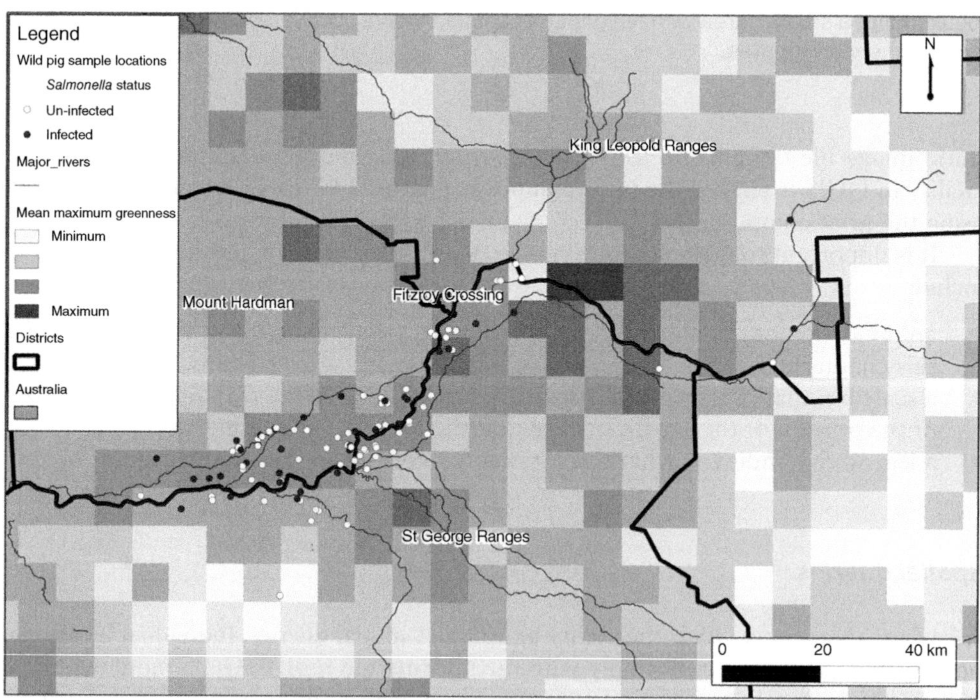

Fig. 15.4. The location of four districts in the study area to assist conceptualization of the spatial query. These districts are Fitzroy Crossing (a town district), King Leopold Ranges, St George Ranges and Mount Hardman.

Table 15.2. The number of pigs sampled in each of the districts of the wild pig study area.

District	Number of pigs sampled
Fitzroy Crossing	0
King Leopold Ranges	5
Mount Hardman	63
St George Ranges	41

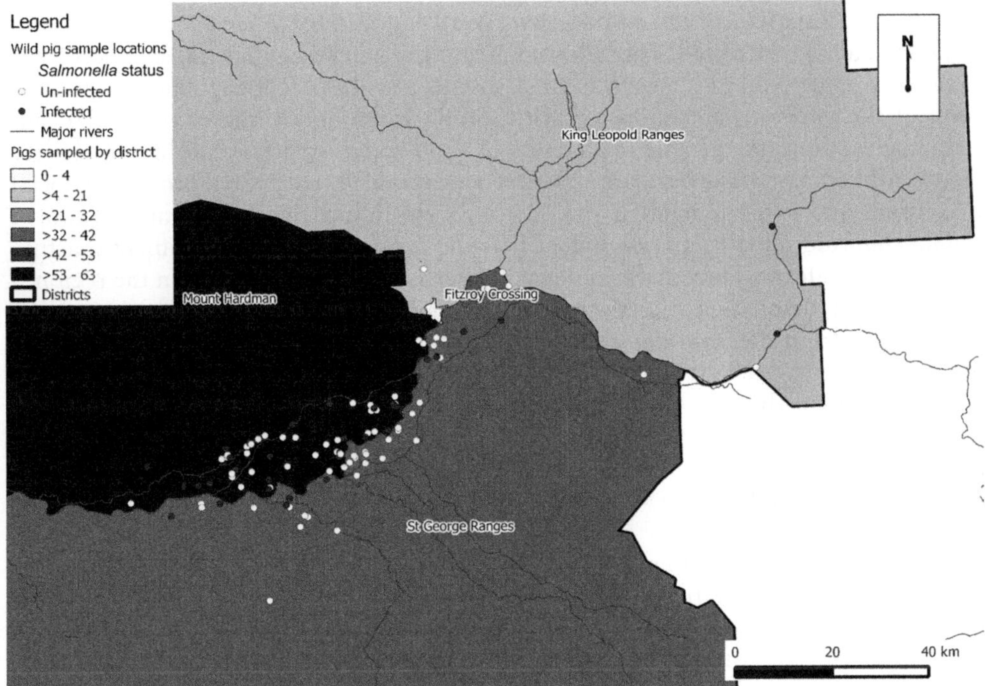

Fig. 15.5. Choropleth map where district polygons are darker based on the number of samples collected. Higher intensity sampling districts are darker and as sampling intensity declines the polygon colour moves from dark grey to white where no samples were taken. King Leopold Ranges has the most samples taken (darkest) and Fitzroy Crossing (white) no samples.

over 150–200 km of river length. It is also apparent that a large proportion of the pigs were infected with *Salmonella*, but that there are more uninfected than infected pigs.

Visualization is also very useful to begin formulating hypotheses, for example, about what may be risk factors for disease or infection. However, care is required because spatial visualization has the potential to mislead the reader due to mapping artefacts (Pfeiffer *et al.*, 2008). Hence spatial visualization as a descriptive means of analysis is best used early in the analysis phase before statistical analyses (Pfeiffer *et al.*, 2008). In the case of the wild pig case study, close examination of Fig. 15.2 reveals that perhaps infection is more common in those wild pigs that are close to major rivers. This is suggested as there are several uninfected pigs a long distance from major rivers, but no infected pigs a long way from rivers. In contrast, there appears to be little discernible relationship between the greenness of a pig's location and infection status. However, these are initial impressions and should only contribute to the formulation of hypotheses that can be tested with more objective means (further spatial statistical analyses).

Further analyses were conducted in this wild pig study and will be discussed conceptually and briefly here to illustrate some applications of spatial epidemiological techniques.

Univariable statistical analyses were used to screen for associations between risk factors and infection status of wild pigs and spatial cluster analyses were used to look for evidence of spatial clusters of infection (Ward *et al.*, 2013). A cluster and significant variable (age) was detected. This allowed a cautious inference that transmission from older to younger wild pigs near water bodies was possibly occurring. Further examination of the dataset was conducted with multivariable modelling of molecular epidemiological data (the genetic relatedness of *Salmonella* isolates) and the presence or absence of infection (Cowled *et al.*, 2012b). This revealed that spatial proximity, social structuring and some individual risk factors were influencing local transmission of *Salmonella*. Additionally, it was evident that the richness of the environment (pasture growth and water resources) was influencing persistence of *Salmonella* in the region.

Spatial epidemiological analyses were thus integral to the interpretation of the information from the wild pig case study. Without considering spatial location and risk factors that were derived through spatial analyses, the data could not have been interpreted correctly.

15.5 Summary

Spatial proximity is very important to the transmission of infection and even for the expression of a non-infectious disease. It is therefore critical that the field veterinarian considers spatial relationships when investigating infection or disease. It is also useful for veterinarians to consider spatial relationships when planning animal health interventions/programmes and when communicating animal health information to others.

Fortunately there has been a rapid expansion in the availability and accessibility of spatial techniques, spatial data and GIS software. It is now possible to download free GIS software and data, record animal health information with a mobile device and create a useful map to visualize disease across a region. It is even possible to begin to develop hypotheses about the cause of disease by simply visualizing the distribution of disease against putative risk factors. Simple queries and spatial analyses are relatively easy to perform such as counting events (e.g. pig samples) within polygons (districts). More complex queries and analyses are possible but are not presented in depth in this chapter.

The ability to undertake these basic spatial epidemiological procedures can be enhanced by an understanding of some relatively simple concepts associated with GIS. Key concepts include the fact that data are imported into a GIS as geographically referenced tables (layers), generally as vector or raster data. These layers can be overlaid, manipulated and queried to produce maps and further spatial data. This can aid understanding through visualization and can assist generation of further hypotheses. These GIS displays can be exported as images to allow insertion of good quality maps into reports. However, it is important to realize that there are some intricacies associated with GIS such as projections that need to be understood and managed effectively to allow valid analyses and visualization.

The case study of wild pigs provides an introduction to the utility of spatial epidemiology. Readers can explore the wild pig dataset and create their own analyses by accessing files and additional resources in the EpiTools website. *Spatial Analysis in Epidemiology* (Pfeiffer *et al.*, 2008) is a useful, concise and readable text for those requiring a greater depth of knowledge than can be provided in this basic introduction.

References

ABARES (Australian Bureau of Agricultural and Resource Economics) (2011) Multi-Criteria Analysis Shell for Spatial (MCAS-S) Decision Support Version 3: DATA - 2011. Department of Agriculture, Fisheries and Forestry, Canberra.

Choquenot, D., Mcilroy, J. and Korn, T. (1996) *Managing Vertebrate Pests: Feral Pigs*. Bureau of Resource Sciences, Australian Government Publishing Service, Canberra.

Cowled, B., Ward, M.P., Hamilton, S. and Garner, G. (2009a) The equine influenza epidemic in Australia: spatial and temporal descriptive analyses of a large propagating epidemic. *Preventive Veterinary Medicine* 92, 60–70.

Cowled, B.D., Giannini, F., Beckett, S.D., Woolnough, A., Barry, S., Randall, L. and Garner, G. (2009b) Feral pigs: predicting future distributions. *Wildlife Research* 36, 242–251.

Cowled, B.D., Garner, M.G., Negus, K. and Ward, M.P. (2012a) Controlling disease outbreaks in wildlife using limited culling: modelling classical swine fever incursions in wild pigs in Australia. *Veterinary Research* 43, 3.

Cowled, B.D., Ward, M.P., Laffan, S.W., Galea, F., Garner, M.G., Macdonald, A.J., Marsh, I., Muellner, P., Negus, K., Quasim, S., Woolnough, A.P. and Sarre, S.D. (2012b) Integrating Survey and Molecular Approaches to Better Understand Wildlife Disease Ecology. *PLoS ONE* 7, e46310.

Elliott, P. and Wartenberg, D. (2004) Spatial Epidemiology: Current Approaches and Future Challenges. *Environmental Health Perspectives* 112, 998–1006.

ESRI (2012) *What is GIS?* ESRI, Redlands, California.

Geoscience Australia (2006) *GEODATA TOPO 250K Series 2 Topographic Data*. Geoscience Australia, Canberra.

Hone, J. (1990) How many feral pigs in Australia. *Australian Wildlife Research* 17, 571–572.

Pfeiffer, D.U., Robinson, T.P., Stevenson, M., Stevens, K.B., Clements, A.C.A. and Rogers, D. (2008) *Spatial Analysis in Epidemiology*. Oxford University Press, Oxford, UK.

Schollmeyer, M. (2013) *GPS Essentials: Getting started*. Michael Schollmeyer Software Engineering, Holzkirchen, Germany.

Ward, M.P., Cowled, B.D., Galea, F., Garner, M.G., Laffan, S.W., Marsh, I., Negus, K., Sarre, S.D. and Woolnough, A.P. (2013) Salmonella infection in a remote, isolated wild pig population. *Veterinary Microbiology* 162, 921–929.

Glossary

Acceptable risk Risk level judged by OIE Member Countries to be compatible with the protection of animal and public health within their country, taking into account epidemiological, social, and economical factors.

Accuracy The degree to which a measurement represents the true value of the attribute that is being measured.

Active surveillance Surveillance that is designed and initiated by the primary user of the data.

Adjusted rates Rates used to compare populations with different structures for a characteristic of interest (such as age, sex or breed). Also known as standardized rates.

Airborne transmission Where infectious material is carried in air to the portal of entry (usually the respiratory tract). Material may be suspended in air as droplet nuclei or dust, and transmission may occur over long distances or long periods of time.

ALOP Appropriate level of protection (see **Acceptable risk**).

Analytical sensitivity The ability of a laboratory assay to detect small amounts of the target substance.

Analytical specificity The ability of a laboratory assay to react only when the particular material is present and not react to the presence of other compounds.

Antagonism A negative interaction between two risk factors.

Association The degree of statistical dependence between two or more events or variables. Association does not necessarily imply a causal relationship.

At-risk population The population that is naturally susceptible to a disease and is potentially exposed – the population at risk.

Attack rate An attack rate is the proportion of a specific population affected during an outbreak. A special form of cumulative incidence.

Attributable fraction The proportion of exposed cases that could have been prevented if the exposure had not been present.

Attributable risk The difference in risk that is explained by the characteristic or risk factor under study.

Bar chart A graph showing the frequency of occurrences of each value for a nominal variable by the height of bars for each value.

Basic reproductive rate (R_0) The expected number of secondary individuals infected by a single infected individual during the entire infectious period for that individual, in a population that is entirely susceptible.

Bayes' theorem A statistical theorem first proposed by Thomas Bayes that allows the calculation of conditional probabilities.

Bias Any systematic error in the design, conduct or analysis of a study which results in estimates that depart systematically from the true value.

Binomial distribution A probability distribution that describes the number of successful outcomes (*x*) from a number of repeated observations or trials (*n*), where the probability of success (*p*) at each observation or trial is constant.

Biocontainment Implementation of measures to prevent the onward transmission of unwanted pathogens from a (potentially) infected livestock (or other) population.

Bioexclusion Implementation of measures to prevent the introduction of unwanted pathogens into a livestock (or other) population.

Biosecurity Protection of the economy, environment, social amenity and public health from negative impacts associated with pests, diseases and weeds.

Box and whisker plot A graph that shows both the frequency and distribution of observations for one or more variables (or for different values of a single variable).

Carrier An animal which is capable of transmitting infection but shows no clinical signs.

Case-control study A study that compares subjects with disease (cases) to subjects without disease (controls) to see if they have different risk factor exposures.

Case definition A set of standard criteria for deciding whether an individual unit of interest in the study has a particular disease or other outcome of interest.

Categorical data A qualitative property or characteristic of an individual or group.

Cause A cause is an event, condition or characteristic that plays an essential role in producing an occurrence of the disease in question.

Chain of infection The series of mechanisms by which an infectious organism passes from an infected to a susceptible host.

Chronic Over a long period of time.

Chronic carrier An animal with long-term infection, which is capable of transmitting infection but shows no clinical signs.

Cluster sampling A form of multi-stage sampling where higher level units (clusters) are selected and then all animals within selected clusters are sampled or measured.

Codex The Codex Alimentarius Commission – responsible for developing food standards, guidelines and codes of practice under the Joint FAO/WHO Food Standards Programme.

Coefficient of variation Relative variation, calculated as the standard deviation divided by the mean.

Cohort A group of subjects with shared characteristics.

Cohort study A study where disease-free subsets are enrolled based on exposure status and followed forward in time to measure onset of disease.

Commodity Animals, animal products, animal genetic material, feedstuffs, biological products and pathological material.

Conditional probability The probability of an event given that another event has occurred.

Confidence interval A confidence interval will, over infinite repetitions of the study, contain the true but unknown parameter value with a frequency no less than the confidence level (often 95%).

Confidence limits The upper and lower end-points of a confidence interval.

Confirmed case A subject that meets criteria defined in a case definition.

Confounding Confounding occurs when part of an apparent association between an exposure and an outcome is in fact due to a third confounding factor that is associated with the outcome and with the exposure.

Consequence assessment A description of the potential consequences of a given exposure and an estimate of the likelihood that each will occur.

Contagious Transmitted by direct contact. See also **Transmission**.

Contamination Presence of an infectious agent(s). See also **Infection**.

Continuous data A variable that may take any value in an interval.

Convalescent An individual who no longer has clinical signs but has not yet returned to full health.

Convenience sampling A sampling technique where units are chosen because they are easy, quick or inexpensive to collect.

Cross-sectional study A study examining associations between risk factors and outcomes in a defined population at a point in time.

Crude rates Rates expressed for the entire population at risk (e.g. crude mortality rate).

Cumulative incidence The number or proportion of animals in a defined population that experience onset of a disease in a defined period of time.

Cyclical fluctuation Variations in disease occurrence that occur at rather regular intervals; these intervals are usually longer than seasons.

Data A collection of facts of any kind, often numbers.

Descriptive study A study describing patterns of a disease or event in a population.

Design prevalence A fixed value for prevalence used for testing the null hypothesis that the population is infected at a prevalence equal to or greater than the design prevalence. Used in disease freedom testing.

Diagnosis The process of determining the health status for an individual or group of subjects.

Diagnostic test A test or procedure applied to an individual to aid in diagnosis.

Dichotomous variable A nominal variable that has only two possible values (e.g. yes/no).

Direct cause A cause with no other factor intervening between it and the outcome of interest.

Direct transmission A mechanism of disease spread, which requires direct transfer of an infectious agent from the exit portal of an infected animal to the entry portal of a susceptible animal.

Disease Literally a physiological dysfunction or state of non-health. May be used to refer to suboptimal or abnormal states of health and of productivity in animal production systems.

Disease control programmes Activities directed at reducing the prevalence or impact of a disease.

Disease eradication programmes Activities directed at elimination of clinical disease or the causal agent from a defined area within an acceptable time frame.

Disease reservoir Any animal, plant or environment or combination of these in which an infectious agent normally lives and multiplies and upon which it depends as a species for survival in nature.

Ecology of disease The relationship among animals, pathogens and their environment in a natural situation without intervention.

Effect modification Variation in the effect of a defined factor across the levels of another factor (also called interaction).

Effective contact Contact between an infectious and susceptible individual that results in infection of the susceptible individual.

Effective reproductive ratio (R) The average number of secondary cases infected by a single infected individual in a population that is comprised of both susceptible and non-susceptible hosts.

Efficacy The extent to which an intervention produces a beneficial outcome.

ELISA Enzyme-linked immunosorbent assay – a type of (usually) serological test.

Endemic The constant presence of a disease or infectious agent within a given geographic area or population group. It also implies a prevalence which is usual in the area or in the population.

Epidemic The occurrence of cases of disease clearly in excess of normal expectancy.

Epidemic curve A graph of the number of cases of disease against the time of onset of each case.

Epidemiology The study of the patterns and causes of disease in populations.

Eradication The extinction of an infectious agent in a time-limited campaign from a defined population or area.

Erratic variations Variations in disease occurrence that occur in a totally unpredictable fashion.

Exposure assessment A description of the biological pathways necessary for the exposure of animals and humans in the importing country to the hazards released from a given risk source, and an estimation of the probability of this occurring.

External validity The extent to which the results of a study can be related to the target population of interest.

False negative When the result of an individual test is negative but the disease or condition is present.

False positive When the result of an individual test is positive but the disease or condition is not present.

FAO Food and Agricultural Organization

Fomites Inanimate objects that transmit infection.

Fraction A fraction where the numerator is a subset of the denominator (see **Proportion**).

Frequency A count or number of occurrences of an event in a specified population and time period.

Frequency distribution A table or graph of the values observed for a variable and the observed frequency of occurrence for each value.

Frequency polygon A line graph representation of a frequency distribution, or a line graph connecting the mid-points of the tops of the columns in a histogram.

GATT General Agreement on Tariffs and Trade.

Gaussian distribution An alternative name for the normal distribution.

General surveillance Surveillance not focused on any particular disease, but rather capable of detecting any disease or pathogen.

Gold standard test Best available or benchmark diagnostic test used for comparative purposes.

Haphazard sampling A sampling technique where units are chosen with no fixed purpose or reason, in an attempt to imitate random sampling.

Harmonization Development of standards such that compliance jurisdiction should be considered to be compliant with international standards.

Hazard In the context of the OIE Code is a pathogenic agent, usually infectious.

Hazard identification The process of identifying relevant pathogenic agents, usually as part of a risk analysis.

Herd immunity The resistance of a group of animals to an infectious agent based on the resistance to infection of a high proportion of (but not all) members of the group.

Herd sensitivity The probability that an infected herd will give a positive result to a particular testing protocol, given that it is infected at a prevalence equal to or greater than the design prevalence (HSE).

Herd specificity The probability that an uninfected herd will give a negative result to a particular testing protocol (HSP).

Histogram A graph of the frequency distribution of a variable, with each value or class represented as a column on the graph.

Homogeneous The situation where all individuals in a group or population are similar in relation to a particular characteristic(s).

Horizontal transmission Direct transmission of infection infected and susceptible individuals in a population by close contact.

Immune Individuals that are resistant to infection.

Import risk analysis The process of assessing and managing the disease risks associated with the importation of animals, animal products, animal genetic material, feedstuffs, biological products and pathological material.

Incidence The proportion of individuals within the population at risk who convert from a non-diseased to diseased state during a specified time period.

Incidence density The number of new cases of disease in a population during a certain period divided by the total number of animal-time-units at risk for all animals in the population at risk (also called incidence rate).

Incubating Individuals that are in the incubation period for the infection.

Incubation period The interval of time from exposure to infection through to when clinical signs are first manifested in an individual.

Index case The first diagnosed case of an outbreak in a herd or other defined group. See also **Primary case**.

Indirect cause A cause that has an intervening direct cause acting between it and the outcome of interest.

Indirect transmission Any mechanism of transmission that is not classified as direct. May be further classified as vehicle-borne, vector-borne or airborne.

Induction period The period from exposure to a disease-causing agent to the onset of clinical signs of disease. Generally applied to non-infectious agents.

Infection Entry, development and multiplication of an infectious agent in a host.

Infective Capable of transmitting infection.

Infective period The longest period during which an affected animal can be a source of infection.

Infectivity The ability of an agent to enter, survive and multiply in a susceptible host. Epidemiologically, it is measured as the proportion of the individuals exposed to an agent who become infected.

Inference The process of drawing generalized conclusions about the reference population from observations undertaken in a sample of the population.

Information The result of processing, analysing and interpreting data.

Information bias Systematic flaws or variation in measuring something.

Interaction See **Effect modification**.

Internal validity The extent to which the results of a study reflect true differences between study groups.

Intervention study A study involving intentional change in some aspect of status of subjects such as assignment to treatments (e.g. randomized clinical trial, experimental study).

IPPC International Plant Protection Convention.

IRA Import Risk Analysis.

Judgemental sampling A sampling technique in which animals are deliberately selected in an effort to achieve a representative or balanced sample. Also called purposive sampling.

Kappa A measure of the relative agreement between two tests.

Latent infection Persistence of an infectious agent within the host without clinical signs of disease.

Latent period The period from exposure to a disease-causing agent to the onset of clinical signs of disease.

Likelihood The probability of an event occurring under given conditions.

Line of identity A line on a graph that passes through the origin and for which $y = x$ for all values (i.e. a line through 0,0; 1,1; etc.).

Long term (secular) trend Long-term changes in disease occurrence.

Mean The arithmetic average of a series of values (the sum of the values divided by the number of values).

Measurement bias See **Information bias**.

Mechanical vector A vector where the infection is carried physically by the vector but does not undergo multiplication or development in the vector.

Median The middle value of an ordered group of observations (i.e. 50% of observations have lower values and 50% have higher values).

Misclassification bias Systematic error due to misclassification of an individual or attributes in different groups being compared, usually associated with errors in measurement or testing.

Mode The most frequent value for a variable.

Monitoring Routine collection of information on disease and other attributes in a population.

Monte Carlo simulation Modelling methods based on multiple iterations with stochastic sampling to represent uncertainties in parameters.

Multi-stage sampling The selection of a sample in two or more stages.

Necessary cause A causal factor that must be present for occurrence of the effect.

Negative predictive value The probability that an animal with a negative test does not have the disease.

Nominal variable A variable classified in unordered, qualitative categories (red, blue, green).

Non-probability sampling Any sampling method where members of the population do not have a known, non-zero probability of being selected in the sample (i.e. any method that is not a probability-sampling method).

Non-representative sample Any sample from a population that is not representative of the population. Non-representative samples result in biased estimates.

Non-systematic error Any error that occurs as a result of chance or random events.

Normal distribution A particular form of probability distribution with a smooth, bell shape, a central single peak and symmetrical tails.

Normally distributed A variable with a frequency distribution that is consistent with a normal distribution.

Observational study A study that does not involve any intervention by the investigator.

Odds The ratio of the probability of an event occurring to that of it not occurring.

Odds ratio The ratio of two odds.

OIE Office International des Epizooties or World Animal Health Organization.

OIE Code International Animal Health Code of the OIE

Option evaluation The process of identifying, evaluating the efficacy and feasibility of, and selecting measures in order to reduce the risk associated with an importation in line with the Member Country's ALOP.

Ordinal variable A type of categorical variable where categories have an inherent order.

Outlier A value that differs so widely from the rest of the data that it may be an error or from a different population.

Pandemic An epidemic occurring over a very wide area, involving many countries and usually affecting a large proportion of the population.

Parallel tests The interpretation of multiple tests where an animal is considered positive if it reacts positively to either or both (or any) tests.

Passive surveillance Secondary use of routinely collected data that was generated for some other purpose.

Pathogenicity The ability of an organism to produce overt disease. Epidemiologically, it is measured as the proportion of infected individuals who develop clinical disease.

Percentage A proportion multiplied by 100.

Percentile A number that indicates the percentage of the distribution that is less than or equal to that number.

Period prevalence The cumulative proportion of individuals within the population at risk that have the disease at the start of a specified time period or develop the disease during the time interval of interest.

Phytosanitary To do with human and animal health.

Pie chart A graph that shows the relative frequency or percentage of occurrences of each value for a nominal variable as segments of a circle.

Point-source epidemic An epidemic resulting from exposure of all (or most) affected animals to a single source of infection or toxicity, with little or no secondary transmission.

Population A defined group whose individual members have the potential to interact with one another and can be distinguished from other groups.

Population coverage The proportion of the population of interest that is included in the surveillance system.

Population immunity See **Herd immunity**.

Population at risk The population that is naturally susceptible to a disease and is potentially exposed.

Positive predictive value The predictive value of a positive test (PPV) is the proportion of test positive animals that have the disease.

Power The probability of rejecting the null hypothesis when it is false.

Precision Lack of random error.

Pre-clinical A stage of infection in which an animal is infected but not yet showing clinical signs.

Prepatent period For parasitic diseases, the period from first exposure to infection until the parasite has reproduced and is capable of further transmission of infection.

Prevalence The proportion of individuals within the population at risk who have the disease at a particular point of time or during a particular period.

Primary case The individual that introduces disease into a herd, flock, or other group under study. Not necessarily the first diagnosed case in that herd.

Primary sampling units The units being sampled at the first stage in a multi-stage sampling approach.

Probability A measure, ranging from 0 to 1, of the degree of belief that an event will occur.

Probability distribution A frequency distribution of a random variable, which may be theoretical or empirical (based on observed data).

Probability proportional to size A multi-stage sampling method where the probability of selection for primary sampling units is proportional to their size.

Probability sampling A sampling technique in which each member of the population has a known, non-zero probability of being selected in the sample.

Propagating epidemic An outbreak or series of outbreaks resulting from animal to animal spread.

Proportion A fraction where the numerator is a subset of the denominator.

Purposive sampling See **Judgemental sampling**.

Qualitative risk analysis An assessment where the outputs on the likelihood of the outcome or the magnitude of the consequences are expressed in qualitative terms such as high, medium, low or negligible.

Quantile plot A graph that plots the percentiles of the distribution of a variable against the corresponding percentiles of a specified probability distribution.

Quantitative risk analysis An assessment where the outputs of the risk assessment are expressed numerically.

Quarantine A state of enforced isolation applied to individuals or areas.

Random Governed by chance.

Random sample A sample of a population assembled so that each member of the population has an equal and non-zero opportunity to be selected.

Range The difference between the largest and smallest observed value for a variable.

Rate An expression of the change in one quantity per unit time.

Ratio The expression of the relationship between a numerator and denominator where the two are separate and distinct quantities.

Record A collection of data for a number of variables that relate to a single unit of interest (individual, herd, pond or farm).

Recovered Individuals that have survived infection and are no longer infected. May be immune or susceptible.

Reference population The population to which it is hoped to generalize or apply the results of an epidemiological investigation. Also called the target population.

Regionalization Procedures implemented by a country under the provisions of the OIE Code with a view to defining subpopulations of different animal health status within its territory for the purpose of international trade, and in accordance with the recommendations stipulated in the relevant Chapters in the Code (also called zoning).

Registered Something for which registration has been completed.

Relative risk The ratio of the risk of an event among the exposed group compared to the risk among an unexposed group (also called risk ratio).

Release assessment A description of the biological pathways necessary for an importation activity to introduce a hazard into a particular environment, and an estimation of the probability (qualitative or quantitative) of the complete process occurring.

Repeatability The ability of a test to give consistent results in repeated tests performed under conditions that are as constant as possible, in the one laboratory, by one operator using the same equipment over a short period of time.

Representative A sample selected in such a way that estimates of population characteristics calculated from the sample are not biased.

Reproducibility The ability of a test to give consistent results in repeated tests under widely varying conditions in different laboratories at different times by different operators.

Resistant Individuals that are less susceptible to (able to resist) infection despite exposure.

Restricted risk estimate The estimated risk associated with the proposed importation after risk management measures have been implemented to reduce the risk to an acceptable level.

Risk The likelihood (probability or chance) of the occurrence and the likely magnitude of the consequences of an adverse event to animal or human health in the importing country during a specified time period.

Risk analysis The process composed of hazard identification, risk assessment, risk management and risk communication.

Risk assessment The evaluation of the likelihood and the biological and economic consequences of entry, establishment, and/or spread of a pathogenic agent within the territory of an importing country.

Risk-based surveillance A form of stratified surveillance, where the population is stratified according to a known or hypothesized risk factor and sampling within strata is not proportional to stratum size.

Risk communication The process by which information about risk analysis is communicated to stakeholders.

Risk estimation An integration of the results of the release assessment, exposure assessment and consequence assessment to produce an overall measure of the risk associated with each identified hazard.

Risk estimation matrix A table combining and summarizing the product of two likelihoods or a likelihood and consequences.

Risk evaluation The process of comparing the risk estimated in the risk assessment with the country's appropriate level of protection.

Risk factor An attribute or exposure that increases the probability of occurrence of disease or other specified outcome. May be a causal or non-causal risk factor.

Risk management The process of identifying, selecting and implementing measures that can be applied to reduce the level of risk.

Risk ratio See **Relative risk**.

Sample A subject selected from all the subjects in a particular group.

Sampling bias See **Selection bias**.

Sampling error The part of total estimation error that is due to random error associated with subject selection.

Sampling frame A list of all the members of the population, from which the sample is chosen.

Sampling interval The number of units between each selected unit when undertaking systematic sampling. Calculated by dividing the study population by the sample size.

Sampling units The units being sampled at each stage in a multi-stage sampling approach.

Sanitary To do with human and animal health.

Sanitary measure Measures such as those described in each Chapter of the OIE Code, which are used for risk reduction and are appropriate for particular diseases.

Scatter plot A two-dimensional graph showing the relationship between two numerical variables.

Screening tests Tests applied to apparently healthy individuals to detect disease. Tests used for this purpose are usually cheap, rapid, easily performed, sensitive but often not very specific.

Seasonal variation Variations in disease occurrence that display a seasonal pattern.

Selection bias Selection bias is due to systematic differences in characteristics between those individuals selected for study and those who are not.

Sensitivity The proportion of animals with the disease (or infection) of interest who test positive.

Sensitivity analysis The process of examining the impact of the variation in individual model inputs on the model outputs in a quantitative risk assessment.

Sentinel herd Usually a small number of immunologically naive animals that are maintained together and sampled on a regular basis to test for seroconversion or examined for clinical signs of target diseases.

Series testing The interpretation of multiple tests where an animal must be positive on both (or all if more than two) tests to be considered positive – this increases specificity at the expense of sensitivity.

Simple random sampling A sampling technique where each member of the population has the same probability of being selected.

Skewed A measure of lack of symmetry of a distribution.

Source population The actual population from which eligible study subjects are drawn for the epidemiological investigation.

Specific rates Rates expressed for a specified sub-population of the population at risk, based on one or more characteristics such as age, breed or sex.

Specificity The proportion of animals without the disease (or infection) of interest who test negative.

Spectrum of disease The full range of manifestations of a disease.

Sporadic A disease occurring irregularly and generally infrequently and without any apparent underlying pattern.

Spread The movement of infection from an infected population or sub-population to a susceptible population or sub-population.

SPS Agreement WTO Agreement on the Application of Sanitary and Phytosanitary Measures.

Standard deviation A standard measure of the variation that exists in a series of values or of a frequency distribution. Calculated as the square root of the variance.

Standard error Estimated as the standard deviation of a sample divided by the square root of the number of samples.

Standard normal distribution The normal distribution with mean = 0 and standard deviation = 1.

Standardized rates Rates used to compare populations with different structures for a characteristic of interest (such as age, sex or breed). Also called adjusted rates.

Statistics The scientific application of mathematical principles to the collection, analysis and presentation of numerical data.

Stem and leaf plot A simple graphical display for numerical data, which shows the distribution of observed values.

Strata One of a series of separate, exclusive groups within the population, categorized on the basis of a specified characteristic(s) such as region or herd size.

Stratified sampling The process of dividing the population into distinct subgroups (strata) according to some important characteristic (e.g. herd size), and selecting a random sample out of each subgroup.

Study population See **Source population**.

Study unit The primary unit of analysis in the investigation and may be an individual animal or a group of animals such as a pen of pigs, a pond or cage of fish, a mob of sheep or cattle, an entire farm or a district or region.

Sub-clinical Where disease is detectable by special tests, but affected animals do not show any clinical signs of disease.

Sufficient cause The complex of component causes that induces a disease. Several different sufficient causes may induce the same disease.

Surveillance Surveillance is the systematic ongoing collection, collation, and analysis of information related to animal health and the timely dissemination of information to those who need to know so that action can be taken.

Susceptible Able to be infected with an agent if exposed – not resistant or immune to infection or already infected.

Suspect case Definition of a disease state where the animal meets some but not all of the confirmed case criteria.

Syndrome A defined collection of clinical signs, usually relating to particular body systems or characteristics of diseases of concern.

Synergism A positive interaction between two risk-factors.

System sensitivity The probability that infection will be detected in the population of interest by the surveillance system, given that it is infected at a prevalence equal to or greater than the design prevalence(s).

Systematic bias/ error Any error due to factors other than chance.

Systematic random sampling The procedure of selecting according to some simple systematic rule, such as every fifth cow in the herd as they enter the milking parlour.

Target population The population to which it is hoped to generalize or apply the results of an epidemiological investigation. Also called the reference population.

Targeted surveillance Surveillance that is focused on a specific disease or pathogen.

Test Any procedure used to assist in determining the cause of disease or whether or not an animal is infected or has been exposed to a particular agent.

Theoretical epidemiology The development of mathematical/statistical models to explain different aspects of the occurrence of a variety of diseases.

Transmission The movement of infection from an infected animal to a susceptible animal within an infected population.

Transparency Comprehensive documentation of all data, information, assumptions, methods, results, discussion and conclusions relevant for an issue or decision. Used in risk analysis.

Trend A long-time movement in an ordered series (e.g. a time series).

Unbiased A parameter estimate that has an expected value equal to the true value of the parameter. Without systematic error or bias.

Uncertainty The lack of precise knowledge of a parameter value due to measurement error or lack of knowledge.

Unit of study The biological unit of primary concern in an epidemiological investigation.

Unrestricted risk estimate The initial estimate of overall risk associated with the proposed importation before risk management measures are implemented.

Validity The extent to which a study or test measures what it sets out to measure.

Variability The range of values for a parameter within a defined population. Reflects natural variation in the real world.

Variable A characteristic or attribute of an animal or group that can have different values for different individuals or groups of interest.

Variance Estimated as the sum of the squares of the deviations from the mean value for the variable divided by the number of degrees of freedom (n–1).

Vector An insect or other living organism that transports infectious material from an infected animal or its wastes to a susceptible animal or its immediate surroundings.

Vector-borne transmission A mechanism of indirect transmission where infectious material is transmitted by a vector.

Vehicle-borne transmission A mechanism of indirect transmission where infectious material is transmitted by contaminated inanimate materials or objects, including animal products.

Vertical transmission Direct transmission of infection between parent and offspring, usually between dam and offspring. May be genetic, trans-ovarial, trans-placental or via milk.

Virulence The degree of severity of disease produced by an agent in a given host. Epidemiologically, it is measured as the proportion of individuals with disease who become seriously ill or die.

WHO World Health Organization.

World Organisation for Animal Health The Office International des Epizooties. Also called OIE.

World Trade Organization (WTO) Global international organization dealing with the rules of trade between nations.

Zoning See **Regionalization**.

Index

Page numbers in **bold** refer to glossary definitions.

Printed and bound by CPI Group (UK) Ltd, Croydon, CR0 4YY

15/03/2026

14843206-0001